A Textbook of Scons

A Textbook of Science for the Health Professions

Second edition

Barry Hinwood

Senior Head Teacher, Department of Biological Sciences,
Sydney Institute of Technology, Sydney, Australia

First published as *Science for the Health Team*
First published in 1987 by:
Chapman & Hall
Second edition 1993
(ISBN 0 412 46730 5)

Reprinted in 1997 by:
Stanley Thornes (Publishers) Ltd

Reprinted in 2001 by:
Nelson Thornes Ltd
Delta Place
27 Bath Road
CHELTENHAM
GL53 7TH
United Kingdom

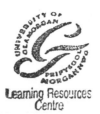

04   05   /   10   9   8   7   6

A catalogue record for this book is available from the British Library.

ISBN 0 7487 3377 9

Page make-up by Best-set Typesetters Ltd

Printed and bound in Great Britain by Athenæum Press

To my daughters, Laura, Justine and Aimée.

Contents

Contents

Acknowledgements

I would like to thank my students, past and present, my colleagues from the Sydney Institute of Technology and the City of Westminster College, London for their constructive comments with particular thanks to Paul Armson. I would also like to thank Desmond Arnold, Philippe Vandervaere and Trevor Hinwood for their suggestions; Lesley Maxwell, Mark Manly and Maria Tordon for their assistance with electron micrographs; Diane Clucas and Margaret Manny for photography, and Theresa Cooper and the staff at Chapman & Hall. I would especially like to thank my wife Danielle for her support, encouragement and suggestions.

The author and publishers are grateful to The John Curtain School of Medical Research, Australian National University for the electron micrographs provided for Figures 26.3, 26.4, 35.6, 36.2 and 37.1. Also, the Sydney Institute of Technology for the electron micrographs in Figures 22.2, 25.2, 26.1, 35.3 and 35.10, and the photographs for Figures 14.3, 15.9, 15.11 and 19.8.

Preface

The increased depth and breadth of knowledge required for the training of persons in the health care professions has been addressed by the expansion of the previous book *Science for the Health Team*. The strands of biology, chemistry, physics, nutrition and biochemistry, medical microbiology and physiology are introduced to demonstrate the relationship between science and health care. The comprehensive scope of this book will enable those entering or re-entering a health care course to use the book both as an introductory text and subsequently as a reference book throughout the remainder of their education and work. The layout of the book is designed to help students overcome any difficulties they have in applying science to their work. The essential features of the earlier book have been retained. These include:

1. The theme of homeostasis is used to link various aspects of science and apply them to health care and body function.
2. The book is divided into units containing a common theme.
3. Each unit is an independent entity, which enables the reader to select the general order of contents to suit individual needs. This is facilitated by extensive cross-referencing.
4. Each chapter contains a list of objectives and a summary.
5. The inclusion of over a hundred applica-

tions and many hundreds of examples is intended to assist the student relate science to health care. The applications supplement the text and can be omitted without influencing the general context of a particular aspect of science.
6. A series of diagrams is used to show how substances combine in chemical reactions.
7. SI units are used with the non-SI unit being placed in brackets beside the corresponding unit. In addition, two tables listing common SI unit conversions and frequently used pathology test conversions are given in Appendixes.
8. A glossary of terms is included.

In addition to these features the following changes have been introduced in order to provide a book that addresses the scope and course patterns required for students entering or re-entering the health care professions in the 1990s.

1. The number of chapters has been expanded from 30 to 40 chapters.
2. The increased chapters have led to a restructuring from 10 units into 13 units.
3. New chapters in chemical interactions and organic chemistry and the expansion of other chapters to form two units 'Chemical properties of matter' and 'Organic chemistry'.
4. The unit energy and the physical properties of matter has been expanded from

three chapters to seven with a chapter for each energy form and the inclusion of magnetism with electricity.

5. The expansion and updating of 'cell structure' to form Chapter 22, 'The cellular basis of life'.

6. Human nutrition has been expanded and restructured into two units (10 and 11). Unit 10, 'Nutritional principles and bio-molecule groups' contains a new chapter 'Nucleotides and nucleic acids' and a comprehensive rearrangement of the other chapters. Unit 11, 'Regulation of biomolecules' expands and integrates information on the metabolism by combining the factors involved in the control of metabolism with the main pathways through which the bodies chemicals are processed to provide energy or other biomolecules. New chapters are 'Enzymes' and 'Metabolism'.

7. Unit 12, 'Medical microbiology' has been restructured and expanded to provide a separate chapter, 'The world of microorganisms'.

8. All chapters have been updated with many containing an environmental health and safety component to address the need for those studying a health care profession to understand the relationship between the environment and the hazards associated with working in health care.

9. A new appendix has been included that lists generic and brand names for drugs referred to in the book.

Unit One
Homeostasis

This unit discusses homeostasis in relation to the health of a patient. The relationship between homeostasis and science is introduced as a principal theme of this book.

Chapter 1   Homeostasis

Homeostasis

Objectives

At the completion of this chapter the student should be able to:

1. define homeostasis;
2. relate homeostasis to the health of a patient;
3. discuss the differences in homeostasis that exist between single-celled and multicellular organisms;
4. relate cell homeostasis to cell membrane function;
5. describe the components of homeostatic mechanisms and relate these to homeostatic mechanisms in the body;
6. explain the relationship between stress and homeostasis.

1.1 Homeostasis

Homeostasis and the health of a patient

Homeostasis is a relative state of equilibrium between the internal environment of an organism and a changing external environment. This stage of equilibrium or optimum conditions usually ranges between an upper and lower limit. Beyond these limits harmful effects can occur. Homeostasis is an essential characteristic of life which controls the processes required for life. Homeostatic mechanisms assist in returning abnormal conditions back to the normal optimum range. A continuation of abnormal conditions usually results in ill health, and in some instances can lead to death. Treatment of a body imbalance generally involves either eliminating the causative factors and/or replenishing deficiencies of substances.

An understanding of homeostatic mechanisms is important in determining the impact of a particular treatment on the entire body. Throughout this book an emphasis is therefore placed on homeostasis and its relationship to scientific principles. Examples of the following aspects of homeostasis are found in the cited chapters.

1. Factors that indicate the health of a person, i.e. normal versus abnormal homeostatic state. EXAMPLES: 'Measurement and units' — Chapter 2; 'Concept of concentration' — Chapter, 3; 'The composition and properties of body fluids' — Chapter 18 and Appendix I.
2. The properties of matter that are involved in homeostatic mechanisms. EXAMPLES:

'Atoms and matter' — Chapter 4; 'Energy and the physical states of matter' — Chapter 9; 'How atoms combine' — Chapter 5; 'Chemical interactions' — Chapter 6; 'Electricity and magnetism' — Chapter 10; 'Properties of pressure' — Chapter 19; 'Diffusion' — Chapter 20; 'Enzymes' — Chapter 32.

3. The properties of matter that influence the care and treatment of patients. EXAMPLES: 'Mechanical properties of matter' — Chapter 15; 'Important biological functional groups' — Chapter 8; 'Properties of fluid mixtures' — Chapter 17; 'Properties of pressure' — Chapter 19.

4. The properties of energy that assist diagnosis and therapy of abnormal homeostatic conditions. EXAMPLE: 'Energy and the physical properties of matter' — Unit Five.

5. The homeostatic mechanisms that maintain a healthy person. EXAMPLES: Acid–base balance in Chapter 16; 'Osmosis and body fluid balance' — Chapter 21; 'The plasma membrane' — Chapter 23. 'Enzymes' — Chapter 32.

6. The effect of abnormal homeostatic mechanisms. EXAMPLES: Genetic abnormalities in Chapter 24; Endocrine malfunction in Chapter 40.

7. Factors that can cause homeostatic imbalances. EXAMPLES: Excess energy in Unit Five; Infections in Chapter 36; Stress in Chapter 38.

8. Inter-relationship of homeostatic mechanisms. EXAMPLES: Blood gases in Chapter 26; 'Metabolism' — Chapter 33; 'General organization and function of the endocrine system' — Chapter 40.

9. Integration and control of homeostatic mechanisms. EXAMPLES: 'General organization and function of the nervous system' — Chapter 38; 'Neuroendocrine connections' — Chapter 39; 'General organization and function of the endocrine system' — Chapter 40.

The examples mentioned above are only intended to indicate a sample of the relationships between homeostasis and health. Many chapters contain information that relate to more than one of the aspects of homeostasis that are listed.

Homeostasis in single-celled organisms

Single-celled organisms such as bacteria and protozoa are capable of withstanding relatively large alterations in their external environment. This is due to their ability to perform all the functions that are necessary for an organism to exist. The ability to obtain all the substances that are essential for their existence eliminates the need for a dependence on other cells. These single-celled organisms are thus able to maintain a relative state of equilibrium within their internal environment.

Homeostasis in multicellular organisms

In complex multicellular organisms such as humans, homeostasis can be divided into that occurring within the cell and that occurring outside the cell but within the body. The latter contains fluid referred to as extracellular fluid.

Cell homeostasis

Cell homeostasis involves the maintenance of an optimum environment for a particular cell to function. This cellular environment consists of optimum concentrations of gases, nutrients, chemical regulators (hormones and enzymes), electrically charged particles (ions) and water. Cell homeostasis is maintained by the cell membrane and the nucleus.

The cell membrane, by acting as a selective barrier between the intracellular and extracellular fluid is able to regulate the movement of substances into and out of cells. All cell membranes have similar homeostatic properties in that they regulate the internal environment according to the needs of a particular cell. The specialized nature and the diversity of function of cell types in the body are described in Chapter 25. This diversity of cell function requires cell membranes to have properties related to the specialized function of a particular cell. EXAMPLE: In nerve cells, a momentary flow of sodium ions into the cell is required for a nerve impulse to occur. The membranes of these cells have the specialized property of allowing sodium to pass through them for brief periods of time. Without this mechanism the function of both the cell and the body functions that it influences would be altered.

Within a cell, chemicals are continually manufactured, broken down or altered. The collective term for these chemical reactions is metabolism. The nucleus maintains optimum concentrations of chemicals by altering the concentrations of enzymes, the regulators of chemical reactions. By so doing the nucleus regulates the production, breakdown or conversion of chemicals within a cell. Malfunctions in the production of key enzymes result in homeostatic imbalances within a cell which can have a generalized affect throughout the body. EXAMPLE: Phenylketonuria (see Application, 29.12).

Body homeostasis

The integrated function of the body is essential for a complex multicellular organism such as humans. The actions of highly specialized cells need to be coordinated for efficient body function.

The maintenance of cell homeostasis in a particular cell usually depends upon the integrated action of other cell types throughout the body. The different needs of specific cells also require coordinated homeostatic mechanisms for the individual cell's needs to be satisfied. EXAMPLE: Nerve cells con-

stantly depend upon a high concentration of glucose in the extracellular fluid, whereas muscle cells only require high concentrations during exercise. An increase in the flow of blood to regions of muscle contraction results in the necessary elevated supply of glucose. A homeostatic mechanism is used to selectively increase the flow of blood to the muscle cells. This mechanism includes:

1. an increase in heart rate and its pumping ability to force blood and thus glucose at a rapid rate to the relevant region;
2. a localized dilation in the blood vessels resulting in an increased flow of blood in the vicinity of the contracting muscles.

Homeostatic mechanisms have therefore increased the supply of glucose to the relevant muscle cells by increasing the volume of blood to the region. Note that the concentration of glucose, that is the quantity of glucose molecules in a certain volume, has not been significantly altered.

Body homeostasis involves the maintenance of a relatively constant concentration of substances in the extracellular fluid. The supply of nutrients to different regions of the body is altered by homeostatic mechanisms according to the needs of particular cells. The composition of extracellular fluid depends upon the integrated action of several different homeostatic mechanisms. EXAMPLE: The concentration of oxygen in the extracellular fluid relies upon the coordinated and efficient function of the respiratory tract, lungs, heart and blood vessels, along with a sufficient quantity of red blood cells for transporting the oxygen. An imbalance between these factors can alter the supply of oxygen to the cells. The integration of these factors is thus necessary for homeostasis to occur.

Body homeostasis differs from cell homeostasis in that it relies upon an intercellular communication network. Without this network an imbalance in body homeostasis would occur. In addition, the coordinated action of various homeostatic mechanisms requires an integrating centre to assess the effects of the actions of any homeostatic mechanism on the entire body.

The brain acts as the integrating centre for most homeostatic mechanisms. It receives information, assesses it and then sends out instructions that regulate homeostatic imbalances. The communication networks that it utilizes are the nervous system and the endocrine system. The role that they play in body homeostasis is described in Chapters 38, 39 and 40.

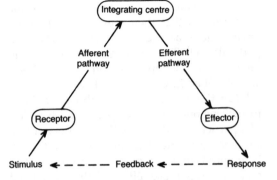

Figure 1.1 Generalized diagram of a homeostatic mechanism.

1.2 Homeostatic mechanisms

Generalized homeostatic mechanisms

In any homeostatic mechanism several essential components are necessary:

1. Receptor — sensor or detector used to inform the body of any imbalances.
2. Integrating centre — used to coordinate sensor information and determine the required response to any imbalance. If the response is insufficient then a further response will occur.
3. Effector — these effect the response. EXAMPLES: glands, muscle.
4. Communication pathways — a pathway is necessary to link the information of the receptor to the integrating centre. This is called the afferent pathway. An efferent pathway connects the integrating centre with the effector.

The relationship of these components is shown in Figure 1.1. This generalized diagram can be superimposed on any homeostatic mechanism. Note that all of these components are essential for a particular homeostatic mechanism to work. A loss of any component will result in an inability of the homeostatic mechanism to function. EXAMPLE: An inability of the effector to function in the blood sugar homeostatic mechanisms results in this mechanism being unable to function. The result is diabetes mellitus.

An understanding of the principle of homeostasis and the mechanisms involved will assist in the understanding of the sites of malfunction and the possible effects of a particular imbalance on body function.

An individual homeostatic mechanism usually involves several parts of the body, and in many cases this results in an overlap with other homeostatic mechanisms. EXAMPLE: The homeostasis of blood pressure involves the heart, arterioles and veins, large arteries, sympathetic and vagus nerves, brain and any factors that either require or cause an altered blood pressure. All of these components can be combined to form a homeostatic mechanism that is based on Figure 1.1.

Application: Homeostasis of blood calcium

The homeostasis of blood calcium consists of a relatively simple mechanism. The general mechanism is shown in Figure 1.2. This diagram indicates that a decrease in blood calcium concentration stimulates the receptor in the parathyroid gland. This gland probably acts as part of the integrating centre which compares this low level of calcium with the normal concentration in order to determine the magnitude of response. An increased quantity of parathormone is secreted from the gland and into the blood. This hormone acts on bone to release the appropriate quantity of calcium into the blood. The elevated concentration of calcium is then detected by receptors and compared with normal values to determine the next response.

Homeostasis of calcium is important, as calcium plays an important role in nerve and muscle function and in the coagulation of blood.

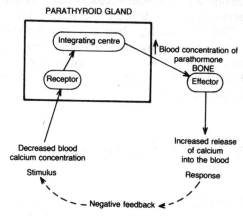

Figure 1.2 Homeostatic mechanism for the regulation of blood calcium concentration.

Feedback controls

Imbalances in the body's homeostasis require carefully monitored adjustments by the integrating centres. The relationship between an imbalance and the response of the integrating centre to this imbalance is called feedback.

There are two forms of feedback, negative feedback and positive feedback. Negative feedback results in the response of the body being opposite to the imbalance. EXAMPLE: Blood sugar levels — a decreased blood sugar level results in negative feedback causing homeostatic mechanisms to raise the blood sugar level, whereas if an increased level exists the mechanisms will cause a decrease in blood sugar levels. Nearly all homeostatic mechanisms involve negative feedback, that is a system that attempts to return imbalances to the normal ranges.

Positive feedback results in the response of the body being the same as the imbalance. Positive feedback therefore acts as an amplifier, that is, it enhances the imbalance which results in the imbalance being further away from the normal range. Clearly, positive feedback is an undesirable mechanism for homeostasis! Some homeostatic mechanisms involve positive feedback but generally its use in the body is limited. EXAMPLE: In the menstrual cycle, an increase in the blood level of the hormone oestrogen stimulates the release of another hormone called luteinizing hormone. Blood oestrogen levels cause a positive feedback on the pituitary gland to increase the levels of luteinizing hormone.

1.3 Stress

Stress was first defined by Hans Selye in 1935. He defined stress as a condition of the body produced by a variety of injurious

Table 1.1   Body's fight or flight response

Organ	Action	Response
Blood vessel	dilates in skeletal muscles and brain	↑ blood flow to essential organs involved in the response
	constricts in non-essential areas such as skin and viscera	↓ blood flow to non-essential areas
Heart	↑ heart rate and pumping capacity	↑ blood flow
Liver muscle	↑ conversion of glycogen to glucose	↑ glucose supply
Lungs	↑ respiratory rate and ↑ dameter of respiratory passages	↑ supply of oxygen ↑ removal of carbon dioxide
Spleen	contracts	↑ releases stored blood

agents or stimuli, referred to as stressors. Stressors can be physical, chemical or psychological factors or a combination of these. They can originate from the external environment or internally. EXAMPLES: External stressors — temperature variation, loud noise, pollution and exposure to harmful microorganisms. Internal stressors — high blood pressure, pain, tumours, emotional upset and endocrine disturbances. Often a combination of external and internal stressors occurs.

Selye introduced the term 'general adaptation syndrome' to describe the changes that occur under the condition of stress. The general adaptation syndrome refers to an initial stage of alarm in which the body is prepared for the fight or flight (Table 1.1). In the second, or resistance stage, the body repairs the damages caused by the stressor and resists its effects. In the third, or exhaustion stage, the body's homeostatic mechanisms have failed to cope with the effects of the stressor. Diseases of stress usually appear in this stage. EXAMPLE: Ulcers. NOTE: Everyday life produces stress from a wide range of factors. Some of this stress in fact prepares us to meet challenges. This 'productive stress' is often referred to as eustress while harmful stress is referred to as distress.

The effect of stress on different people will vary according to their individual homeostatic abilities to cope with it. The greater the stressor, the greater the demands placed on the body's homeostatic mechanisms to counteract the effects of the stressor. The ability of the body to withstand and correct imbalances will depend upon the overall state of health of the patient. EXAMPLE: An ill person may have a lower capacity to cope with an emotional problem or an infection than a healthy person. Both symptoms may therefore ensue from stressors that a healthy person has little difficult in coping with.

The relationship between psychological stressors and physicals stressors and their mechanism of action is discussed in 40.5. Table 1.1 describes the main body responses in the alarm stage.

1.4   Biofeedback

Biofeedback is a conscious homeostatic mechanism that relies upon signals to act as the feedback mechanism. It is an attempt to override the subconscious automatic homeostatic mechanisms of the autonomic nervous system.

Biofeedback is the process whereby a patient is taught to consciously control some actions of the autonomic nervous system such as heart rate or muscle tension. This is achieved by monitoring the action with visual or auditory evidence such as sounding a tone when the blood pressure reaches a certain point.

The steps involved in biofeedback are:

1. Detection of subconscious physiological activity and the connection of a transducer that converts the activity into a visual or auditory signal. This signal must be a representative signal of the physiological activity, that is, variations in the physio-logical activity must result in a relative alteration in the signal.
2. The patient is then instructed on how to respond to the signal. EXAMPLE: Increased muscle tension produces an elevated volume of sound. The patient is asked to reduce this volume by perform-ing the previously shown methods of relaxation.

Biofeedback is presently used in an attempt to control many stress-related physiological imbalances. EXAMPLES: Tension headache, anxiety, essential hypertension and gastro-intestinal disorders. Its application and effec-tiveness is certain to increase in the future as an understanding of body homeostatic mechanisms increases.

Summary

Homeostasis is a relative state of equilibrium between the internal environment of an organism and a changing external environ-ment. It is essential for life. Stressors can cause imbalance in the normal homeostatic state. These imbalances can result from factors in either the external or internal environments.

Homeostatic mechanisms return any imbalance to the normal optimum range of conditions. The greater the stressor and the resulting imbalance, the greater is the extent to which a homeostatic mechanism is required to function. The condition of stress occurs in three stages: the alarm stage, the resistance stage in which body homeostatic mechanisms attempt to return the body to normal function, and the exhaustion stage in which the homeostatic mechanisms fail to cope with the effects of the stressor. When the homeostatic mechanism is unable to cope with the stressor, ill health can result. The inability to cope with a particular stressor may be due to the following factors.

1. The level of the stressor is greater than the capabilities of the homeostatic mech-anisms of an individual, and these capa-bilities vary between individuals.
2. Continued stress may result in a decrease in the efficiency of a homeostatic mech-anism to correct an imbalance.
3. The state of health of the patient may decrease the ability to cope with any addi-tional stresses.
4. A malfunction in the homeostatic mech-anism prevents the mechanism from functioning.

Treatment of a particular body imbalance will usually involve eliminating the causative factors and/or correcting abnormal levels of substances. Both these approaches assist homeostatic mechanisms in returning the body to normal function.

In single-celled organisms such as bacteria the cell performs all the vital functions for the organism, whereas in multicellular organisms such as humans a coordinated action of many cells is required for the organism to live. Single-celled organisms depend upon the cell membrane for their homeostasis whereas humans rely upon both cell homeostasis and the coordinated action of cells or body homeostasis.

Homeostatic mechanisms require the following components for the mechanism to function: receptor, integrating centre, effector and communication pathways linking these. The integrating centre relies upon these pathways for feedback on the effect of its instructions on the body. In most homeostatic mechanisms negative feedback is used, that is, a system that attempts to return imbalances to the normal ranges.

Biofeedback is the process whereby a patient is taught to consciously control some actions of the autonomic nervous system.

Unit Two
Measurement

This unit introduces the methods of measuring matter, with emphasis on the use of SI units as a system of measurement.

Chapter 2

Measurement and units

Objectives

At the completion of this chapter the student should be able to:

1. differentiate between qualitative, semi-qualitative and quantitative measurements;
2. name the fundamental SI units;
3. express numbers in scientific notation;
4. express measurements of weight, volume, size, temperature, pressure and energy in SI units.

2.1 Measurement and matter

The universe consists of matter, energy and space. **Matter** is defined as anything that occupies space and has mass. It stores energy in a variety of forms. The measurement of matter and energy plays an important role in patient care, as any variation in the health status of a person represents a change in the quantity or interrelationship between different forms of matter or of energy.

The term **mass** is simply the quantity of matter that a substance contains when compared with a standard piece of platinum kept at the International Bureau of Weights and Measures in France. This standard has a mass defined as 1 kilogram (kg) in the international units known as SI units. A substance with half as much matter as the standard mass, has a mass of 0.5 kg, whereas a substance of 2 kg mass has twice as much matter as the standard mass.

The mass of an object or the quantity of matter in an object is the same wherever the object is taken in the universe. This book has the same mass in water as it does in a classroom or on Mars. The amount of matter or mass does not change. The relationship between mass and volume is called density. **Density** is the amount of mass in a given volume (15.3 Gravity).

A knowledge of the fundamental structure of matter is important in understanding its physical properties, such as how matter moves, and its chemical properties, such as how the structural units of matter interact. All matter consists of fundamental building blocks of different distinct sizes called particles. The three particles, known as protons, neutrons and electrons, combine to form larger particles called atoms. **Atoms** are the chemical building blocks of matter. They can be altered by gaining or losing electrons to form ionic particles. Atoms can be combined to form particles consisting of tightly bound units called molecules. The atoms within molecules are arranged in specific proportions. EXAMPLE: A water molecule (H_2O) consists of two hydrogen atoms for each oxygen atom.

Correctly observing, recording and interpreting a patient's condition is essential for the effective functioning of a health team. The recording of observations often relies on the need to measure what you are observing. EXAMPLES: Blood pressure, urine output, fluid intake and temperature. The recorded measurement relies on the experience and training of the person who is observing a sign and interpreting it. The recorded measurements need to be written in a manner that other hospital staff can interpret. There are three categories of measurement.

Qualitative measurements

Qualitative measurements are based on the presence or absence of signs. Signs are the evidence of a disease to an observer who records the signs in acceptable terms such as pale, very pale. A combination of descriptive signs can assist in the understanding of a patient's problems.

Semi-qualitative measurements

A semi-qualitative measurement records information on a relative scale. The recorded information is usually in the form of + or relative words. The relative number of + indicates the extent of the sign. EXAMPLE: +++, ++, +, 0 is used to indicate the sensitivity of microorganisms to antibiotics, and also the presence of glucose with clinistix tests. Descriptive words such as absent/moderate/severe are used to indicate the extent of shock. Semi-qualitative measurements are estimates of an observation.

Application: Apgar score

A relative scale indicating the condition of a newborn infant is usually recorded 60 seconds after birth. Values of 0, 1 and 2 are given for the signs listed in the chart. The apgar score is the sum of the points recorded for each sign and is a general expression of the newborn's condition.

Apgar scoring chart

Sign	Score		
	0	1	2
Heart rate	Absent	Slow (below 100)	Over 100
Respiratory effort	Absent	Slow, irregular	Good, crying
Muscle tone	Flaccid	Some flexion of extremities	Active motion
Reflex irritability	No response	Grimace	Cry
Colour	Blue, pale	Body pink, extremities blue	Completely pink

Quantitative measurements

Quantitative measurements use numbers to express the quantity of a variable. These measurements require the use of instruments which enable a precise numerical measurement to be recorded. The observed number that is recorded by an instrument is a precise measurement as long as the instrument is operating and functioning correctly. A number is often useless by itself unless an indication is given of what the number is referring to! EXAMPLE: A pulse rate of 50 fails to indicate whether there are 50 pulses per second, per 15 seconds, per 60 seconds, etc. Most quantitative measurements require an additional piece of information which is referred to as a unit.

2.2 Units of measurement

A unit is a standardized, descriptive word which specifies the dimension of a number. Traditionally there have been seven properties of matter that were measured independently of each other. The terms used to describe such measurements were referred to as fundamental units. These seven fundamental physical properties of matter are:

1. duration of measurement or time;
2. the physical size of an object or length;
3. the mass of an object or mass;
4. the amount of electric current passing through an object or current;
5. the temperature of an object or temperature;
6. the amount of substance present;
7. the brightness of an object or luminous intensity.

Each of these fundamental units is standardized by a term which is defined by a precise physical phenomenon that can be measured. Any measurement of a fundamental unit is based on a reference to the standardized physical phenomenon. EXAMPLE: The universal term for time is the second. A second is defined as the duration of 9 192 631 770 cycles of radiation associated with a specified transition of the caesium-133 atom. The time of any watch or clock in the world is based upon this definition. Clearly an individual is unable to determine a second directly by measuring the cycles of radiation associated with a caesium-133 atom. An individual can measure seconds indirectly by checking his or her watch with the standard time which is announced over telephones, radios and television sets.

The number of properties that are expressed independently of each other has decreased in recent years as technology and our understanding of matter has increased. Currently, only **mass**, **time** and **length** are considered to be fundamental units although texts often use for convenience the seven units previously described.

All other physical properties of matter can be distinguished from each other by derivation from a combination of fundamental units. A derived unit can always be written as a combination of several fundamental units. EXAMPLE: The SI unit of force is the newton. It is derived by combining the units mass, length and time. Unfortunately over the past few centuries the development of scientific knowledge in different parts of the world has led to the formation of several distinct measurement systems. The two principal systems that were formed are commonly referred to as the Imperial/US system and the metric system. Problems were encountered when information was reported in one system but was required to be converted into the other, and often a lot of unnecessary time was spent converting measurements from one system to another. (Some SI unit conversions are given in Appendix II.) Also, no uniform progression exists in the Imperial/US system. EXAMPLE: converting yards to inches requires two different multiplications of ×3 to feet and ×12 to inches.

2.3 SI and US unit systems

What is an SI unit?

Several years ago an international system of units was agreed upon by most major countries. This Système International d'Unités or SI units is a modern system of units that relates present scientific knowl-

Table 2.1   Fundamental SI units

Quantity	Name	Symbol
Length	metre	m
Mass	kilogram	kg
Time	second	s
Current	ampere	A
Temperature	Kelvin	K
Amount of substance	mole	mol
Luminous intensity	candela	cd

Table 2.2   Common derived SI units

Physical quantity	Name	Symbol
Force	newton	N
Energy	joule	J
Pressure	pascal	Pa
Potential difference	volt	V
Frequency	hertz	Hz
Volume	litre	L

edge to a uniform simplified system of units. The introduction of the SI units will bring uniformity of terminology, simplicity and a trend towards more uniform practice.

The fundamental SI units are listed in Table 2.1. In addition to the fundamental units there are a number of derived units such as litre, joule and pascal that are used in hospitals (Table 2.2).

US system

The US system is used in everyday life in the United States of America and is based on the English imperial system. The fundamental units are the **foot**, **pound** and **second**. Scientific measurements are usually described in the SI system although it is important for persons working in health care to be aware of the main US units described in Tables 2.4, 2.5 and 2.6 and Appendix II.

Multiples and submultiples

The magnitude or size of a measurement may result in an extremely large number for a specified unit. EXAMPLE: 3600 seconds is difficult to comprehend in terms of time. Other submultiples and multiples of a unit are used to eliminate cumbersome aggregates of numbers. EXAMPLE: The multiples of time are the minute, hour, day, week and year. These are useful to use, as one hour represents 3600 seconds. Imagine how unwieldy it would be writing 86 400 seconds when referring to one day! Subdivisions of a second include milli- (one thousandth) and micro- (one millionth).

The SI system is based on multiples of ten, that is, multiples and submultiples of each unit are used when describing the magnitude of a measurement. The names of these multiples and submultiples are listed in Table 2.3.

The expression of a number such as one millionth, which is one divided by a million, can be written as either 1/1 000 000 or 0.000001. Both of these forms of expressing numbers appear unnecessarily large and complex. Since sophisticated pathology equipment can measure quantities as low as one millionth of a millionth, a simplified form of numerical expression is used to record all medical results. This simplified expression is known as scientific notation.

Scientific notation

Very large and very small numbers are often encountered when describing chemical and biological measurements. When these numbers are written in their ordinary way a visually large set of numbers occurs. EXAMPLES: There are 8 500 000 000 white

Table 2.3 Names and abbreviations of SI unit multiples and submultiples

Prefix	Symbol	Meaning	Scientific notation
tera	T	one million million	10^{12}
giga	G	one thousand million	10^{9}
mega	M	one million	10^{6}
kilo	k	one thousand	10^{3}
hecto	h	one hundred	10^{2}
deca	da	ten	10^{1}
deci	d	one tenth	10^{-1}
centi	c	one hundredth	10^{-2}
milli	m	one thousandth	10^{-3}
micro	μ	one millionth	10^{-6}
nano	n	one thousandth of a millionth	10^{-9}
pico	p	one millionth of a millionth	10^{-12}
femto	f	one thousandth of a pico	10^{-15}
atto	a	one millionth of a pico	10^{-18}

$$25 = 2.5 \times 1000 \qquad\ = 2.5 \times 10^1$$
$$2500 = 2.5 \times 1000 \qquad = 2.5 \times 10^3$$
$$2\,500\,000 = 2.5 \times 1\,000\,000 \qquad = 2.5 \times 10^6$$

The accepted form of scientific notation is to place only one numeral to the left of the decimal point. The number of numerals that are on the right of the decimal point is written above the ten, e.g. 5400 is 5.4×10^3 since three numbers are to the right of five.

Numbers that are less than one are written the following way. Place a decimal point to the right of the first non-zero digit. Multiply this number by ten and place above the ten the number of digits that have been moved past the original position of the decimal point. A negative sign is placed in front of the raised numeral to indicate that the powers of ten are being divided into the digit.

EXAMPLES:

$$0.1 = 1.0 \times 10^{-1} \quad \text{or} \quad 1/10$$
$$0.01 = 1.0 \times 10^{-2} \quad \text{or} \quad 1/100$$
$$0.001 = 1.0 \times 10^{-3} \quad \text{or} \quad 1/1000$$
$$0.0065 = 6.5 \times 10^{-3} \quad \text{or} \quad 6.5/1000$$
$$0.000084 = 8.4 \times 10^{-5} \quad \text{or} \quad 8.4/100\,000$$

blood cells per litre of blood in a normal person. The amount of insulin in a fasting patient is in the range 0.0000000001 to 0.00000000001 mole per litre of serum. These numbers are difficult to write without making mistakes, hard to understand and almost impossible to say. The use of submultiple and multiple prefixes can assist in describing a number, but a simplified system of numbers is necessary when mathematical calculations are required.

Scientific notation is the writing of numbers in terms of a power of ten. EXAMPLES:

$$100 = 10 \times 10 \qquad\qquad\qquad\qquad = 10^2$$
$$1000 = 10 \times 10 \times 10 \qquad\qquad\qquad = 10^3$$
$$1\,000\,000 = 10 \times 10 \times 10 \times 10 \times 10 \times 10 = 10^6$$

Note that with large numbers, the figure placed above the ten is equal to the quantity of zeros.

When a number contains other numerals the number is written as follows:

Important SI units

Kilogram

The kilogram is the unit of weight and is represented by the symbol kg. Table 2.4 shows the relationship between other units and the kilogram. There are 1000 grams to a kilogram. The gram is often used as a base unit in hospitals. One milligram is thus 10^{-3} of a gram and not 10^{-3} of a kilogram. The symbol g refers to grams.

Litre

The SI unit for volume is the litre which is represented as L (note L is the preferred symbol although l is often used). The relationship between the litre and other units is shown in Table 2.5.

Table 2.4 Comparative measures of weight

1 kilogram	=	100 gram
1 gram	=	1000 milligram
1 milligram	=	10^{-3} gram
1 microgram	=	10^{-6} gram
1 pound	=	0.454 kilogram
1 pound	=	454 gram
1 ounce	=	28.35 gram
25 gram	=	0.9 ounce
1 ounce	=	8 dram

Table 2.6 Comparative measures of length

1 metre	=	10^{-3} kilometre
1 centimetre	=	10^{-2} metre
1 millimetre	=	10^{-3} metre
1 square metre	=	10^{2} metre
1 metre	=	39.37 inch
1 mile	=	1.6 kilometre
1 yard	=	0.9 metre
1 foot	=	0.3 metre
1 inch	=	25.4 millimetre

Table 2.5 Comparative measures of volume

1 litre	=	100 millilitre
100 millilitre	=	1 decilitre
1 millilitre	=	1000 microlitre
1 UK gallon	=	4.5 litre
1 US gallon	=	3.8 litre
1 pint	=	568 millilitre or 500 mL (US)
1 fluid ounce	=	28.42 millilitre or 30 mL (US)
1 fluid dram	=	4 mL
1 teaspoon	=	5 mL
1 tablespoon	=	15 mL

Metre

The metre or m is the SI unit of length. There are 39.37 inches in one metre. The common measures of length are shown in Table 2.6.

Kelvin

The Kelvin (K) is the SI unit of temperature. Absolute zero or 0 K is equal to $-273°C$ (7.6). A change of 1 K is identical to a change of 1°C. Note that Kelvin is not preceded by a ° degrees symbol. To determine K temperature from a Celsius temperature, simply add 273 to the Celsius temperature. EXAMPLE: A body temperature of 38°C is equal to 311 K as 38°C + 273 = 311 K. For practical purposes degrees Celsius will continue to be used for the present time.

The Fahrenheit scale of 32 to 212°F en- compasses the same temperature range as 0 to 100°C (Appendix B). A change of 1°F is not equal to 1°C. The conversion of a reading in Fahrenheit into Celsius is performed by subtracting thirty-two, multiplying by five and dividing by nine. EXAMPLE: 97°F − 32 = 65 × 5 = 325 ÷ 9 = 36.1°C. The conversion of a reading in Celsius into Fahrenheit is performed by reversing the above procedure, that is multiply by nine, divide by five and add thirty-two. EXAMPLE: 36.1°C × 9 = 325 ÷ 5 = 65 + 32 = 97°F.

Pascal

The pascal or Pa is the SI unit of pressure. The kilopascal or kPa is being introduced as the unit in blood gas estimations. A kilopascal is determined by multiplying the old units of millimetres of mercury (mm Hg) by 0.133. The old method of recording blood pressure in mm Hg will continue to be used until practical considerations permit the use of kPa sphygmomanometers.

The British unit of pounds per square inch (lb/in^2) or psi is converted into kPa by multiplying by 6.88.

Joule

A joule or J is described as the potential energy which is released when 1 kg weight falls through 1 metre by the force of gravity. The joule is to replace the calorie as the unit

Table 2.7   Comparative measures of energy

1 calorie	=	4.184 joules
1000 calories	=	1 dietary Calorie or kilocalorie
1 dietary Calorie	=	4184 joules or 4.184 kilojoule
1000 Calorie	=	4184 kilojoule
1 kilojoule	=	0.238 Calories

of energy. Since the joule is smaller than the dietary Calorie, the larger kilojoule is preferred. A Calorie is converted into a kilojoule by multiplying by 4.184. The common comparative units are listed in Table 2.7.

Mole

The mole is the SI unit for the amount of substance present. This unit is discussed in Chapter 3.

Summary

Three types of measurement of a patient's condition can be made.

1. Qualitative measurement is used to describe the presence or absence of signs.
2. Semi-qualitative measurement records information on a relative scale using + or relative words. This measurement relies on experience and training for the estimation of an observation.
3. Quantitative measurement records information in terms of numbers. This measurement usually requires the use of an instrument.

The SI unit systems are now being used in many major countries and are the preferred units for reporting scientific measurements. The US system is used for everyday life measurements in the United States of America.

The three fundamental physical properties of matter and their SI units are: time — second, length — metre, mass — kilogram. A further four physical properties are often also considered as fundamental units. These are: current — ampere, temperature — Kelvin, amount of substance present — mole, luminous intensity — candela.

Important SI units that can be derived from the seven fundamental units are: force — newton, energy — joule, pressure — pascal, potential difference — volt, frequency — hertz and volume — litre.

A simplified system of expressing numbers is used in the SI system. Prefixes such as micro- and nano- can be used to describe a number. Alternatively, numbers are expressed as multiples of ten. EXAMPLE: One million is written as 10^6 and one millionth as 10^{-6}.

Chapter 3

Concept of concentration

Objectives

At the completion of this chapter the student should be able to:

1. explain the term concentration;
2. express concentration in SI units;
3. define the terms mole, molar and atomic weight;
4. convert other concentration expressions into moles per litre;
5. explain the difference between SI units and international units of concentration.

3.1 Concentration and the body

Concentration refers to the quantity of substance present in a given volume. In SI units this volume is one litre. The concentration of substances within different healthy individuals is approximately the same, even though the amount of substances may be different. A large person generally contains more substances than a small person. However the large person also contains a proportionately greater volume which results in both people containing approximately the same concentration.

Body function relies upon a balanced concentration of many different body substances. These substances form the basis of the biochemical tests that are performed by pathology laboratories. Within a population, a normal concentration range has been determined for many body chemicals. Variations in the concentration of a particular substance from the normal range usually indicates

abnormal body function. Biochemical tests are used to assist diagnosis and in addition they can be used for monitoring the response of a patient to treatment.

3.2 SI unit for concentration

Moles/litre

The SI unit termed moles per litre has resulted in a uniform expression of concentration. Prior to the introduction of moles per litre and millimoles per litre many forms of expressing the concentration of chemicals were found in hospitals. EXAMPLES: Milliequivalents per litre, percentage solutions, gram per litre, gram per decilitre, gram per 100 millilitre, volume per cent, Bessey units, etc. In most cases these units have been abolished. The confusion in understanding biochemical results was compounded by the use of several units for the same substance. EXAMPLE: Plasma calcium was measured in either milligram per 100 millilitre or milliequivalents per litre, the latter being twice the former.

Determining concentration

Concentration refers to the number of particles present in a given volume. The following methods are used to determine the quantity of particles in a container.

1. Determine the total weight of the particles and divide this weight by the weight of one particle. ANALOGY: A box of eggs has a weight of 600 g and the weight of each egg is approximately 50 g. The number of eggs present is calculated by dividing 50 into 600, that is, the box contains 12 eggs.
2. Count the total number of particles present. ANALOGY: If the eggs could be counted in the container the quantity of eggs is easily determined.

With these methods it is necessary to either weigh or count the particles in order to determine the concentration of a substance.

Often in the past, the person dealing with chemicals had to calculate the particle concentration, since the units of concentration were not uniform and did not represent the total particle concentration. With the introduction of SI units a uniform and precise system of representing particle concentration has been introduced. This system has the advantage of eliminating the need for calculating the true concentration from units that express a relative concentration such as grams per litre (3.3). With the SI system the particle concentration in a container is stated and thus the number of particles is known. ANALOGY: At a supermarket, the number of eggs in a carton is printed on the container which eliminates the need to count the

number of eggs or to weigh the total contents and divide by the weight of one egg. The major advantage of this system is that the true particle concentration of different substances can be compared without the need for calculations.

In chemistry, a very large number of molecules exists in any small sample of a substance. Instead of labelling chemical containers with very large confusing numbers a simplified system is now used. The enormous number 6.023×10^{23} is replaced in chemistry by the term one mole which is abbreviated to mol. This large, convenient number is referred to as Avogadro's number. In a container there is one mole of molecules present for every 6.023×10^{23} molecules. ANALOGY: When referring to large quantities of paper it is convenient to use the term ream. A ream represents 480 sheets of paper whereas in chemistry a mole represents 6.023×10^{23} molecules. Three reams of paper indicate a quantity of 3×480 whereas three moles of substance represent $3 \times 6.023 \times 10^{23}$ molecules.

A container with three moles of a particular substance contains the same number of molecules as another container with three moles of another substance. ANALOGY: A package with three reams of foolscap paper contains the same number of pages as a package with three reams of a different size paper. The term mole is also used to indicate the number of ions present in a solution. The concentration of molecules refers to the number of molecules of a substance that is present in a volume of one litre. The relationship between moles and concentration is as follows: **the concentration of a solution is determined by the number of moles of substance present in one litre of that solution**. This concentration is referred to as molar. EXAMPLE: A one molar solution contains one mole of substance in one litre of the solution, whereas a two molar solution contains two moles of substance in one litre of the solution. Note that a solution consists of substances dissolved in a liquid. A more detailed description is given in 17.2.

The concentration of substances within the body and in solutions added to the body is generally lower than one mole. This results in the use of other units such as millimole per litre, micromole per litre and nanomole per litre. The most frequently used unit is the millimole (one thousandth of a mole).

So far we have determined that the mole represents a specific number of particles in any substance. The total number of particles in a mixture of substances can be determined by adding the moles of each substance. EXAMPLE: The intravenous amino acid solution 'synthamin 17' contains 100 mmol/L of amino acids, 70 mmol/L of acetate and 40 mmol/L chloride. The total quantity of substances present is 100 + 70 + 40 = 210 mmol/L. Every litre of 'synthamin 17' contains 210 mmol of molecules and ions. A solution of 500 mL contains half the volume and thus half the quantity of these substances, i.e. 105 mmol. The term molarity refers to the number of moles of a substance or substances present in one litre of a solution. EXAMPLE: 'Synthamin 17' has a molarity of 210 mmol.

The number of millimoles in a bottle may not be the required quantity that has to be administered to a patient. The volume of solution that represents the required amount of millimoles can be determined by using the following equation:

volume of solution needed

$$= \frac{\text{required moles substance}}{\text{molarity of solution}}$$

EXAMPLE: A patient requires a quantity of 200 mmol of sodium chloride from a one litre bottle that contains 308 mmol/L (1.8%) sodium chloride. Volume of solution required = 200 mmol/308 mmol = two-thirds of a litre. The volume required is therefore approximately 670 mL.

Sometimes it is necessary to calculate the total quantity of moles of a substance that has been administered for a given volume. The total number of moles can be calculated as follows:

millimoles of substance
  = solution molarity × volume in litres.

EXAMPLE: How many millimoles of sodium chloride has been administered in 500 mL of a 150 mmol sodium chloride solution? The number of millimoles of substance = 150 × 0.5 = 75 mmol.

Preparing a molar solution

Most preparations are labelled with the quantity of millimoles present. To assist in the understanding of molarity it is necessary to explain how a solution has been prepared. Clearly a person is unable to count a given number of molecules and make up a one litre solution.

Initially it is necessary to weigh an amount of a substance. The required weight will vary according to the weight of one molecule. There is an enormous variation in the weight of the molecules of different substances. For a given quantity of molecules, a substance that consists of a relatively heavy molecule will require a greater amount than a substance that is composed of a lighter molecule. ANALOGY: A cherry weighs less than an orange. Therefore if one takes ten of each fruit, a greater weight is observed with the ten oranges.

Both atoms and molecules are extremely small and may not be weighed on a balance. The weight of an individual molecule is determined by adding the weights of the constituent elements. The weight of each element varies according to the number of protons and neutrons present since the mass of an atom results from its protons and neutrons (4.2). The weight of each proton is defined as one, as is the weight of each neutron. Nearly all carbon atoms contain six protons and six neutrons, although a very small percentage contain six protons and eight neutrons. The carbon atom is defined as having an atomic mass of twelve.

The atomic mass of any atom is the weight of that atom relative to an atom of carbon. This means that atomic mass is not an actual, but a comparative weight and it therefore lacks a unit. EXAMPLES: Hydrogen mainly consists of one proton and therefore has an atomic mass of one. Oxygen contains a total of sixteen protons and neutrons which results in an atomic mass of sixteen. The atomic mass of each element is listed in the Periodic Table (see inside back cover). An element such as chlorine exists mainly as two isotopes, one of which contains two additional neutrons. The atomic mass of chlorine is 35.5 which is derived by averaging the proportions of the mass of each isotope.

The atomic mass is a useful chemical term as it indicates the relative mass of an atom compared to another element. When twelve grams of carbon are weighed a total of 6.023×10^{23} atoms are present, that is, one mole of atoms is present. Note that a sample of a pure element only contains one type of atom. A mole refers to the number of atoms and not molecules in these situations. **Whenever the atomic weight of an element has the same number as the number of grams, one mole of atoms is present**. EXAMPLES: One mole of hydrogen atoms is present in one gram of hydrogen, whereas sixteen grams of oxygen forms one mole of oxygen atoms since the atomic mass of hydrogen is one and oxygen is sixteen.

The weight of a molecule is termed the molecular weight. It is the total weight of all the constituent atoms. EXAMPLE: A glucose molecule is composed of six carbon, twelve hydrogen and six oxygen atoms. The molecular weight of glucose is calculated as follows:

carbon	6×12	=	72
hydrogen	12×1	=	12
oxygen	6×16	=	96
total		=	180

One mole of glucose molecules is present in 180 g. A one molar solution of glucose contains 180 g of glucose in one litre of solution. A one millimolar solution of glucose contains 0.180 g or 180 mg of glucose in one litre of solution. A 0.5 millimolar solution is prepared from 90 mg of glucose.

The SI unit of concentration is moles per litre. This unit can only be expressed if the molecular weight of a particular molecule is known, since the molar solution can only be prepared by using the atomic and molecular weights. There are numerous substances for which the molecular weight has not been obtained. EXAMPLE: Many proteins. These substances require other forms of expression to indicate their concentration.

3.3 International units

With some substances where the molecular weight is unknown the concentration is reported in terms of international units. An international unit is a measure of the effect of a concentration of a particular substance upon a standard solution with which that substance reacts. These units have been standardized by an International Conference for the Unification of Formulae. The substances where the biological effect is the unit of concentration, are usually either biological substances such as enzymes, hormones, vitamins, or drugs such as penicillin. EXAMPLE: The international unit of insulin is 1/22 of a milligram of the pure crystalline product. International units differ from substance to substance, and thus the international units from two substances cannot be compared or added.

3.4 Other expressions for concentration

Prior to the introduction of SI units several methods existed for expressing concentrations. These methods were replaced by millimoles per litre, except where the molecular weight of a substance was unknown.

Milliequivalents

These units have been replaced by the millimole. A milliequivalent is determined by relating the ability of an element to combine with, or displace, hydrogen. Unlike millimoles, one milliequivalent (meq) of one substance does not necessarily contain the same number of particles as one milliequivalent of another substance. EXAMPLE: One milliequivalent of calcium ions contains half the number of particles that one milliequivalent of sodium ions does.

Care must be taken when converting plasma calcium (Ca^{2+}) and magnesium (Mg^{2+}) into mmol/L since 1 meq/L of these substances represents 0.5 mmol/L. With most of the other chemicals that were expressed in meq/L, the concentration in mmol/L is represented by the same number. EXAMPLE: 1 meq/L of sodium ions equals 1 mmol/L.

Weight–volume

Prior to the introduction of SI units, the concentration of a substance was sometimes expressed as the number of grams per 100 mL of water. A concentration expressed in this form is a percentage solution. EXAMPLE: A 5% dextrose (glucose) solution indicates that there are five grams of dextrose in a solution of 100 mL. This form of concentration does not indicate how many glucose molecules are present. A 10% dextrose solution indicates that there are twice as many glucose molecules present than in the 5% solution.

A 5% solution of sodium chloride does not contain the same quantity of molecules as a 5% dextrose solution as sodium chloride has a molecular weight of 58.5 and dextrose one of 180. The sodium chloride molecule is approximately one-third the weight of a dextrose molecule, and thus 5 g of sodium chloride will contain approximately three times the number of molecules of 5 g of glucose. ANALOGY: In a purchase of 5000 g of oranges and 5000 g of cherries a far greater quantity of cherries would be expected since the weight of a cherry is less than that of an orange.

No comparison can be made between percentage solutions of different substances without taking into account the molecular weight of each substance. Percentage solutions fail to indicate the concentration of molecules in a solution, and for this reason they have been replaced by molar solutions wherever the molecular weight of a substance is known.

The use of weight–volume solutions is now restricted to substances whose molecular weight is unknown. EXAMPLES: Pathology reports — plasma proteins, enzymes, hormones; intravenous solutions such as intralipid (10 and 20%) and various dextran solutions. In addition, the introduction of SI units has resulted in an alteration in expression of percentage solutions from grams per 100 millilitre to grams per litre. EXAMPLE: A total protein concentration of 7.0 g/100 mL is now recorded as 70 g/L.

Ratio solutions

Ratio solutions express concentration in the terms of a ratio. EXAMPLE: A ratio of 1:1000 represents the number of grams per volume of solution. The one is in grams and the 1000 in millilitres. Ratio solutions lack a unit. These solutions can also be expressed in terms of the proportion of one substance to another. EXAMPLE: Dextrose–nitrogen ratio represents the ratio between dextrose and nitrogen in the urine. Different ratio solutions cannot be compared.

Summary

Concentration refers to the quantity of substance present in a given volume. In the body, a balanced concentration of substances is necessary for homeostasis.

The SI unit of concentration is moles per litre. This unit represents the number of particles present in one litre of solution, with one mole being 6.023×10^{23} particles (Avogadro's number).

The total number of particles in a mixture of substances can be determined by adding the moles of each substance.

The term molarity refers to the number of moles of a substance or substances present in one litre of solution.

The atomic mass of an element is the weight of an atom compared with that of another element. The atomic mass is approximately equal to the number of protons and neutrons present in the most abundant isotope of an element. When the atomic mass of an element is the same number as the number of grams, one mole of atoms is present.

The molecular mass is the total atomic mass of the constituent atoms of a molecule.

The molarity of a solution can only be determined if the atomic and molecular masses are known. When these masses are not known the concentration can be expressed as the number of grams per litre.

Some substances with an unknown molecular mass have their concentration expressed in international units. An international unit is a measure of the effect of a particular substance on a standard solution. International units will differ from substance to substance, and thus the international units of two substances cannot be compared or added. This method of expressing concentration can be used for hormones, enzymes, vitamins and drugs.

Unit Three
Chemical Properties of Matter

This unit describes the structural and
chemical properties of matter.

Chapter 4

Atoms and matter

Objectives

At the completion of this chapter the student should be able to:

1. define the terms matter, mass, element, isotope, atomic number, energy level, energy sublevel, ground state, electron affinity, ionization energy, atomic mass unit, electronegativity;
2. describe the structure of an atom and relate this structure to the properties that identify a particular element;
3. explain how cations and anions are formed;
4. list the main elements used by the body;
5. describe the toxic effects of elements.

4.1 Matter and chemistry

A knowledge of the interaction of particles is necessary to understand the mechanisms of body function and how these mechanisms can be altered by disease and trauma. The study of structure and composition of matter and the interactions within matter is called chemistry. The characteristics of a substance during its interaction with another substance and any resulting changes following the interaction are referred to as chemical characteristics or properties. EXAMPLES: The rusting of iron, the interaction of drugs with body chemicals, and the formation and breakdown of glucose within the body. Chapter 5 describes how atoms are combined to form substances.

4.2 Atoms

Matter is mainly composed of three sub-atomic particles known as protons, neutrons and electrons. These particles are arranged to form a structure called an atom which acts as the building block or structural unit of matter. All atoms are composed of a central region of relatively large mass known as a nucleus which contains protons and neutrons, and an outer cloud of orbiting particles with little mass called electrons (Figure 4.1).

Protons

The nucleus consists of positively charged subatomic particles called protons. Each proton has a charge of +1, and thus five

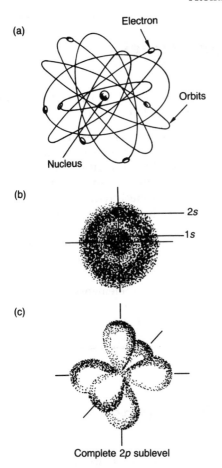

Figure 4.1 (a) Bohr solar system model of an atom. (b) Electron cloud view of an atom. (c) The 2p sublevel.

protons would have a charge of +5. To date, the maximum number of protons found in a nucleus is 109. The properties of an atom are determined by the number of positive charges within the nucleus, that is, the number of protons.

Electrons

All atoms contain negatively charged sub-atomic particles called electrons. Each elec-tron contains approximately 1/2000th the mass of a proton. These minute amounts of mass each have a charge of −1, and thus five electrons would have a charge of −5.

Electron distribution

Neils Bohr in 1913 described the electron dis-tribution in atoms as similar to that of planets revolving around the sun. This 'solar system model' of electrons forming orbits around the nucleus has been an important step in leading to the current understanding of electron distribution.

Electrons are believed to spin around the nucleus. Each electron occupies a certain region of space called an electron cloud or electron shell. When there are many elec-trons, more than one electron cloud exists. A cloud represents the space where there is usually at least a 95% chance of finding a particular electron. Each electron cloud represents an amount of energy as energy is required to hold electrons within the cloud. Electron clouds are often referred to as energy levels.

The maximum number of electrons that can be held in a shell is limited by the amount of energy present. The quantity of energy in each shell varies with its distance from the nucleus. Since a shell close to the nucleus has less energy to support electrons than a shell further away from the nucleus, it follows that shells further away from the nucleus contain more electrons than inner shells.

Another property of energy levels is that the maximum number of electrons that can be carried by the outermost shell is inde-pendent of the inner shells. The first shell will have a maximum of two electrons even when it is the only shell. If more than one shell exists the outermost shell will contain a maximum of eight electrons.

A general property of electrons is that they occupy the lowest available energy level first, in order to obtain the most stable electron distribution. The first energy level or electron shell is thus filled before electrons begin to fill the second shell. Whenever possible, electrons orbit the nucleus in pairs.. The maximum number of electrons for the first four energy levels are: first (2e), second (8e), third (18e) and fourth (32e).

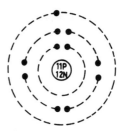

Figure 4.2 Sodium contains eleven electrons which requires the formation of a third electron shell.

Filling electron shells

To determine the distribution of electrons in atoms that contain more than ten electrons (two in the first shell, eight in the second) it is necessary to combine the property of holding a maximum of eight electrons in the outermost shell and the property of filling successive energy levels. When an atom has eleven electrons (sodium) two will be in the first orbit, eight in the second and one in the third (Figure 4.2).

If the third shell is the outermost shell a maximum of eight electrons can be held. However, if an atom contains more than eighteen electrons (first shell — two; second shell — eight; outermost — eight) a fourth shell is formed which automatically becomes the outermost shell. Now the third shell is not restricted to the rule governing outermost shells and thus it can hold a greater number of electrons. EXAMPLE: Iron (Figure 4.3). When four or more shells exist, the third shell contains eighteen electrons. Likewise, when a fifth shell is present the fourth level contains enough energy to hold up to thirty-two electrons.

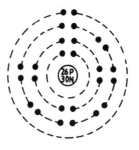

Figure 4.3 Iron contains twenty-six electrons which results in the third orbit containing fourteen electrons.

Energy sublevels

Within each energy level electrons are arranged in sublevels of energy or 'sublevels'. These sublevel arrangements are important as they influence the ability of an atom to combine within another atom. The sublevels within an energy level are known as *spdf* with s being the lowest sublevel energy. ANALOGY: The energy content of an atom changes by steps which can be compared with the floors of a building which represent energy levels and the steps between floors being the sublevels. Each sublevel can only carry a maximum of two electrons which must be spinning in opposite directions. Electrons are believed to spin like tops with some spinning in one direction while other electrons spin in the opposite direction. This property of pairing electrons is an important factor in combining atoms (5.2). The number of orbitals per sublevel increases from one for s to seven in f (Table 4.1).

Table 4.1   Energy sublevels

Energy sublevel	s	p	d	f
Number of orbitas	1	3	5	7
Total electrons per sublevel	2	6	10	14

Table 4.2   Order of electron filling

Start with bottom left hand corner and follow the arrows upward until the total electron number

2	6	10	14
7s2	7p6	7d10	7f14
6s2	6p6	6d10	6f14
5s2	5p6	5d10	5f14
4s2	4p6	4d10	4f
3s2	3p6	3d	
2s2	2p6		
1s²			

Filling electron subshells

Electrons fill the lowest energy level and sub-levels first which is abbreviated as 1s where the superscript indicates the number of electrons per sublevel. Hydrogen has one electron ($1s^1$) whereas Helium has 2 electrons ($1s^2 2s^1$). Remember that the first energy level can contain only two electrons. Lithium has three electrons and therefore forms two energy levels. Lithium is represented as $1s^2 2s^1$ whereas Oxygen with 8e has the distribution ($1s^2 2s^2 2p^4$). The order of filling electrons and therefore the electron distribution follows the pattern 1s, 2s, 2p, 3p, 4s, 3d, 4p (Table 4.2). The order for an atom can be found by following the diagonal arrows.

Sodium and potassium are two important body substances that have similar properties, yet different numbers of electron. Sodium (Na) has eleven electrons which are represented as $1s^2 2s^2 2p^6 3s^1$ whereas potassium contains nineteen electrons distributed as $1s^2 2s^2 2p^6 3s^2 3p^6 4s^1$. The electrons in the outermost energy level are often given a specific name since the number of outermost electrons represents the ability of an atom to combine with another atom. These outermost electrons are known as valence electrons and will be discussed in 5.8.

Ground state

The addition of energy such as heating to an electron will result in the electron changing from its resting energy level called ground state to a higher energy level. The ground state of an atom is when all electrons are occupying their normal lowest possible energy levels. The addition of external energy such as heat results in an electron jumping to a higher energy level. The atom is now in an unstable excited state. The excited unstable electron quickly returns to its normal energy level. This electron releases the same amount of energy as was used to place it in the higher energy level.

The amount of energy released is fixed for an electron. The energy emitted is in the form of electromagnetic radiation (11.1). The specific length of the electromagnetic waves identifies an atom. EXAMPLE: A sodium street lamp emits waves the same length as those of red light whereas a mercury lamp emits waves the same as blue light.

4.3   Ions

General properties

A fundamental property of nature is that all atoms attempt to have a full outer shell of electrons. This property confers important physical and chemical effects on matter and is thus of great importance in body function.

Many atoms gain or lose electrons in an attempt to form a complete outer electron shell. This change in electron number and

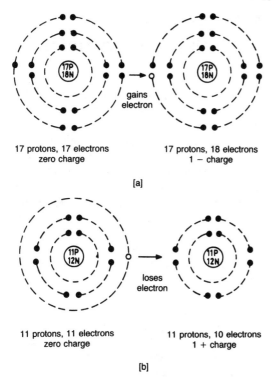

17 protons, 17 electrons
zero charge

17 protons, 18 electrons
1 − charge

[a]

11 protons, 11 electrons
zero charge

11 protons, 10 electrons
1 + charge

[b]

Figure 4.4   (a) Chlorine gains one electron to complete the outer shell. (b) Sodium loses one electron to complete the outer shell.

Not all atoms form ions. The atoms of boron, carbon and silicon are relatively small atoms which require the loss or gain of a large number of electrons (Chapter 5). The noble gases contain completed outer shells and thus do not require the loss or gain of electrons.

Anions

Generally atoms with more than four electrons in their outer shell gain or accept electrons in order to fill the outer shell (Figure 4.4a). Less energy is involved in gaining one, two or three electrons than in losing seven, six or five electrons respectively.

An atom with seven electrons in the outer shell will gain one electron so that the outer shell is complete with eight electrons. This extra electron results in the atom now having an excess of electrons with respect to protons, that is, the atom has a charge of −1. Likewise, an atom with six electrons in the outer orbit has a charge of −2 when the outer shell is completed. An anion is any atom or group of atoms that has a negative charge of at least 1.

Cations

Generally, atoms with less than four electrons in their outer shell find it easier to lose these outer shell electrons than to gain five or more electrons. These atoms are referred to as electron donors. When these atoms lose the outer shell electrons the second outermost orbit (which is usually full) becomes the outer orbit. EXAMPLE: Sodium (Figure 4.4b). The loss of electrons results in the atom containing a relative excess of protons and thus becoming positively charged. The loss of one electron results in a charge of +1 whereas the loss of two electrons results in a charge of +2. A cation is an atom or a group of atoms that has a positive charge of at least 1.

thus electrical charge results in the formation of charged atoms which are now referred to as ions.

An ion is an atom or group of atoms that contain a charge of at least +1 or −1. An ion formed from a metal (4.9) has the same name as the element plus the word ion. EXAMPLE: Sodium forms a sodium ion. An ion formed from non-metals has a name ending in ide. EXAMPLE: Chlorine forms a chloride ion. Ions have different properties to an atom. EXAMPLE: Sodium and lithium both react in water whereas the sodium ion is an important constituent of human body fluids and the lithium ion is administered for the treatment of manic-depressive conditions.

Electron affinity

The amount of energy released when an atom gains an electron to form a negative ion is referred to as the electron affinity. The larger the electron affinity the greater is the attraction of an atom for additional electrons. Atoms with more than four electrons in the outermost shell have a relatively high electron affinity and so gain electrons to complete the outer shell (Figure 4.4a).

Ionization energy

The amount of energy that must be added to an electron to remove one electron from the outermost shell is called the ionization energy. Atoms with greater than four electrons in the outermost shell have relatively high ionization energies. There is little likelihood of those atoms losing electrons to complete the outermost shell. Atoms with less than four electrons have lower ionization energies thereby releasing electrons and forming positively charged ions.

Electrons are released more readily from atoms with less than four outermost electrons. More energy is required to remove additional electrons as the nucleus has a greater attraction for the remaining electrons. The energy added to remove one electron is called the first ionization energy whereas the energy required to remove a second electron is called the second ionization energy. EXAMPLE: Calcium (Ca) has two outermost electrons, the first ionization energy is 596 kJ/mole whereas the second ionization energy is 1151 kJ/mole. Removing a third electron from Calcium requires a large amount of ionization energy 4938 kJ/mole as the loss of an electron from the second energy results in an incomplete shell. Therefore, calcium only forms ions by losing at the most two electrons.

4.4 Attraction of charged particles

A fundamental property of nature is that all matter attempts to have neutral or zero charge. This results in opposite charges attracting and like charges repelling in an attempt to neutralize the charges. Positively-charged particles are thus attracted to negatively-charged particles in an attempt to become neutral, whereas the positively-charged particles are repelled by other positively-charged particles. EXAMPLE: A charge of $+1$ combines with a charge of -1 to produce 0 or no charge. This force of attraction is important in determining properties of matter (Chapter 5), e.g. how substances combine with other substances, electricity and body electrolyte composition.

In an atom this force results in the atom containing the same number of protons (charge $+1$) as electrons (charge -1). The number of electrons orbiting a nucleus, and thus the number of shells, is determined by the quantity of protons fixed in the nucleus.

4.5 Atomic number

The properties of an atom are determined by the number of protons located in the nucleus. An atom with one proton (hydrogen) differs in its properties to an atom with eight protons (oxygen). The importance of the number of protons present in an atom has resulted in the need for a term to describe the quantity of protons that are contained in an atom. This is referred to as atomic number, that is, all atoms with an atomic number of one contain one proton, whereas atoms with an atomic number of eight, contain eight protons.

Table 4.3   Symbols of elements cited in this text

Element	Symbol	Atomic number	Element	Symbol	Atomic number
Aluminium	Al	13	Molybdenum	Mo	42
Arsenic	As	33	Nickel	Ni	28
Barium	Ba	56	Nitrogen	N	7
Bromine	Br	35	Oxygen	O	8
Calcium	Ca	20	Phosphorus	P	15
Caesium	Cs	55	Platinum	Pt	78
Carbon	C	6	Plutonium	Pu	94
Chlorine	Cl	17	Potassium	K	19
Chromium	Cr	24	Radium	Ra	88
Cobalt	Co	27	Radon	Rn	86
Copper	Cu	29	Selenium	Se	34
Fluorine	F	9	Silicon	Si	14
Gold	Au	79	Silver	Ag	47
Helium	He	2	Sodium	Na	11
Hydrogen	H	1	Strontium	Sr	38
Iodine	I	53	Sulfur	S	16
Iron	Fe	26	Technetium	Tc	43
Lead	Pb	82	Tin	Sn	50
Lithium	Li	3	Uranium	U	92
Magnesium	Mg	12	Yttrium	Y	39
Manganese	Mn	25	Zinc	Zn	30
Mercury	Hg	80			

4.6   Elements and Health

What is an element?

The term element describes all atoms with the same atomic number, that is, number of protons. If the number of protons is altered a new element is formed. An element is normally not capable of being broken down into a different element by ordinary chemical means, but can be changed by physical means such as radioactivity. All matter is derived from one of the 108 known elements. Each element is represented by a one or two letter symbol. The symbols of the elements used in this text are listed in Table 4.3.

Of the 108 elements 90 occur naturally in nature with the remainder being created in laboratories by nuclear reactions (12.2).

The earth's crust and atmosphere mainly consist of the five elements oxygen (O), silicon (Si), aluminium (Al), iron (Fe) and calcium (Ca) with oxygen accounting for 49.2% of the total composition. In contrast the human body has the four elements oxygen (O), carbon (C), hydrogen (H) and nitrogen (N) as the main elements. These four represent over 95% of a human body (Table 4.4).

Elements and the human body

The functions of the main mineral elements are described in Table 4.4. A balanced diet is an important means of maintaining the correct concentrations of elements necessary

Atoms and matter

Table 4.4 Elements and the human body

Element	Approx. % mass in body	Function	Toxic effects
Oxygen — O	65	Cellular respiration (33.3)	Damage to eyes, nervous system and lungs in neonates or at high pressure
Carbon — C	18	Forms backbone of organic compounds (Chapter 7)	Inhaled as particulate matter causing lung disease
Hydrogen — H	10	Component of all organic compounds (Chapter 7) acid–base balance (16.5)	In ionic form, acidosis, burns
Nitrogen — N	3	Component of all proteins, amino acids (30.1), nucleic acids (31.2) and cell membranes	Respiratory irritant in oxide forms
Calcium — Ca	1.5	Bone and teeth (1.2); important in muscle contractions (23.3); nerve impulses (23.3); blood clotting (26.2) and membrane function (23.3)	Nausea, lethargy hypertension, formation of bone cysts
Phosphorus — P	1.0	Component of nucleic acids (31.2); bone; cell membranes (23.1) and energy transfer (33.7)	Gastrointestinal bleeding and liver damage
Potassium — K	0.4	Important ion within cells (18.1) assists electrical balance of body fluids (23.2)	In medicinal overuse causing hyerkalemia
Sulphur — S	0.3	Enzyme activity (32.1); essential component most proteins (30.3)	Respiratory irritant and asthma causing agent
Sodium — Na	0.2	Fluid balance (21.3); nerve function (10.5); main extra cellular positive ion (18.1)	Medicinal overuse
Chlorine — Cl	1.5	Main extra-cellular anion (18.1)	Lung irritant in gas form
Magnesium — Mg	0.1	Required by many enzymes assists nerve and muscle action	Medicinal
Iodine — I	trace	Thyroid hormones	Lung irritant when inhaled in gas form
Iron — Fe	trace	Haemoglobin (30.3) myoglobin and some enzymes	Inhaled as a dust causes lung irritation
Chromium — Cr	trace	Increases insulin effectiveness, oxidative enzymes	Toxic to nerve function
Copper — Cu	trace	Oxidative enzymes	Vomiting hypotension, coma and possible death
Fluorine — F	trace	Reduces dental cavities	Lung irritant in gaseous form, hypercalcification

Table 4.4 *Continued*

Element	Approx. % mass in body	Function	Toxic effects
Manganese — Mn	trace	Enzymes required for some	Affects central nervous system liver cirrhosis
Molybdenum — Mo	trace	Required for some enzymes essential for normal growth	Anaemia, poor growth rate and diarrhoea, joint deformities
Zinc — Zn	trace	Required for many enzymes (32.5)	Gastrointestinal upset, diarrhoea
Selenium — Se	trace	Component of some enzymes essential for growth and fertility	Toxic to nerve function gastrointestinal disorders, liver and spleen damage
Cobalt — Co	trace	Component of Vitamin B_{12}	Goitre, cardiac and respiratory effects

for body homeostasis (Chapter 27). Some elements produce harmful effects when higher than normal concentrations occur in the body. EXAMPLE: Aluminium, magnesium (4.11). Other elements not normally found in the body can produce toxic effects. EXAMPLE: Lead (4.11).

4.7 Atomic mass

Dalton first proposed that atoms of the same element had the same weight whereas atoms of different elements had different weights. The term atomic mass is now usually used instead of atomic weight (Eqn 4.1). An understanding of relative atomic masses is important for performing chemical calculations.

The nucleus contributes most of an atom's mass. Within the nucleus the mass results from the two subatomic particles known as protons and neutrons. A neutron has no charge associated with it since it is composed of a bound proton (+1) and a bound electron (−1) so its effective mass is approximately the same as a proton. The bound electrons in a neutron are unable to exhibit the chemical properties of free electrons orbiting the nucleus. Atoms in an element always contain the same number of protons whereas the number of protons can vary without affecting the element's chemical properties. Atoms with different numbers of neutrons but the same number of protons are called isotopes (4.10). EXAMPLE: Hydrogen consists of the following isotopes, one proton and no neutrons (prontium), one proton plus one neutron (deuterium) and one proton plus two neutrons (tritium).

A relative scale has been developed which uses as the standard the most abundant isotope for Carbon. The six protons and six neutrons of this isotope have been assigned the value of twelve atomic mass units (amu). This isotope of carbon called carbon-12, has a very small mass of 1.992×10^{-23} g. This system represents a simplified approach to dealing with extremely small weights. An isotope with one-third the total of protons and neutrons has a mass of four amu whereas an isotope with twice as many protons plus neutrons has a mass of 24 amu.

The atomic mass or weight of an element is not a whole number in contrast to the whole numbers found with isotopes. Examination of the atomic mass (weight) of elements in the Periodic Table reveals that nearly all elements are not whole numbers. This difference with isotopes is due to averaging the masses of each isotope to produce an average mass for the element. Since isotopes exist in different proportions the final average mass of an element is the weighted average of the isotopes expressed in amu. EXAMPLE: Chlorine mainly occurs as two isotopes. One isotope has a mass of 35 amu and represents 75.53% of the atoms in a container of chlorine whereas the second isotope has a mass of 37 amu and represents the remaining 24.47% of the chlorine.

Chlorine average mass

$$= \left(\frac{75.53}{100} \times 35\right) + \left(\frac{24.47}{100} \times 37\right)$$

$$= 35.5 \text{ amu} \qquad \text{Eqn 4.1}$$

4.8   The Periodic Table

Periodic Table arrangement

The Periodic Table lists all the 108 known elements (see inside back cover). The table provides information about each element. The characteristics of an element can be determined by the information contained within the element's box (Figure 4.5). The position of an element in the Table enables a person to predict various properties about that element.

The Periodic Table is arranged so that elements with similar properties are grouped together in vertical columns (Periodic Table) with the elements being referred to as

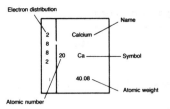

Figure 4.5   Periodic Table key.

a **group** or family of elements. The atoms in a group contain the same number of outer shell electrons. Elements in the same horizontal row are all members of the same **period** and contain the same number of electron shells.

Different systems have been used to identify groups. The system used in this book identifies the eight main groups of elements as IA to VIIIA. Roman numerals represent the number of electrons in the outer shell. EXAMPLE: Group IIA elements such as Calcium (Ca) have two outer shell electrons. The number of outer shell electrons identifies an atom's relative ability to combine with other atoms (4.3).

The middle groups are known as the transition elements as they display similar chemical properties both within groups and along periods. These chemical features result from an incomplete second outermost electron shell. Electrons are not added to the outermost shell but to the incomplete second outermost shell. EXAMPLE: Iron (Fe), Cobalt (Co) and Nickel (Ni) are located in the fourth row and contain two outermost electrons. These elements have different total numbers of electrons but similar chemical properties. Certain groups are also described using common names that represent a chemical property. The alkali metals (Group IA) react with water to produce an alkaline solution (16.2). The alkaline earth metals (Group IIA) are commonly found in earthy substances such as limestone. The halogens (Group VII) are named after the Greek word representing salt forming. EXAMPLE: Chlorine (Cl) combines with sodium (Na) to form table salt (NaCl). The noble gases (Group VIIIA) or inert gases have a completed outer shell which results in an inability to react with most substances.

Size of atoms

The size of an atom is an important factor in determining the structure and function of molecules (5.11). Smaller atoms hold electrons closer to the nucleus. The closer the outer electrons are to the central positive nucleus the greater is the ionization energy required to remove the electrons when compared with larger atoms where the outermost orbits are more distant from the nucleus.

The increase in the number of protons across a period results in a greater attraction for the oppositely charged electrons. This increased attraction results in a corresponding decrease in the diameter of atoms from left to right across a period. EXCEPTION: Noble gases.

Ionization energy

The closer the outermost electrons are to the nucleus the greater is the amount of energy required to remove one of these electrons. Therefore the ionization energy increases from left to right across a period. The increase in the number of electron shells down a group results in a corresponding decrease in ionization energy down a group. EXAMPLE: Caesium (Cs) requires less energy to lose an electron than sodium (Na).

Electron affinity

The electron affinity of an atom indicates the ability of an atom to attract additional electrons. The greater the electron affinity the larger is the attraction of the atom for additional electrons. Electron affinity increases across a period and decreases down a group.

Two atoms with the same number of shells but with different numbers of protons will therefore differ in their ability to pull electrons closer to the nucleus. EXAMPLE: Lithium has a diameter of 3.0 nm whereas oxygen's diameter is 1.3 nm. The increase in the number of electron shells down a group results in an increase in diameter of atoms. EXAMPLE: Sodium has a smaller diameter (37 nm) than potassium (4.6 nm).

Electronegativity

A property of elements associated with their ability to attract electrons is called electronegativity. This property assists our understanding of how and why different elements combine (5.3). Electronegativity is the relative ability of an atom to attract electrons in a bond to itself. Generally electronegativity increases from left to right across a period (except for the noble gases). EXAMPLE: Oxygen has a greater electronegativity than lithium. Electronegativity increases up a group. EXAMPLE: Lithium has a greater electronegativity than potassium. The most electronegative elements occur in the top right hand corner (except the noble gases) with fluorine being the most electronegative element.

4.9 Metals and non-metals

Metals and non-metals differ as a result of the number of electrons in the outer shell. Most metals contain one, two or three electrons in the outer shell and are thus electron donors. Most elements are metals. The non-metals occur in the upper right hand corner of the Periodic Table. Non-metals usually contain four, five, six or seven electrons in their outer orbit and are thus electron acceptors

Table 4.5   Characteristics of metals and
non-metals

Metals	Non-metals
Conduct heat and electricity	Poor conductors of heat and electricity
Donate electrons	Accept electrons
Usually solid	Solid, liquid or gas
Shiny surface when cut	Dull surface when cut

Table 4.6   Common metals and non-metals found
in the body

Metals	Non-metals
Calcium	Carbon
Potassium	Chlorine
Sodium	Hydrogen
	Nitrogen
	Oxygen
	Phosphorus
	Sulphur

(see Periodic Table). Hydrogen exhibits properties of both metals and non-metals. The characteristic physical properties of metals and non-metals are listed in Table 4.5. The common metals and non-metals found in the body are listed in Table 4.6.

Some elements exhibit properties of both metals and non-metals. These elements are located at the border between metals and non-metals in the Periodic Table. These metalloids or semi-metals conduct electricity less effectively than metals and are known as semiconductors. EXAMPLES: Silicon (Si). Chips use the property of semi-conduction in computers.

4.10   Neutrons and isotopes

Neutrons

The nucleus also contains subatomic particles known as neutrons. A neutron has no charge associated with it since it is composed of a bound proton (+1) and a bound electron (−1). Electrons within a nucleus always form part of a neutron and thus they do not exert the properties of an orbiting electron. Since neutrons have a neutral charge, they are unable to alter the number of free protons in the nucleus and the quantity of electrons in the shell. Neutrons therefore do not influence the chemical properties of an atom and thus matter. Neutrons can influence the physical properties of atoms by emitting radiation (11.1).

Isotopes

Isotopes are elements that contain the same number of protons but a varying number of neutrons. An element may therefore have several isotopes without changing the atomic number. Since isotopes of the same element only vary according to the number of neutrons present, they are both chemically and physiologically indistinguishable. EXAMPLE: There are 23 isotopes of iodine; of these, 3 contain 74, 78 or 82 neutrons. These three isotopes all have similar chemical characteristics and they each exist in a fixed proportion in nature.

Mass number

As all isotopes of a given element have the same atomic number, they cannot be identified by this means. The term mass number is used to identify isotopes. Mass number represents the number of protons plus neutrons present in an atom. EXAMPLE:

Table 4.7 Elements and toxicity

Element	Source	Toxic effect
Aluminium — Al	Oral aluminium hydroxide	Alters gastrointestinal function and nervous system function
Lead — Pb	Pollution	Alters nervous system function
Platinum — Pt	Industrial and jewellery	Allergenic reactions such as dermatitis
Mercury — Hg	Industrial waste, water and air	Altered respiratory, nerve and muscle function

Iodine contains 53 protons and either 74, 78 or 82 neutrons. These are 3 of the 23 isotopes of iodine. The mass numbers of these 3 isotopes are therefore 127, 131 and 135.

The mass number and atomic number of any element can be represented as follows:

mass number
(protons and neutrons)

ELEMENT

atomic number
(protons)

EXAMPLE: Iodine is represented by the symbol I and the three isotopes above are represented as:

$$^{127}_{53}I \qquad ^{131}_{53}I \qquad ^{135}_{53}I$$

4.11 Environmental health and safety

Toxicology

Some useful elements are harmful in high concentrations (Table 4.4) while other elements not normally found in the body may be toxic (Table 4.7). Care must be taken to minimize exposure to these elements.

Summary

Matter is anything that occupies space and has some mass. It is composed of three subatomic particles known as protons, neutrons and electrons. These particles are arranged to form a structure called an atom which acts as the building block of matter.

An atom consists of a positively charged nucleus and an outer cloud of orbiting electrons. The nucleus contains protons with a positive charge and neutrons with no charge. Electrons have a negative charge, and the number orbiting the nucleus equals the number of protons in the nucleus. The equal number of protons and electrons results in atoms having no net charge.

Electrons are distributed around the nucleus in electron clouds or energy levels. These clouds consist of spdf sublevels containing pairs of electrons spinning in opposite directions. Clouds are filled from the lowest energy level and sublevel to the highest. Adding energy to an atom causes an electron to move momentarily from its ground state to a higher energy level.

The properties of atoms that determine their ability to combine with other atoms are:

1. The number of electrons in the outer shell. All atoms with more than one shell attempt to have a completed outer shell

of eight electrons. Atoms with less than four electrons in the outermost shell have a low attraction for electrons (low electron affinity) and a high ability to lose electrons (high ionization energy). These atoms lose electrons and form a positively charged ion called a cation. When atoms contain four or more electrons, the opposite conditions exist resulting in the attraction of electrons to form negatively charged ions called anions.

2. All atoms attempt to have a neutral charge. When ions are formed the oppositely charged ions are attracted to each other in an attempt to become neutral.

Atoms at present are known to contain up to 109 protons. An element consists of atoms with the same proton number or atomic number since these atoms all have identical chemical properties.

The body requires a variety of elements for normal function. Abnormal increases in these levels alters body function as does the exposure to a range of other toxic elements from the environment.

The characteristics of each element are summarized in the Periodic Table. This table consists of elements arranged into groups and periods according to their atomic number.

Most elements contain less than four electrons in the outermost shell and are called metals. Non-metals usually contain four or more electrons in the outermost shell.

The number of neutrons in a particular element can vary between atoms. Atoms of an element that have different numbers of neutrons are called isotopes.

Chapter 5

How atoms combine

Objectives

At the completion of this chapter the student should be able to:

1. describe the chemical classification of matter;
2. describe how the structure of atoms relates to the formation of compounds;
3. explain the differences and function of ionic bonds, covalent bonds, metallic bonds and hydrogen bonds;
4. explain the differences between ionic and covalent compounds;
5. relate the structure of polar molecules to their ability to form dipole–dipole interactions;
6. explain the difference between structural and molecular formulae;
7. explain the relationship between electronegativity and bond formation;
8. define the terms mixture, compound, molecule, polyatomic ion, resonance, electro-negativity, alloy, van der Waal forces, coordinate covalent; polar molecule, valence and;
9. draw structural formulae.

5.1 Chemical classification of matter

To achieve the variety of matter that supports life and the environment it is obvious that a mechanism must exist where the 90 naturally occurring elements are combined to form other chemicals. Matter can be classified according to its composition into pure substances and mixtures. Pure substances can further be divided into **elements** (4.6) and **compounds**. The latter being a combination of different elements in a fixed proportion whereas **mixtures** exist as a variable composition of different substances (Figure 5.1). Mixtures can be broken down by physical means whereas compounds cannot.

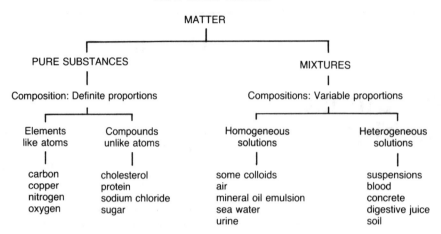

Figure 5.1 Chemical classification of matter.

Compounds

A compound is a combination of atoms in a fixed proportion which confers definite physical and chemical properties. EXAMPLE: Water (H_2O), carbon dioxide (CO_2). Compounds can be broken down chemically whereas elements cannot. A compound exhibits properties totally different to those of its constituent elements. EXAMPLE: When the two highly inflammable elements hydrogen (H) and oxygen (O) are combined in the fixed proportions of two hydrogens: one oxygen the compound water (H_2O) is formed which has the completely opposite effect in fires.

A **molecule** is the smallest combination of atoms that can combine together and still exhibit the properties of a compound. EXAMPLE: One molecule of water consists of two hydrogen atoms and one oxygen atom, which is written as H_2O. Six molecules of water would be written as $6H_2O$ whereas two molecules of water is $2H_2O$. Compounds can be broken down by chemical means into simpler substances whereas elements cannot. EXAMPLE: H_2O forms Hydrogen and Oxygen. When a compound is broken down

the constituent substances will occur in fixed proportions. The **Law of Definite Proportions** states that **a compound is composed of specific elements in a 'definite' proportion by weight**. EXAMPLE: A litre of water will always contain two hydrogen atoms for every oxygen atom.

Mixtures

Mixtures contain two or more elements that are not bound to each other and which may exist in variable proportions. EXAMPLE: The constituents of air such as oxygen, nitrogen and carbon dioxide are not bound to each other and the proportion of these elements in a sample of air would vary in different environments. A mixture's properties result from a combination of the mixture's constituents. A uniform distribution of constituents is called a homogeneous mixture. EXAMPLE: Sugar in tea. Non-uniform distribution of substances is referred to as a heterogeneous mixture. EXAMPLE: Oil in water forms two separate layers.

Mixtures of solids usually consist of one metal uniformly dispersed in another. These metal mixtures or **alloys** are formed while the constituent metals are in a molten state. Atoms of transition elements have similar chemical properties, are approximately the same size and readily form alloys. Cooling of the molten mixture results in a solid being formed with special properties. EXAMPLE: Brass (copper and zinc).

Alloys can be designed to provide specific properties by including non-transition elements and/or increasing the range of elements used. EXAMPLE: Stainless steel (iron, chromium, nickel and carbon).

Application: Prosthetic appliances

The ability of alloys to be designed to meet specific needs has led to their use as surgical implants. These implants or **prosthetic appliances** are used to replace defective or missing parts of the body such as the weight bearing hip and knee joints. The alloy can be designed to take into account corrosion, comfort, structural requirements and the wearing of the appliance. EXAMPLE: Aluminium based alloys.

Fluid mixtures play an important role in body function and health care. The properties of fluid mixtures are explained in Chapter 17.

5.2   Chemical bonds

What is a chemical bond?

Atoms are considered stable when the outer electron shell is complete as found in the noble gases (4.3). This property is often referred to as the **octet rule**. Atoms with incomplete outer shells attempt to complete their outer electron shell by several different processes. These processes depend on the atoms relative position in the Period Table (see inside back cover) and the nature of other nearby atoms as an association needs to be formed between atoms for the octet rule to be satisfied. Atoms can satisfy the octet rule by losing, gaining or sharing their outer shell electrons with other atoms. This association or interaction of the nuclei and electrons of different atoms or ions is referred to as a **chemical bond**. A chemical bond is simply the attractive force that holds atoms together. This interaction results in the formation of different atoms or ions that are more stable than the atoms themselves. The formation of chemical bonds results in the release of energy that was previously contained within the atoms.

Atom + atom → atom − atom + energy

Eqn 5.1

It is apparent from observing the characteristics of different compounds that more than one bonding mechanism exists. EXAMPLE: Dissolved table salt (NaCl) conducts electricity whereas dissolved table sugar (sucrose) does not. Atoms can satisfy the octet rule by losing, gaining or sharing their outer shell electrons with other atoms. The combining power of atoms is known as valence (5.8). As the number of outer shell electrons determined the combining power of atoms, these electrons are called **valence electrons**. The process of rearrangement of the valence electrons causes atoms to undergo chemical reactions to form new compounds (Chapter 6).

Ionic bonds

Electrovalency is the number of electrons an atom needs to gain (or lose in order to attain the electron distribution of a noble gas) i.e. a completed outer orbit. EXAMPLE: Electro-

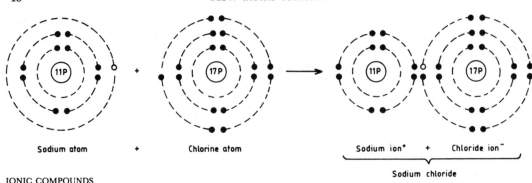

Sodium atom   +   Chlorine atom   Sodium ion⁺   +   Chloride ion⁻

                                                                              Sodium chloride

IONIC COMPOUNDS

valency requires the loss of one electron whereas an electrovalency of −1 requires the addition of one electron. When electrons are transferred from one atom to another ions are formed. The resulting differences in electrical charge result in an attraction of the oppositely charged ions towards each other (4.4). This attraction between negative and positive ions is known as an **ionic bond** or **electrovalent bond**. EXAMPLE: NaCl (Figure 5.2).

Covalent bonds

A second type of chemical bond involves the sharing of valence electrons with compatible adjacent atoms. When two non-metal atoms are in close proximity to each other an overlapping of the two atoms occurs. When the electron of one atom senses the presence of a second atom it becomes attracted to the second atom's nucleus even though it retains its attraction to the original atom's nucleus.

The other electron has the same experience resulting in the pair of electrons sharing a simultaneous attraction to both nuclei. The electrons become established in a new common region that encompasses both nuclei. These atoms are now able to partially satisfy the octet rule. EXAMPLE: The hydrogen molecule consists of two hydrogen

Figure 5.2   Formation of an ionic bond. A sodium atom donates an outer shell electron (○) to a chlorine atom, resulting in a positively-charged sodium ion and a negatively-charged chloride ion. These two ions contain complete outer orbits. The oppositely charged ions are attracted and held together.

atoms each sharing an electron in order to achieve two electrons in the outer shell of each atom (Figure 5.3a).

The force of attraction that holds the atomic nuclei near each other as a consequence of the overlapping electrons is referred to as a **covalent bond**.

Three forms of covalent bonds can be formed between two atoms. These forms depend upon the number of electrons that are shared between two atoms.

Single covalent bonds

In a single covalent bond, one pair of electrons is shared between two atoms. EXAMPLE: Two hydrogen atoms (Figure 5.3a).

Double covalent bonds

This bond involves the sharing of two pairs of electrons between two atoms. As a result the outer electron shell of each atom is complete for a proportion of time. EXAMPLE: Two oxygen atoms (Figure 5.3b).

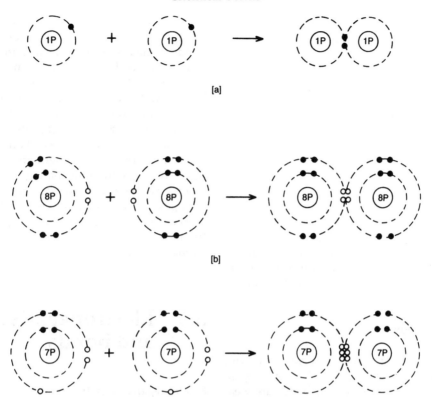

[a]

[b]

[c]

Figure 5.3 Formation of covalent bonds.
(a) Two hydrogen atoms combine to complete their outer shell by sharing their electrons to form a single covalent bond which is symbolized as H··H or H—H.
(b) A double covalent bond is formed between two oxygen atoms when a pair of electrons from one oxygen atom is shared with the other oxygen atom to form eight electrons in the outer shell; symbolized as O::O or O=O. (c) In a triple covalent bond three pairs of electrons are used to complete the outer shell; symbolized as N:::N or N≡N.

Triple covalent bonds

Some elements such as nitrogen, are capable of sharing three electrons with another atom in order to complete the outer shell for a proportion of time. A triple bond is formed when two atoms share three pairs of electrons between them. EXAMPLE: Nitrogen (Figure 5.3c).

Coordinate covalent bonds

A less common way of forming a covalent bond occurs where one atom supplies two electrons and the other none. This coordinate covalent bond is important in the formation of polyatomic ions (5.7). EXAMPLE: NH_4^+ and compounds from transition elements. Once a coordinate covalent bond is formed it acts the same as other covalent bonds.

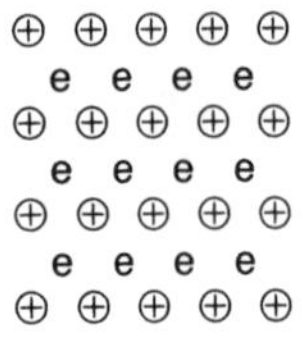

⊕ ⊕ ⊕ ⊕ ⊕
  e e e e
⊕ ⊕ ⊕ ⊕ ⊕
  e e e e
⊕ ⊕ ⊕ ⊕ ⊕
  e e e e
⊕ ⊕ ⊕ ⊕ ⊕

Figure 5.4   Metal lattice with electron sea.

Metallic bonds

A third important bond involves forming pure metallic solids. Metal atoms form a lattice sharing a sea of electrons (Figure 5.4). This arrangement is explained further in 5.6.

Hydrogen bonds

Hydrogen bonds are linkages involving hydrogen between molecules or regions within a large molecule. The bonds are weak as they result from a weak attraction between the slightly positively charged hydrogen and a slightly negatively charged region. The bonds are relatively weak and are approximately one-tenth the strength of the **true** covalent bonds described above but are stronger than van der Waals forces (5.5). Bonds formed between molecules are referred to as hydrogen bonds and play an important role in life and the environment. EXAMPLES: Linking water molecules (17.2), DNA strands (24.7), polypeptides in proteins (30.3) and enzymes binding to biochemicals (32.1). An important property of these bonds is the relationship between strength and direction. Bonds resulting from the joining of the donor atom, hydrogen and the acceptor atom are strongest when in a straight line and become weaker as the angle of the acceptor atom from the line joining the donor and hydrogen atoms increases.

5.3   Electronegativity and bonds

Electronegativity is the relative measure of the electron attracting power of an atom when it is in a chemical bond. An atom with a high electronegativity is likely to gain an electron from an atom with a low electronegativity and form an ionic bond. A covalent

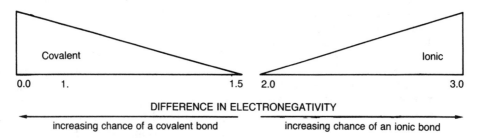

Figure 5.5   Relationship of difference in electronegativity to ionic and covalent bond formation.

bond is more likely to occur when a low difference in electronegativity exists. The relative difference in electronegativity can therefore be used to predict whether an ionic (electrovalent) bond or a covalent bond will occur (Figure 5.5). The relative electronegativity of elements is described in 4.8.

5.4   Ionic compounds

General features

Ionic compounds are formed by the exchange of electrons between an electron donor or cation and an electron acceptor or anion. Electrons are donated or accepted in order that the fundamental force in nature of completing the outer shell of electrons is satisfied. The donation and acceptance of electrons results in the formation of oppositely charged ions. The difference in potential developed between the ions causes the oppositely charged ions to combine as a result of the fundamental force of opposite charges attracting. When atoms combine because of differences in electrical charge ionic bonds are formed. The formation of ionic bonds combines the positive and negative charges so that no difference in charge remains, that is, the compound has zero charge.

Crystals

The combination of ions results in the formation of a crystal. Each crystal is composed of a fixed arrangement between the cations and anions. EXAMPLE: In sodium chloride or common salt each sodium ion is always surrounded by six chloride ions and similarly each chloride ion is surrounded by six sodium ions. An individual sodium atom can donate one electron to any chloride atom

of equal distance from the sodium ion. The sodium atom is now a positively charged ion and the chloride atom, having accepted an extra electron, is negatively charged. The two ions attract one another to form an ionic bond. The resulting array of sodium and chloride ions is called a crystal. The crystal can grow by the addition of more sodium and chloride ions to the established arrangement. Sodium chloride is unable to form a definite structural unit or molecule as each chloride ion belongs to six adjacent sodium ions.

The formula NaCl does not represent a sodium chloride molecule: it simply represents the ratio of sodium ions to chloride ions in the compound. This ratio of one sodium ion to one chloride ion indicates that sodium has lost one electron and one of the surrounding chloride ions was formed from gaining this electron. The interaction between a sodium atom and one of the adjacent chloride atoms is shown in Figure 5.1.

When ionic compounds are placed in water they break up or dissociate into cations and anions. This process is referred to as **dissociation or ionization**.

Note that some crystals are composed of molecules. EXAMPLE: Sucrose (sugar). These molecules are formed from covalent bonds.

5.5   Covalent compounds

General features

Atoms are able to satisfy the force of completing the outer electron shell without the necessary number of electrons being present 100% of the time. This property allows electrons to be shared between two atoms. The shared electrons spend a proportion of their time under the influence of each of the atoms.

Covalent compounds consist of atoms that complete their outer orbit by sharing electrons with other atoms. Elements with four outer orbit electrons such as carbon find it easier to share electrons than attempt to either gain or lose four electrons. The bonds that are formed by sharing electrons between two atoms are termed covalent bonds. These bonds can be formed between atoms of the same element such as oxygen, which forms molecular oxygen, or between atoms of different elements such as carbon and oxygen which form carbon dioxide. Generally covalent compounds are formed from elements with four, five, six or seven electrons in the outer orbit, as these elements attract electrons.

The metals, with one, two or three electrons in the outer orbit tend to lose electrons and thus are generally unable to share electrons and form covalent compounds. Hydrogen has unique properties and is able to gain or lose its electron or share it with other atoms.

A covalent compound may consist of a mixture of single, double and triple bonds. Each individual atom can form any permutation of covalent bonds as long as the total number of shared electrons does not exceed eight in the outer orbit. EXAMPLE: A carbon atom contains four electrons in the outer orbit and therefore requires four electrons for a proportion of time for the outer shell to be complete. The carbon atom can achieve this by any permutation of covalent bonds as long as an additional four electrons are shared. The possible covalent bond permutations for carbon are:

	4 single bonds	= 4 electrons
	2 double bonds	= 4 electrons
1 double bond plus	2 single bonds	= 4 electrons
1 triple bond plus	1 single bond	= 4 electrons

Polar molecules

Polar molecules result from an unequal sharing of electrons between atoms. These molecules lie between the extremes of equal sharing of electrons (covalent bonds) and ionic bonds. Some atoms that share electrons with other atoms will have a greater affinity for the shared electrons. The affinity is insufficient to cause the electrons to spend 100% of their time under the influence of these atoms but is of sufficient strength to hold the electrons in their influence for more than 50% of the time. These electrons are disproportionately shared but not donated to these high electron affinity atoms. Atoms can contain a complete outer shell for less than 50% of the time and still satisfy the force of completing outer orbits.

An atom that gains one electron forms an anion with a charge of 1^-, since each electron has a charge of 1^-. An atom that gains a number of electrons to complete the shell for 50% of the time and loses an equal number of its electrons for the other 50% of the time has a net charge of zero. An atom that contains the correct number of electrons for greater than 50% of the time but less than 100% of the time must have a charge that is smaller than zero but less than 1^-. These atoms contain a slightly negative charge which is represented as δ^-. Similarly an atom that contains a completed outer shell for less than 50% of the time has a slight positive charge which is represented as δ^+.

Polar molecules contain atoms that share electrons disproportionately and therefore contain a separation of charge. This separation of charge is termed a **dipole**.

Highly polar molecules have a greater difference in electron sharing (electronegativity) than molecules with a low polarity. EXAMPLE: In hydrogen fluoride, the electron from the hydrogen atom spends a greater proportion of its time (about 70%) in the sphere of influence of the fluoride atom (Figure 5.6) as fluoride is highly electro-

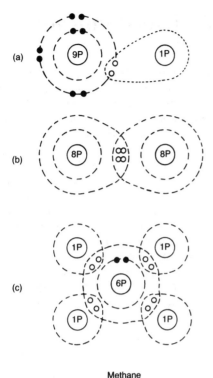

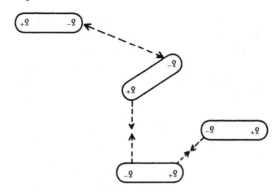

Figure 5.7 Dipole–dipole interaction occurs between oppositely charged portions of different polar molecules. The regions of polar molecules that have like charges, repel one another.

Methane

Figure 5.6 Hydrogen fluoride (a) shares electrons disproportionately and is highly polar. Molecular oxygen (b) and (c) methane (CH_4) share electrons approximately equally and are non-polar.

negative. The greater the difference in sharing between two atoms, the greater is the dipole and thus the polarity of the molecule.

Non-polar molecules contain atoms that share electrons for approximately 50% of the time and thus lack a dipole. All molecules that consist of the same element are non-polar. EXAMPLES: Oxygen (O_2), hydrogen (H_2), chlorine (Cl_2) (Figure 5.6). Sometimes different elements have a similar electron affinity which also results in the formation of non-polar molecules. EXAMPLE: Carbon and hydrogen (Figure 5.6).

The degree of polarity of a substance determines its ability to dissolve in water. Generally polar substances dissolve in water, which is a polar molecule. Non-polar substances are unable to dissolve in water. Non-polar substances however will dissolve in non-polar solvents such as acetone (17.2).

Polar molecules are able to form weak bonds with other polar molecules. These weak bonds or loose linkages are known as **dipole–dipole interactions**. Since opposite charges attract, then the small opposite charges from different polar molecules can be attracted to each other (Figure 5.7). This ability of oppositely charged parts of different polar molecules to form dipole–dipole interactions is of great importance in determining the structure and function of substances such as enzymes, antibodies, genetic molecules and pharmacological agents. When hydrogen is one of the atoms involved in the dipole-interaction, the linking is referred to as a hydrogen bond (5.2).

Non-polar molecules

Non-polar molecules are linked primarily by **van der Waals forces**. This type of bonding is based mainly on the proximity of adjacent atoms. A strong attraction occurs at certain distances, but as the atoms get closer, the electron clouds overlap resulting in a repulsive force balancing the attractive force. Van der Waals forces are more apparent with non-polar molecules than with polar, as polar molecules can form other stronger bonds.

In general, the greater the number of protons and electrons in a molecule the stronger are the van der Waals forces. The forces are therefore influenced by the number of atoms in a molecule as well as the nature of each atom. Van der Waals forces can be important when several large molecules are closely associated.

5.6   Metals

Metal atoms are able to combine with each other to form pure compounds. EXAMPLES: copper and aluminium. As pure metallic substances lack anions, the metallic atoms cannot be linked by ionic bonds. Metal atoms prefer to donate electrons instead of accepting or sharing them, and they therefore do not form covalent bonds, but use an alternative form of binding which involves the loss of outer shell electrons. These electrons form a highly mobile cloud between adjacent cations which acts as a buffer preventing repulsion of the adjacent cations. The resulting structure forms a lattice (Figure 5.4). The free electrons are able to move throughout the lattice. The capacity of electrons to move freely throughout the lattice has important ramifications in the movement of electricity in solids (7.3). The ability of the cations to be held in a fixed position is due to the metallic bonds or metallic binding, which results from the attraction between positive ions and the cloud of electrons. These bonds are weaker than either ionic or covalent bonds.

5.7   Polyatomic ions

A **polyatomic ion** is a group of atoms which acts as a unit within a molecule, and when that molecule undergoes a chemical change the polyatomic ion remains as an intact unit. A polyatomic ion cannot exist by itself since it contains either a net positive or negative charge and thus is required to combine with other atoms to neutralize its charge. A polyatomic ion therefore acts as if it were an individual ion. These ions are also referred to as **radicals**. EXAMPLE: The bicarbonate polyatomic ion (HCO_3^-) always acts as a separate entity. When sodium bicarbonate ($Na^+HCO_3^-$) is involved in a reaction with hydrochloric acid (HCl), the bicarbonate ion combines with the H to form carbonic acid (H_2CO_3):

$$Na^+ HCO_3^- + HCl \rightleftharpoons H_2CO_3 + NaCl$$

$$\text{Eqn 5.2}$$

The importance of polyatomic ions in body function is summarized in Table 5.1. NOTE: The (HCO_3^-) ions formal name is hydrogen carbonate but is commonly referred to in health care as bicarbonate. The symbols in the table will be described in 5.9.

5.8   Valence

A system is required to determine which element will combine with another element to form a compound. In addition, a system is needed to determine the proportion of atoms of an element that are required to combine with atoms of another element to form a particular compound. **Valence** refers to an atom's ability to combine with other atoms. It therefore relates to an atom's attempt to achieve a completed outer electron shell by

Table 5.1 The main polyatomic ions in the body

Name	Formula and charge	Function
Ammonium	NH_4^+	Breakdown chemical of amino acids and is used in the regulation of urine acidity
Bicarbonate (Hydrogen carbonate)	HCO_3^{2-}	Important in acid/base balance and carbon dioxide transport in the blood
Hydroxide	OH^-	Important factor in alkaline solutions and in neutralizing acids
Phosphate	PO_4^{3-}	Important acid control mechanism in blood cells and the kidneys
Sulphate	SO_4^{2-}	Neutralizing acids in urine
Nitrate	NO_3^-	Source of nitrogen smooth muscle relaxants
Hydronium	H_3O^+	Acid

sharing electrons or by either gaining or donating electrons.

In ionic compounds, the valence of an atom is the number of electrons gained or lost by the atom in order to complete the outer electron shell. An atom with seven electrons in the outer orbit requires one electron to complete the outer shell and therefore has a valence of 1^-. The minus sign is due to the atom gaining one electron. Similarly an atom with six outer shell electrons has a valence of 2^- and an atom with five outer electrons has a valence of 3^-. The valence of an atom that donates its electrons to form a cation, with a completed outer shell, is determined by the number of outer orbit electrons. An atom with one outer shell electron has a valence of 1^+ as one electron has been lost. In the same way an atom with two outer orbit electrons has a valence of 2^+ and an atom with three outer electrons has a valence of 3^+.

A compound has no net charge and thus the number of electrons gained and lost must be equal within a compound. EXAMPLE: An element with a valence of 2^- requires either two atoms of 1^+ valence or one atom of 2^+ valence to form a stable compound with no net charge.

In covalent compounds, the valence of the constituent atoms is determined by the number of shared electron pairs that are present. An atom with seven electrons in the outer orbit can achieve its eight electrons by forming a single covalent bond, that is, one electron pair. This atom has a valence of 1. Similarly an atom with six outer orbit electrons has a valence of 2 since two electron pairs are necessary to complete the outer orbit. An atom that requires three electron pairs to complete the outer shell has a valence of 3. Note that no minus or plus sign is used since electrons are shared and not gained or lost. When determining the valence required to combine two atoms to form a covalent compound, it is necessary to match numerically the valence of each atom. EXAMPLE: An atom with a valence of 2 requires either two atoms with a valence of 1 or one atom with a valence of 2 to form a covalent compound.

Throughout this book a system of diagrams is used to show how valence relates to the ability of an atom to combine with other atoms (Figure 5.8). Each atom, or in some cases a radical group, is represented by a square. The addition of each electron to an atom is represented by an individual peak. EXAMPLE: Two peaks indicate an anion which contains two additional electrons. The removal of each electron from an atom is shown by a triangular indentation. EXAMPLE: Two indentations indicate a cation which has a valence of +2. The sharing of each electron pair between two

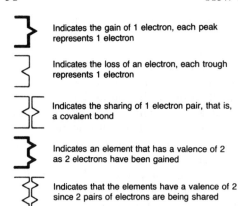

Indicates the gain of 1 electron, each peak represents 1 electron

Indicates the loss of an electron, each trough represents 1 electron

Indicates the sharing of 1 electron pair, that is, a covalent bond

Indicates an element that has a valence of 2 as 2 electrons have been gained

Indicates that the elements have a valence of 2 since 2 pairs of electrons are being shared

Indicates that the elements have a valence of 2 since 2 electrons have been either gained or lost, that is, an ionic bond exists

Figure 5.8   Schematic representation of valence. This system is used throughout this book to show how valence relates to the ability of an atom to combine with other atoms. An anion is identified by (−) outline where each peak represents one extra electron. A cation has a (−) outline and each lost electron is represented by a triangular indentation. Where covalent bonds exist, each shared electron pair is indicated by a triangular indentation in each atom.

atoms is indicated by a triangular indentation in each atom.

5.9   Expressing chemical combinations

When atoms are combined, it is necessary to use a system of symbols that identifies their combination. A formula conveys information about the structure and composition of any specific combination of atoms. An under-

standing of how formulae are used is necessary for understanding how substances are formed and broken down in the body, and for understanding their chemical and physiological action. The two forms of chemical formulae used in this book are the molecular formula and the structural formula.

Molecular formulae

A molecular formula states the actual number of atoms of each element present in either a molecule or group of atoms in a polyatomic ion. The number of atoms of an element is represented as a subscript. EXAMPLE: H_2O indicates that two hydrogen atoms are present and one oxygen. When no subscript is present, such as with oxygen, only one atom is present. The molecular formula for glucose is $C_6H_{12}O_6$. This formula informs us that there are six carbon atoms, twelve hydrogen atoms and six oxygen atoms present in every molecule of glucose.

In a polyatomic ion such as the bicarbonate ion, which is represented as HCO_3^-, the 3 refers to the number of oxygen atoms and the minus indicates that the radical group contains a charge of −1. Similarly, the hydroxyl ion or OH^- is a polyatomic ion with a charge of −1. The minus refers to the OH and not the H alone.

A number in front of a molecule indicates the number of molecules present. EXAMPLE: Two water molecules would be represented as $2H_2O$ and five water molecules would be $5H_2O$.

In many cases the molecular formula represents a specific structure since the constituent elements can only be combined to form one unique structure. EXAMPLES: H_2O, CO_2, NH_2 (ammonia). In the case of $C_6H_{12}O_6$, there are sixteen different ways that the atoms can be arranged. These sixteen different structures all have unique chemical and physiological properties. An alternative

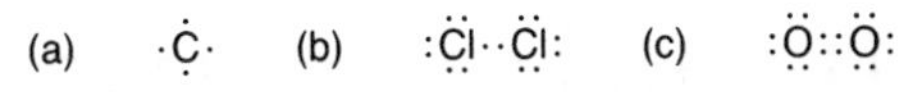

(a)   ·Ċ·   (b)   :Ċl··Ċl: (c)   :Ö::Ö:

Figure 5.9   Electron dot formula (a) the two
energy levels of carbon, (b) single
covalent bond. EXAMPLE: Chlorine
and (c) double bond. EXAMPLE:
Oxygen.

formula is required for indicating which substance is being represented.

Structural formulae

A structural formula shows the actual
number of atoms of each element present
along with the structural composition of the
molecule. There are several different systems
for representing a structural formula. The
Lewis structure or **electron dot structure** represents the valence electrons as dots. The
nucleus and the core electrons are represented
by the elements symbol (Figure 5.9a). NOTE:
Only the four valence electrons are shown as
only the valence electrons are involved in
forming bonds. A single bond is represented
as two dots (Figure 5.9b). A double bond
consists of two pairs of dots (Figure 5.9c).
Compare this representation of oxygen with
the electron arrangement in Figure 5.3b.

It is often simpler and more accurate to
represent a pair of electrons in a bond by a
straight line. EXAMPLES: Cl_2 as $Cl—Cl$; O_2
as $O=O$. In larger molecules such as most
organic compounds (Chapter 6) the relative
arrangement of bonds between atoms is important. EXAMPLE: The molecular formula
$C_6H_{12}O_6$ is represented by 16 different structural formulae. Substances that have the
same molecular formula but a different
structural formula are termed **isomers** (7.4).
EXAMPLE: The two different sugars glucose
and galactose are isomers of $C_6H_{12}O_6$. The
difference in chemical and physiological

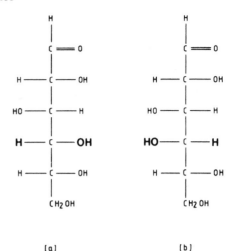

[a]   [b]

Figure 5.10   The molecular formula $C_6H_{12}O_6$ is
represented by sixteen isomers. The
structural formulae of (a) glucose,
and (b) galactose are shown.
Glucose and galactose differ only in
the relative position of H and OH
about a single carbon atom.

action in the body of these two sugars is due
to the relative difference in the position of an
H and an hydroxyl ion (OH) about a single
carbon atom, with respect to the other atoms
in the molecule (Figure 5.10). A structural
formula also indicates the type of bonds that
are present within a molecule, that is, the
presence of single, double and triple covalent
bonds.

The arrangement within a compound can
be represented as a condensed structure
which is often referred to as the compounds
structure (Figure 5.11).

5.10   Resonance

In some compounds more than one electron-
dot structure can be drawn. The SO_3 mol-

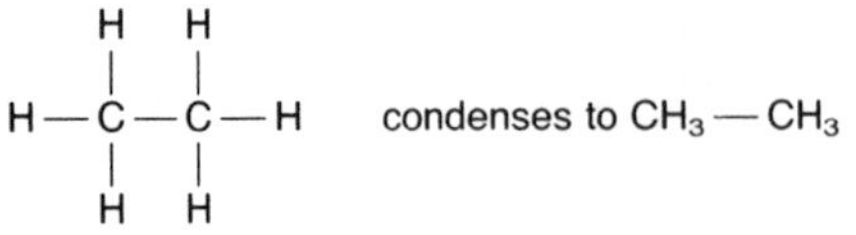

Figure 5.11   Condensing the structure of ethane.

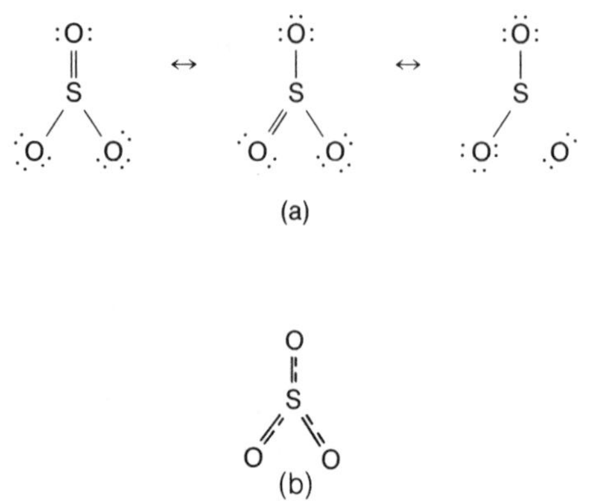

(a)

(b)

Figure 5.12   Resonance structures of SO_3 (a) three possible resonance structures, (b) single resonance structure using broken lines.

ecule can be represented as three different electron dot structures which are referred to as being in **resonance** (Figure 5.12a). These three structures are called resonance structures. The inclusion of double arrows is often used to represent resonance.

Resonance results from electrons moving around the entire molecule instead of pairing. The SO_3 structure is a single structure which can only be represented as an average of the various resonance structures. A method of indicating resonance is to condense the various forms into a single structure which uses a broken line to indicate that the S—O bonds are all equivalent (Figure 5.12b).

Resonance is an important characteristic of organic compounds especially those based on the benzene ring (7.7) and is a factor involved in determining the shape of a structure.

5.11   Molecular shape and life

The properties of a molecule depends on the combination of atoms as previously described in this chapter as well as the physical shape resulting from this combination. Each molecule has a definite shape, as atoms are not free to position themselves in any location within a molecule. Factors such as electrical charge and the nature of the bonds restrict the position of an atom.

Physical shape influences the ability of two substances to lock together. This property results in substances only locking onto complementary shaped structures thereby enabling molecules to act only on a specific structure.

Many processes in the human body can only operate by a process of selection of the correct molecule. That is, life is dependent on the ability of many molecules to act on a specific structure. This specific action or **specificity** is determined by the shape of a molecule. EXAMPLES: Immune system identifying foreign cells and other structures (37.2); enzymes and hormones acting on specific chemical processes (Chapter 32 and Chapter 39 respectively), cell membranes determining the chemicals that can be transported into and out of cells (23.2) and neurotransmitters acting on specific cells (25.5).

The selective alteration of body function through drugs follows the same basic mechanism of a particular substance locking onto a complementary shaped molecular structure. The potency of drugs can be changed by altering their shape (8.1). Any factor that can influence the shape of a substance therefore performs a fundamental role in influencing the processes that maintain life.

Table 5.2 Central atom electron arrangement for predicting shapes

Number of electron pairs	Shape that minimizes repulsion
2	Linear
3	Trigonal planar
4	Tetrahedral
5	Trigonal bipyramidal
6	Octahedral

5.12 Predicting molecular shapes

The relative location of valence electron pairs influences the location of the bonds and therefore, other atoms. The location of an electron pair results from a pushing apart of the pairs by the force of repulsion that acts between like charges (Chapter 10).

The number of pairs of valence electrons repelling each other determines the extent of repulsion, which in turn, controls the relative location of bonds. This information can be used to predict the approximate shape of many molecules by using the valence shell electron pair repulsion model (VSEPR). The shape is determined by:

1. Counting the number of electron pairs in a Lewis dot structure. Double and triple bonds are counted as one pair.
2. Use Table 5.2 to identify the arrangement that minimizes electron pair repulsions.

Figure 5.13 displays the predicted shapes of molecules according to this method. EXAMPLE: Carbon dioxide is a linear molecule as it contains two multiple bonds which according to the method are each considered as one pair (Figure 5.14).

Another approach to predicting shape

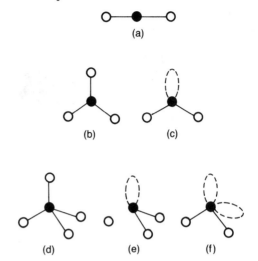

Figure 5.13 Predicted shapes of molecules using the VSEPR method. (a) Two electron pairs-linear; three electron pairs can occur with (b) no unattached pairs-trigonal planar or (c) one unattached pair-bent; four electron pairs can occur with (d) no unattached electrons–tetrahedral, (e) one unattached pair–trigonal pyramidal and (f) two unattached pairs–bent.

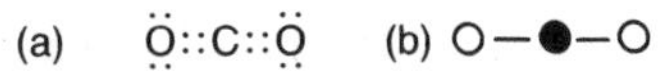

(a) $\ddot{O}::C::\ddot{O}$ (b) $O-\bullet-O$

Figure 5.14 Shape of carbon dioxide (a) Lewis structure and (b) linear shape.

involves those molecules where the central atom forms single covalent bonds. The formation of single covalent bonds from the central atom from groups IV to VII of the Periodic Table results in the formation of a definite shape for each group (Figure 5.15). The larger the molecule, the more complex and unique is the shape. The study of large molecules as described in Chapter 7 and unit 10 requires therefore an understanding of the basis of shape formation.

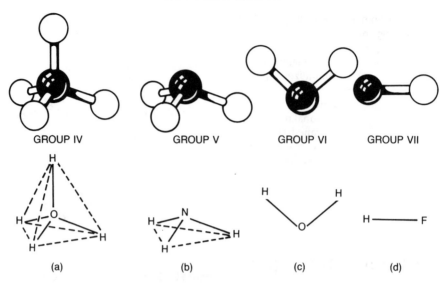

GROUP IV   GROUP V   GROUP VI   GROUP VII

(a)   (b)   (c)   (d)

Figure 5.15   Simple shapes from Group IV–VII.
(a) Methane; tetrahedral. (b)
Ammonia; triangular pyramid. (c)
Water; bent. (d) Hydrogen fluoride;
linear.

5.13 Environmental health and safety

The specific properties of compounds as described in this chapter provide a basis for understanding the potential environmental and occupational hazards of different substances. EXAMPLES: Non-polar substances such as organic solvents are easily absorbed through the surfaces of the body. The shape of particles can stimulate the immune system into an allergic reaction (37.3). The sea of electrons in metals allows electrons to move through a metal and as a result conduct electricity whereas non-metal solids can protect against electric shock as electricity (electrons) is unable to pass through them (10.7).

Summary

Matter is classified according to its composition into compounds and mixtures.

Compounds are combinations of atoms in fixed proportions whereas mixtures are combinations in variable proportions. The smallest combination of atoms that can exhibit the properties of a compound is called a molecule.

Compounds are formed in order that atoms can satisfy two fundamental forces of nature, that is, that atoms can attain a neutral charge and that they have a completed outer orbit. Two mechanisms exist by which atoms can form compounds.

1. Ionic compounds result from the combination of oppositely charged ions. These ions are formed by atoms with a high electronegativity gaining electrons while atoms with a lower electronegativity lose electrons in order that the outer orbit is complete. Each addition or loss of an electron results in an alteration of charge by -1 or $+1$ respectively and a change

in valence of 1. In order for a net charge of zero to exist, the number of positive charges must equal the number of negative charges. The bonds that link these ions are called ionic or electrovalent bonds. These bonds can only be formed between anions and cations, that is, oppositely charged ions. The combination of ions results in the formation of a crystal.

2. Covalent compounds result from the sharing of outer orbit electrons between adjacent atoms. The sharing of electrons results from low differences in electronegativity between the atoms. As a consequence the atoms are 'reluctant' to accept electrons and so are able to complete their outer orbit without the need to donate or accept electrons. Covalent compounds can be formed from either like atoms or different atoms. When different atoms combine, one atom may have a greater attraction for shared electrons than another. In such cases, the shared electrons spend more than 50% of the time with the former atom, which results in this atom becoming slightly negatively charged (δ^-). For a net charge of zero to exist, the other atom must have a slight positive charge (δ^+). Polar molecules are molecules that are formed from a dispro-portionate sharing of electrons resulting from differences in electronegativity.

The slight difference in charge or dipole that exists between atoms in a polar molecule enables these molecules to form weak bonds with other polar molecules. When one of the atoms is hydrogen, the loose linking or dipole–dipole interaction is referred to as hydrogen bonding.

Metal atoms combine by metallic bonds to form pure compounds. The metallic lattice is formed from the buffering action of the mobile electron cloud.

A polyatomic ion is a group of atoms which acts as a unit within a molecule, and when that molecule undergoes chemical change the polyatomic ion remains as an intact unit.

Chemical combinations can be expressed in a molecular formula and/or structural formula. The former represents the relative proportions of atoms whereas the latter shows the structural relationship of each atom.

Resonance structures represent the movement of electrons around an entire molecule. The molecular shape influences the function of a molecule. The molecular shape can be predicted as the repulsion of valence electron pairs influences a molecule's shape.

Chapter 6

Chemical interactions

Objectives

At the completion of this chapter the student should be able to:

1. explain how a reaction occurs and describe the different reaction categories;
2. explain the differences between an exothermic and endothermic reaction;
3. describe the factors that influence the rate of a reaction;
4. explain *Le Chatelier's Principle*;
5. determine the oxidation number of compounds;
6. write and balance chemical equations and half equations;
7. describe the following: reactants, products, basal metabolic rate, activation energy, reaction rate, catalyst, enzyme, chemical equilibrium, oxidation, reduction, oxidation number, reducing agent, oxidizing agent.

6.1 Interactions between substances

Chapters 4 and 5 explained the composition and properties of atoms and compounds respectively. Chemistry also involves the study of interactions between substances which can result in the formation of new substances. It is important to understand how different compounds are formed from interactions that can occur between compounds. EXAMPLE: The body is continually forming new compounds from food or from recycling substances already within the body.

Unit 11 will describe in detail the chemical interactions within the body which are referred to as metabolism.

This chapter explains how substances react with each other to bring about changes in matter and the approaches used to describe these changes.

Reaction terms

The original substances or **reactants** are involved in a **chemical reaction** which results in the formation of a new substance/s called **product/s**. The reactant has different properties to those of its products. EXAMPLE: The products hydrogen and oxygen combine to form the reactant water. The relationships between chemicals within a chemical reaction are described by a **chemical equation**.

How a reaction occurs

Reactions result from collisions between substances. In most collisions the substances simply bounce apart without a reaction taking place. A reaction results from a collision where one of the following has occurred.

1. Sufficient energy is released following a collision to break bonds. The breakage of bonds exposes atoms from each substance. A reaction takes place by new bonds being formed as each atom is required to complete its electron orbits. The amount of energy required to activate a chemical reaction is called the **activation energy**. Raising the temperature of substances increases the energy within atoms and molecules resulting in their increased speed. The increase in energy within these substances results in more violent collisions and an increased release of energy. This provides a greater chance of a reaction taking place.
2. The orientation of a molecule at the time of a collision is also important as all molecules possess a shape (5.11). The collision has to take place between atoms that can complete their electron distribution by forming a new bond. EXAMPLE: A reaction can only occur between water and a positively charged region of a molecule if the positive charge collides with the oxygen atom and not a hydrogen atom of a water molecule. Figure 17.1 shows the positively charged region of a polar molecule being attracted to the negatively charged oxygen region in water and conversely being repulsed by the positively charged hydrogen regions of a water molecule.

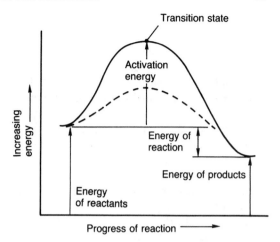

Figure 6.1 Typical reaction energy diagram showing the effect of a catalyst on activation energy.

Activation energy

Activation energy has to be greater than the energy stored in the bonds of the reactants in order to effect a breakage of an existing bond. The relationship between activation energy and a reaction is shown in Figure 6.1.

Every reaction has a different energy diagram. When one or more of the original bonds is in the process of being broken the maximum amount of energy has been imparted. This short period is referred to as the **transition state** and the combination or complex of reacting substances is called the **activated complex**.

The higher the activation energy the greater is the energy required to break a bond and cause a reaction to take place. It therefore becomes more difficult for a reaction to take place. The greater the activation energy the slower the reaction and conversely the lower the activation energy the faster the reaction (Figure 6.1).

Exothermic reactions

Breaking bonds requires energy, but forming new bonds releases energy which is most commonly in the form of heat. EXAMPLE: The release of heat during the breakdown of glucose in the body. The human body is dependent on the intake of energy from food such as glucose as the body is dependent on exothermic reactions for the release of energy to support the necessary activities associated with life. These reactions are described in more detail in Chapter 33.

Chapter 13 describes the relationship between heat and other forms of energy. Most reactions that occur spontaneously are exothermic. EXAMPLE: Explosions.

Application: Body temperature

The body generates heat mainly from exothermic reactions. This heat is distributed throughout the body by blood. An increase in exothermic reactions results in an increase in body temperature. An increase or decrease in reactions within a region of the body results in a corresponding change in heat produced in that region. These changes can be identified using heat detecting equipment (13.4). Such changes can be due to normal activity such as muscles during exercise or abnormal activity such as cancer.

Endothermic reactions

When a continuous supply of heat is required an endothermic reaction is taking place. Endothermic reactions take in more energy than previously existed in the reactants resulting in the products containing a greater amount of energy than the reactants. These reactions are an important means of storing energy in the body. EXAMPLE: Formation of fat in the body.

6.2   Factors affecting reaction rates

The rate at which a reaction takes place is simply the speed of the reaction per unit of time. This is measured by observing the rate at which a product appears or that a reactant disappears, that is, a change in concentration of one of the participants. Changes in reaction rates are an important means of controlling body function whether through natural homeostatic mechanisms or through intervention by health personnel. EXAMPLES: Drugs, intravenous fluid administration sets and lowered temperature.

The **Basal Metabolic Rate** (BMR) is the rate of metabolism at rest as indicated by the amount of energy produced from the exothermic metabolic reactions. BMR provides a general reference for observing the general metabolic status of the body. A more detailed discussion of reaction rates in the body is described in Chapter 33.

Several different factors can influence the rate at which a reaction takes place. These factors include: the nature of the reactants; concentration of the reactants; temperature, catalysts and phase of reactants and products.

Nature of reactants

Simple substances such as sodium ions and chloride ions react quickly compared to more complex substances as more complex substances usually require more bonds to be broken.

Concentration of reactants

Increasing the concentration of reactants increases the rate of formation of the products. The greater the increase in concentration, the greater are the number of collisions between reactants thereby resulting in more product being formed. The relationship between reactant and product concentration is further discussed in 6.5 (reversible reactions).

Application: Use of pure oxygen

Pure oxygen (100% oxygen) is used in oxygen tents, inhalation by patients from cylinders or special oxygen lines within a hospital. Such uses present a potential fire hazard and require the utmost care in maintaining the absence of all flames, sparks and cigarettes as substances burn more readily in the presence of pure oxygen than in air. Sparks can occur from static electricity (10.4). Pure oxygen contains approximately five times the oxygen concentration of air thereby resulting in a far greater reaction rate between oxygen and other surrounding reactants.

Temperature

Increasing the temperature of a reaction results in the reactants being more active (9.9). The more active the reactants the greater is the chance of a collision occurring and the greater the likelihood that a reaction will take place. The violence of collisions also increases with increasing temperature thereby creating a greater chance that any one collision will result in a reaction occurring. These two factors result in temperature effecting large changes in reaction rates. EXAMPLES: An increase of 10°C results in a doubling or tripling of reaction rates.

Application: Raised body temperature

A rise in body temperature of 1°C increases the reaction rates of metabolism to such an extent that 7% more oxygen is required by the body.

A fever allows the body to kill germs by mobilizing the immune system. Temperatures above 40°C (104°F) increase reaction rates to dangerous levels that can lead to convulsions and ultimately death if the body temperature is maintained at temperatures above 42°C (107.6°F). A high fever requires the supply of more oxygen to the tissues in order that the high reaction rates can be maintained. The signs of increased reaction rates are an increased pulse rate and faster breathing.

Catalysts

A **catalyst** is a substance that alters the speed (rate) of a reaction without itself being permanently changed. This is achieved by lowering the activation energy (Figure 6.1). The minute quantities of catalyst used within a reaction are not consumed and can be recovered following the reaction. A catalyst does not change the net energy released in a reaction.

Catalysts play an important role in industry by improving the efficiency of processes such as producing sulphuric acid and refining petroleum. EXAMPLES: Pure metals such as platinum and molecules such as manganese dioxide.

To identify the involvement of a catalyst in a chemical reaction the catalyst is usually shown above or on the arrow. EXAMPLE: Hydrogen peroxide is rapidly decomposed to water and oxygen in the presence of manganese dioxide. Note the formula for a catalyst is not included in the equation.

$$2H_2O \xrightarrow{MnO_2} 2H_2O + O_2 \quad \text{Eqn 6.1}$$

Enzymes

Life as we know it, cannot exist without the assistance of catalysts as the rate at which most chemical reactions occur is far too slow to support life. The major catalysts in living organisms are a group of proteins called enzymes.

Enzymes are responsible for speeding up reactions by many thousands of times to provide the required reaction rates to support life. There are thousands of different enzymes within the body. A particular enzyme will catalyze a specific chemical reaction. EXAMPLE: The enzyme ptyalin in saliva increases the rate at which starch is broken down. The action of a specific enzyme can be enhanced or diminished by the action of drugs since most drugs achieve their effect by altering enzyme function (32.1). The importance of enzymes in maintaining body function is also shown by the impact of deficiencies of specific enzymes in genetic disorders such as phenylketonuria (24.12). Chapter 32 describes in more detail the structure and function of enzymes.

Phase of reactants

When the reactants and products are all in the one phase or state of matter (9.4) a **homogenous reaction** occurs. EXAMPLE: All substances are dissolved in a liquid. Homogenous reaction rates are determined by the above factors. Where more than one phase exists in a reaction the reaction is

referred to as a **heterogenous reaction**. EXAMPLE: Solid in an acid such as solid food in the stomach where hydrochloric acid (HCl) is present. Reactions only take place at the surface of the solid. As the surface area increases the rate of the reaction increases.

Application: Efficiency of digestion

The rate of breakdown of solid materials in digestion is increased by the presence of enzymes that break down large structures into smaller structures causing an increased surface area for other enzymes to act. Overcoming this factor is an important part of the process of digestion. Any factor that reduces this process will result in a decrease in the efficiency of digestion and therefore lead to possible nutritional deficiencies as discussed in Unit Nine.

6.3 Chemical equations

These are used to show which substances are used (reactants) and which substances are formed (products) in a chemical reaction. An equation assists a person in understanding the nature of a chemical reaction. The reactants and products can be separated by either a single arrow →, a double arrow ⇋, or an equal sign.

A single arrow indicates that the reaction is predominantly a one way reaction, that is, products are formed in the direction of the single arrow.

A double arrow indicates that the conversion of reactants into products is always incomplete. Double arrows indicate reversible reactions which can operate in either direction (6.5).

An equal sign between reactants and products is often used instead of double arrows when chemical equilibrium exists.

A chemical equation has to be consistent. Elements cannot be changed into other elements by chemical means. If charges are involved, the net charge on both sides of a chemical equation must be equal. All equations must be balanced, with the amount of reactants and their charges being equal to the amount of products and their charges.

6.4 Balancing equations

Balancing an equation may require altering the quantity of molecules, as the ratios of elements within a molecule are fixed for a specific molecule. EXAMPLE: In Eqn 6.2a, the first point to note is that two Cl^- are required to combine with the Zn^{2+} so that all compounds have a net charge of zero. Eqn 6.2a is rewritten to form Eqn 6.2b. In Eqn 6.2b an excess of Cl^- ions now occurs on the right hand side of the equation. An excess of H^+ ions also occurs on the same side. To balance the equation an increase of H^+ and Cl^- is required on the left hand side. This balance can only be achieved by increasing the quantity of HCl. Increasing the quantity of Cl^- or H^+ in the molecule will result in a different compound being formed. Eqn 6.2c shows the balanced equation for this reaction. The amounts of each substance and their charges are equal on both sides of the equation.

$$Zn^{2+}O^{2-} + \quad H^+Cl^- \quad \rightarrow Zn^{2+}Cl^- + H_2^+O^{2-}$$
zinc   + hydrochloric → zinc   + water
oxide   acid   chloride   Eqn 6.2a

$$Zn^{2+}O^{2-} + \quad H^+Cl^- \quad \rightarrow Zn^{2+}Cl_2^- + H_2^+O^{2-}$$
zinc   + hydrochloric → zinc   + water
oxide   acid   chloride   Eqn 6.2b

$$Zn^{2+}O^{2-} + \quad 2H^+Cl^- \quad \rightarrow Zn^{2+}Cl_2^- + H_2^+O^{2-}$$
zinc   + hydrochloric → zinc   + water
oxide   acid   chloride   Eqn 6.2c

A balanced equation can be used to determine:

1. the amount of reactants required to form a specific amount of product;
2. the chemical result of combining two substances;
3. the valence of an element or radical.

In a balanced equation the number of charges on each side of the equation are equal. A compound contains no net charge and therefore the valence of most elements and radicals can be determined by knowing the valence of only one element or radical. Since the valence of many elements and radicals can be determined from a small number of elements, it is only necessary to remember the valence of a small number of common elements and radicals!

In Eqn 6.3 the valence of all the elements and the radical OH is determined from knowing that hydrogen has a valence of 1^+. Firstly, only one Cl is required to form a zero net charge with H^+ on the left hand side. This indicates that Cl has a valence of 1^-. Similarly, the radical OH must have a valence of 1^- since one H^+ combines with one OH. The valence of Na must be 1^+ as only one Na ion is used to combine with the Cl^- ion.

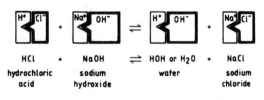

HCl   +   NaOH   ⇌   HOH or H_2O +   NaCl
hydrochloric   sodium   water   sodium
acid   hydroxide   chloride

Eqn 6.3

Table 6.1 Types of chemical reactions

Type	General equation	Example	
Combination	$A + B \rightarrow AB$	Carbon + Oxygen $\rightarrow$ Carbon Dioxide $C \quad + O_2 \quad \rightarrow CO_2$	Eqn 6.4
Decomposition	$AB \rightarrow A + B$	Water $\rightarrow$ Hydrogen + Oxygen $2H_2O \rightarrow 2H_2 \quad + O_2$	Eqn 6.5
Single displacement	$A + BC \rightarrow AC + B$	Zinc $\quad$ + Copper + Zinc $\rightarrow$ Zinc $\quad$ + Copper Sulphate $\qquad\qquad\qquad$ Sulphate	Eqn 6.6
	or		
	$A + BC \rightarrow AB + C$	Chlorine + Sodium $\rightarrow$ Sodium + Bromine $\qquad\qquad$ Bromide $\quad$ Chloride $Cl_2 \quad + 2NaBr \rightarrow 2NaCl \quad + Br_2$	Eqn 6.7
Double displacement	$AB + CD \rightarrow AD + AC$	Sodium + Silver $\rightarrow$ Silver $\quad$ + Sodium Chloride $\quad$ Nitrate $\quad$ Chloride $\quad$ Nitrate $NaCl \quad + AgNO_3 \rightarrow AgCl \quad + NaNO_3$	Eqn 6.8
Reversible reactions	$A + B \rightleftharpoons C + D$	Hydrochloric + Sodium $\quad \rightarrow$ Carbonic + Sodium Acid $\qquad$ Bicarbonate $\quad$ Acid $\qquad$ Chloride	Eqn 6.9

NOTE: The physical state of the substance is included where a change in the physical state is considered important. The symbols used are; s, solid; aq, aqueous; g, gas.

6.5 Types of chemical reactions

Chemical reactions can occur in a variety of combinations. The combinations can be divided into the following categories according to the nature of the reaction: combination or synthesis reactions; decomposition reactions; single displacement or substitution reactions; double displacement or metathesis reactions; reversible or equilibrium reactions and oxidation–reduction or redox reactions. Examples of each equation are listed in Table 6.1 apart from redox reactions which are described in more detail in 6.6.

Combination or synthesis reactions

Two or more substances combine to form a single substance. These reactions provide the mechanism for growth and repair within the body where smaller molecules are combined into larger molecules. EXAMPLE: Proteins are assembled from building block molecules called amino acids.

Decomposition reactions

These reactions involve the breakdown of one substance to form two or more products. This reaction is particularly important in the breakdown of food into smaller molecules that can be used by the body (28.3) and in the decomposition of organic matter by microbes in the carbon cycle (28.1).

Single displacement reactions

These reactions are also referred to as substitution reactions as one element is substituted by another usually as a result of the second element being more **reactive**. This process is important in the formation of many new organic compounds where hydrogen atoms are displaced by other elements (8.2).

Double displacement reactions

In double displacement reactions substitution of elements between compounds results in the formation of more than one new compound.

Reversible reactions

Reversible or equilibrium reactions are reactions where the products can unite to reform the original reactants. Such reactions are called two-way reactions and are represented by double arrows ⇌ to indicate that the reaction can occur in both directions (Eqn 6.9). The activation energies for both the reactants and products must be similar as a low activation energy in one direction results in a high activation energy in the reverse direction. The direction of the high activation energy would not proceed for the reasons described in 6.1. The direction of the reaction is also dependent upon conditions such as the concentration of each substance. The direction can be influenced by catalysts as they alter the rate (speed) at which the chemical reactions proceed on each side of the equation. Reversible equations play a major role in the maintenance of homeostasis in the body. EXAMPLE: Maintenance of acid/base balance which is achieved through balances in the formation of carbonic acid, bicarbonate and CO_2.

The rates of formation of and decomposition of a reversible reaction become equal over a period of time. A **chemical equilibrium** then exists. It is important to note that chemical equilibrium does not result in equal concentrations on both sides of an equation. It means that a balance now exists between formation and decomposition. No net increase now occurs in the formation or de-composition of substances even though the reaction has not stopped since the rate of the forward reaction now equals the rate of the reverse reaction.

When a stress such as a change in concentration or temperature is applied to a reaction at equilibrium, the equilibrium will be displaced in such a direction as to relieve that stress. This principle is referred to as **Le Chatelier's Principle**. EXAMPLE: An increase in the concentration of carbonic acid will result in the decomposition of carbonic acid until the proportion of carbonic acid to bicarbonate is again 1:20 (see Application). Chemical equilibrium is discussed further in Chapters 17 and 33.

Application: Ratio of carbonic acid to bicarbonate

Carbonic acid and bicarbonate exist in a proportion of 1:20 in our body. This chemical equilibrium is shown in Eqn 5.2.

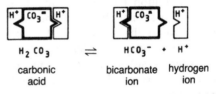

$$H_2CO_3 \quad \rightleftharpoons \quad HCO_3^- \quad + \quad H^+$$

carbonic acid — bicarbonate ion — hydrogen ion

Eqn 6.10

An elevation of carbonic acid would cause an alteration to the fixed proportion. This results in a proportionate amount of HCO_3^- and H^+ being formed from the H_2CO_3. A ratio of one carbonic acid to twenty bicarbonate is maintained. Similarly, an alteration to the amount of bicarbonate will cause a proportionate change in the amount of carbonic acid. This maintenance of a ratio of one to twenty is important in maintaining the acid/base balance in blood (16.5).

6.6 Oxidation and reduction

Oxidation and reduction reactions are involved in a wide range of important chemical reactions. EXAMPLES: Bleaching of clothes, digestion of food, corrosion of metals and the burning of petrol in a car. They play a particularly important role in the body as they are responsible for the breakdown of glucose and the subsequent production of energy for the body to use (8.3).

Oxidation and reduction definitions

Originally oxygen was used in a chemical classification system as its reactive nature enables it to combine with most elements. **Oxidation** was defined as a reaction in which a substance gained an oxygen or lost a hydrogen.

This definition has been found to be too restrictive as similar chemical reactions could occur without the involvement of oxygen. **Oxidation is now also defined as the process where a substance loses one or more electrons whereas reduction is the gaining of electrons**.

Oxidation can never occur without reduction as a loss of electrons from an atom, ion or compound requires a substance to pick up the electrons since electrons cannot remain free and the reaction has to be balanced. Reactions involving oxidation therefore result in the transfer of electrons from one substance to another. These reactions are called **oxidation–reduction reactions or redox reactions**.

Oxidation and reduction of covalent compounds

In covalent compounds it is often difficult to determine which atom has gained or lost an electron. An important category of covalent compounds are organic compounds which represent 95% of all substances (Chapter 7). In organic compounds it is often convenient to use the original oxidation and reduction definitions which relate to oxygen and hydrogen. That is, **oxidation** is a reaction in which a substance gains an oxygen or loses a hydrogen. EXAMPLE: The oxidation of alcohol involves the loss of hydrogen resulting in the formation of acetic acid. This reaction represents wine 'going off' (oxidizing). NOTE: The oxidant product is of no interest regarding the outcome of the reaction and is written above the arrow.

$$CH_3CH_2OH \xrightarrow{K_2Cr_2O_7/H^+} CH_3COOH$$
$$\text{Eqn 6.11}$$

ethanol $\longrightarrow$ acetic acid

Reduction of covalent compounds usually involves the addition of hydrogen. EXAMPLE: Reduction of methanal to methanol

$$CH_2O + H_2 \xrightarrow{Ni} CH_3OH \quad \text{Eqn 6.12}$$
$$\text{methanal} \qquad\quad \text{methanol}$$

Oxidation number

Redox reactions always involve a change in valence (5.8) for at least some of the atoms or ions in the reaction. **Oxidation number** is used to identify the relative loss or gain of electrons and is equal to the number of electrons gained or lost. EXAMPLE: Sodium has an oxidation number of +1 as each sodium atom donates one electron in a chemical reaction resulting in the formation of Na^+. NOTE: The oxidation number and charge are the same. As chlorine gains one electron each chlorine atom has an oxidation number of −1.

A **loss** of electrons represents oxidation and also an increase in oxidation number. **An increase in oxidation number therefore indicates that the substance has been oxidized while a decrease in oxidation number represents a reduction of a substance**.

The correct formula for a compound requires no net charge (5.4) so the sum of oxidation numbers must be zero. EXAMPLE: Calcium chloride is not represented as $Ca^{+2}Cl^{-1}$ since the sum of the oxidation numbers is not zero but as $Ca^{+2}Cl_2^{-1}$. Uncombined elements have an oxidation number of zero

$$2\,Na^0 + Cl_2^0 \rightarrow 2Na^{+1} + 2Cl^{-1} \quad \text{Eqn 6.13}$$

where the upper number represents the respective oxidation number.

The above information can now be combined to identify what happens in a more complex reaction such as the breakdown of glucose to produce energy.

$$\underset{\text{glucose}}{C_6H_{12}O_6} + \underset{\text{oxygen}}{6O_2} \rightarrow \underset{\substack{\text{carbon}\\\text{dioxide}}}{6C^{+4}O^{-2}_2} + \underset{\text{water}}{6H_2O^{-2}} + \text{ENERGY}$$

$$\text{Eqn 6.14}$$

The oxidation number of carbon in glucose is zero whereas the oxidation number of the carbon atom in carbon dioxide is +4. The carbon atom in glucose was oxidized as a gain in oxidation number has occurred. Alternatively, the glucose molecule was oxidized as the carbon within it has been oxidized. In this example oxygen (O) has decreased its oxidation number to −2. Oxygen has in fact been **reduced**!

Determining the oxidation number

Determining the oxidation number in simple ionic compounds is straight forward as the oxidation number is the same as the charge (Table 6.2). In molecules containing covalent bonds the oxidation number is not as apparent.

The following rules are used to determine the oxidation number for covalent compounds where electrons are shared and not transferred.

1. All elements in their free state have an oxidation number of zero.
2. Oxygen has an oxidation number of −2. EXCEPTION: Peroxides where it is −1.
3. Hydrogen has an oxidation number of +1. EXCEPTION: Metal hydrides where it is −1.
4. In compounds the sum of all oxidation numbers is zero.
5. Group IA elements have an oxidation number of +1.
6. Group IIA elements have an oxidation number of +2.

In a polyatomic ion (5.7) oxygen always has a charge of −2. This information assists the calculation of the oxidation number of other elements within the ion. EXAMPLE: The phosphate ion PO_4^{3-}. The oxidation number of phosphate is determined as follows.

Step 1
Determine the oxidation number of PO_4^{3-} which is indicated by the overall charge. Therefore the oxidation number is −4.
Step 2
Separate the ion into its components.
Phosphate + 4(Oxygen) = −4

Table 6.2 Frequently used oxidation numbers

Oxidation number	Where found
0	All free elements such as Al, O_2
+1	H^+ (most cases), Na^+, K^+
+2	Ca^{2+}, Mg^{2+}
+3	Al^{3+}
−1	F^-, C^-, I^-
−2	O^{2-} or in polyatomic ions

Step 3
  Replace oxygen by -2
  Phosphate $+ 4(-2) = -4$
Step 4
  Complete the equation
  Phosphate $-8 = -4$
  Phosphate $= +4$

Reducing and oxidizing agents

It is often necessary when describing oxidation to refer to the agent causing the oxidation. An **oxidizing agent or oxidant** is a substance that accepts electrons from another substance causing an oxidation of that substance. NOTE: The oxidizing substance has now gained electrons and so has been **reduced**.

A **reducing agent or reductant** is a substance that donates electrons to another substance causing a reduction of that substance and as a consequence is itself **oxidized**. The relationship between the agent and the reactant being changed can be summarized as:

  substance oxidized = reducing agent
  substance reduced = oxidizing agent

Half equations

Redox reactions can be written in the form of half reactions. This is useful for balancing redox reactions and describing reactions where the physical separation of the products is important. EXAMPLE: Electrolysis (10.2). **Half reactions** are hypothetical descriptions of part of the overall reaction. One half reaction will describe the process of oxidation while the other half describes the reduction. EXAMPLE: Copper placed in silver nitrate solution. NOTE: The nitrate ion is not involved in the reaction described below and therefore is not included in the equation.

General reaction
$$Cu(s) + Ag^+(aq) \rightarrow Cu^{2+}(aq) + Ag(s)$$
                                           Eqn 6.15

Oxidation reaction
$$Cu \rightarrow Cu^{2+} + 2e \text{ (electrons)}$$ Eqn 6.15a

Reduction reaction $Ag^+ + e \rightarrow Ag$
                                           Eqn 6.15b

In order to balance this reaction the following have to be taken into account:

1. The total number of atoms on both sides must be equal.
2. The net charge on each side must be equal.
3. The total increase in oxidation number of the reducing agent must equal the total decrease in the oxidizing agent's oxidation number. This is achieved by balancing the number of electrons for both agents.

Balancing the equation involves multiplying each half reaction by the number required to make the increase in electrons equal the decrease. Cu has to be multiplied by 1 as the RHS contains two electrons.

Balanced $Cu \rightarrow Cu^{2+} + 2e$ Eqn 6.15c

Ag has to be multiplied by 2 to match the number of electrons above.

Balanced $2Ag^+ + 2e \rightarrow 2Ag$ Eqn 6.15d

Balanced redox equation
$$Cu + 2Ag^+ \rightarrow Cu^{2+} + 2Ag$$ Eqn 6.15e

In summary **oxidation** can be described as an increase in oxidation number, a loss of electrons, a gain of oxygen or a loss of hydrogen

6.7   Environmental health and safety

Fires are one of the main hazards associated with chemical reactions. As a fire is a reaction our understanding of the mechanisms of a reaction can be applied to extinguishing a fire. A fire can be extinguished by removing oxygen, the reactant or by lowering the heat which is providing the activation energy for the reaction to take place. It is important that the correct fire extinguisher is selected for a fire as a range of fire extinguishers exist. EXAMPLES: Foam, dry chemical powder, carbon dioxide and BCF. The nature of the fire can differ according to the materials involved. Particular care should be taken in selecting an extinguisher for an electrical fire as there exists the possibility of electrocution.

The carbon dioxide extinguisher is a common extinguisher found in hospitals. It acts by both lowering the temperature and eliminating the oxygen. Carbon dioxide is extremely cold and as it is heavier than oxygen, the carbon dioxide is able to surround the burning area as long as the fire extinguisher is directed at the base of the fire. Carbon dioxide fire extinguishers are used for electrical fires and oil fires.

Some chemical reactions involve the rapid release of large amounts of energy. These reactions are called explosions.

Application: Explosions

Explosions occur when a flammable substance receives sufficient energy to meet the low activation energy for the reaction to take place. The small amount of energy could come from a spark or match. Great care is required when working in an environment which contains flammable substances as sparks can arise from faulty electrical equipment or the build up of static electricity.

Summary

The formation of new substances results from interactions between chemicals. These interactions are described with the aid of chemical equations. A chemical reaction involves the combination of reactants to form products. The amount of each substance and their charges must be the same on both sides of the equation, that is, the equation must be balanced.

For a reaction to take place the reactants must collide and produce an activation energy greater than the energy stored in the bonds and/or the molecules collide with the correct orientation. Catalysts assist this process without themselves being permanently changed. The higher the activation energy the lesser is the chance that a reaction will take place. When the reaction releases a net quantity of energy it is referred to as an exothermic reaction. A reaction requiring more energy than previously existed in the reactants is called an endothermic reaction. In the body, an exothermic reaction is required to provide the energy for the body whereas an endothermic reaction is required to store energy.

The rate at which a reaction occurs is influenced by the: concentration of reactants, temperature, catalysts and phase of the reactants. The main biological catalysts are the specialized protein group known as enzymes.

The type of chemical reaction varies according to the reactants. The different types are: combination or synthesis reactions; decomposition reactions; single displacement reactions; double displacement reactions; reversible reactions and oxidation and reduction reactions. In reversible reactions the reaction takes place in both directions until a chemical equilibrium exists. Oxidation and reduction reactions have to occur together as oxidation involves the losing of electrons whereas reduction gains electrons. These reactions are often called redox reactions. The relative number of electrons gained or lost is identified by the oxidation number. The agent causing an oxidation is called an oxidizing agent and conversely a reducing agent reduces a substance. A useful method of balancing a redox reaction is to write the half equations for the reaction.

The principles of chemical reactions can be applied to extinguishing fires. As the properties of fires vary, care should be taken to use the appropriate fire extinguisher.

Unit Four
Organic Chemistry

This unit describes the structure and chemical properties of biologically important organic compounds.

Chapter 7

Introduction to organic compounds

Objectives

At the completion of this chapter the student should be able to:

1. explain how organic and inorganic compounds differ;
2. explain the difference between saturated and unsaturated organic compounds;
3. describe an alkane, alkene and alkyne;
4. describe the difference between straight chain hydrocarbons and cyclic hydrocarbons;
5. define conformation, isomer, homologous series, hydrocarbon;
6. describe the different forms of isomerism;
7. describe the approaches used to identify and name organic compounds;
8. explain the safety precautions relating to the use of organic compounds.

7.1 Organic and inorganic compounds

All chemical compounds are divided into two categories; organic compounds and inorganic compounds. Organic compounds always contain carbon whereas inorganic compounds generally lack carbon. EXCEPTION: Compounds such as carbonic acid (H_2CO_3) and carbon dioxide are classified as inorganic compounds.

Carbon has a valence of four which enables carbon atoms to link with each other to form large and complex covalent compounds. The study of carbon and its compounds is a separate branch of chemistry known as organic chemistry. Carbon compounds form 95% of the total number of known chemical compounds. Most carbon compounds contain large quantities of hydrogen. The molecular structure of humans is based on organic compounds. EXAMPLES: Proteins, lipids and carbohydrates. Most pharmacological substances and all plastics also contain carbon.

Inorganic compounds are generally smaller than organic compounds. They also serve an important role in the human body by acting independently or with organic compounds. EXAMPLES: Electrolytes (such as sodium and potassium ions), carbon dioxide, and inorganic acids such as hydrochloric acid.

Organic compounds differ from inorganic compounds in the following ways:

1. organic compounds are covalent whereas inorganic compounds can be ionic or covalent;
2. organic compounds are mainly incapable of dissolving in water whereas most inorganic substances can dissolve in water;
3. organic compounds form the main molecular framework of tissue whereas inorganic compounds assist in strengthening skeletal tissues and aid body metabolism.

7.2 Saturated and unsaturated organic compounds

Carbon has a valence of four since the outer electron orbit contains four electrons. Carbon can form single, double or triple bonds with other carbon atoms. The presence of these bonds confers individual properties to a carbon molecule.

When carbon atoms are linked by single bonds the molecule is referred to as a saturated compound. These compounds always contain a chain of carbon atoms that are linked by the sharing of one pair of electrons. The remaining bonds are usually formed with hydrogen (Figure 7.1a) although oxygen and nitrogen can be present. In Figure 7.1a all of the carbon atoms contain four covalent bonds since carbon has a valence of four.

An unsaturated compound contains some carbon atoms that are linked to other carbon

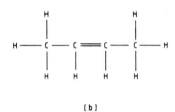

[a]

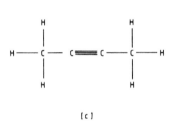

[b]

[c]

Figure 7.1 (a) Saturated compounds contain carbon atoms linked by single bonds whereas unsaturated compounds contain some carbon atoms that are linked by (b) double bonds or (c) triple bonds.

atoms by either double or triple bonds (Figures 7.1b, 7.1c). Note that all of the carbon atoms still contain four covalent bonds. A polyunsaturated compound contains many double or triple bonds linking carbon atoms. The word poly is a frequently used prefix in organic chemistry. It simply means 'many'. EXAMPLE: Most animal fats are polysaturated and thus contain a predominance of single bonds whereas many plants contain polyunsaturated fats.

7.3 Describing organic compounds

Structural formulae

Carbon has the ability to form long chains of carbon atoms. These atoms can form straight chains, often with a network of side chains or branches (Figure 7.2a). Carbon atoms can also form cyclic chains which may have straight chains attached (Figure 7.2b). The structural formulae of carbon compounds can be abbreviated by indicating each carbon atom and its covalent bonds, but not the large number of hydrogen atoms. Unless otherwise indicated a hydrogen atom is inferred as existing at the end of any covalent bond (Figure 7.2c).

With inorganic compounds a particular substance can be described with a molecular formula (5.9). EXAMPLE: H_2O will always represent water. With organic compounds, owing to the formation of isomers, a molecular formula is usually not representative of a unique compound. EXAMPLE: $C_6H_{12}O_6$ represents sixteen different compounds (5.9 and Figure 5.9). The existence of isomers requires the use of a structural formula.

Limitations of structural formulae

Because organic molecules are often large and complex, the use of structural formulae on labels of containers or in textbooks presents problems. An alternative system uses words to describe specific organic compounds. In the past, common names were used to identify individual organic compounds. EXAMPLES: Acetic acid, xylene, acetone and aspirin. Unfortunately, an infinite potential exists for forming new organic compounds thereby resulting in the need to memorize an enormous number

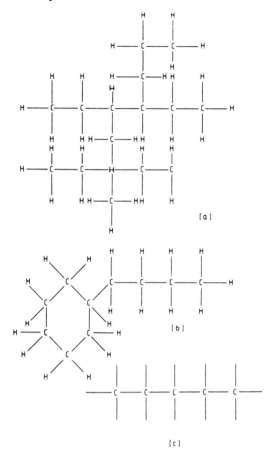

Figure 7.2 Carbon can form either (a) long open ended chains with numerous side chains, or (b) closed carbon chains. (c) The structural formula for carbon compounds can be abbreviated by implying the presence of hydrogen at the end of each incomplete covalent bond.

of substances. A system devised by the International Union of Pure and Applied Chemists (IUPAC) is now generally accepted throughout the world.

The IUPAC system establishes a word picture for each compound and a mechanism for converting the word picture into the structural formula. This removes the need to memorize a large number of common names. A limitation of the IUPAC system is the possible formation of extremely long words. EXAMPLE: 2-bromo-2-chloro-1,1,1,-trifluoroethane (Figure 8.8). The use of generic words overcomes this limitation, e.g. the above substance is usually called halothane.

The word picture system can result in extremely long and complex words. These are purely descriptive and, if broken down into the constituent parts, enable a person to draw the structure of a compound. It is necessary to have a general understanding of this system in order to study the fundamental components of organic and cell chemistry.

7.4 Conformation and isomerism

Shape

Life is dependent on the unique shape that exists with many organic molecules as this uniqueness enables specific body processes to occur (5.11). Changes in shapes can arise from atoms connected by a single bond as one of the properties of a single bond is that atoms can freely rotate about the bond. Shapes arising from these rotations are called **conformations**. NOTE: The basic structure of a molecule does not change with rotation as the atoms are still arranged in the same order but the function can change with the change in shape. **Conformational change** is an important process in biological reactions and will be discussed in Chapter 32.

Isomers as described in 5.9 reflect the possible different arrangements of atoms and the resulting shape that can exist for a given molecular formula. There are four different categories of isomer: structural, functional, geometric and optical. Geometric and

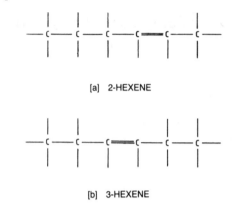

[a] 2-HEXENE

[b] 3-HEXENE

Figure 7.3   The location of the double bonds in two hexene structural isomers.

optical isomerism are also referred to as **stereoisomerism** or **spatial isomerism** as they represent molecules where the bonding sequence is the same but a relative difference exists in the positions of the atoms in space.

Structural isomers

These isomers contain the same molecular formula, same groups of atoms attached to the carbon chains but have different structural formulae. EXAMPLE: 2-hexene and 3-hexene (Figure 7.3). The number of structural isomers increases rapidly with increasing carbon chain length as the number of potential positions for double and triple bonds increases. There are only three structural isomers for C_5H_{12} whereas there are 75 structural isomers of $C_{10}H_{22}$ and 366 319 for $C_{20}H_{42}$.

Functional isomers

Functional isomers are compounds that contain the same molecular formula but contain different functional groups (Chapter 8). EXAMPLE: Propanoic acid and 2-hydroxypropanal (Figure 7.4).

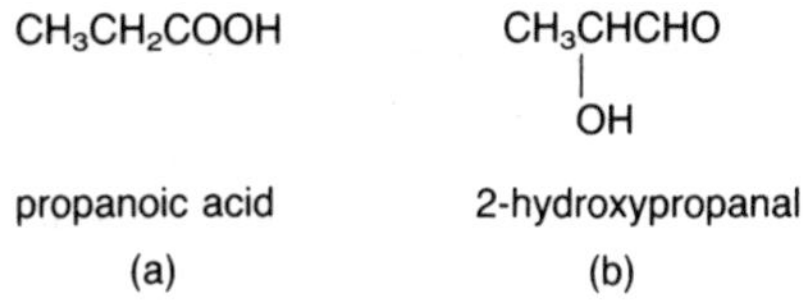
CH3CH2COOH
CH3CHCHO
OH
propanoic acid
2-hydroxypropanal
(a)
(b)

Figure 7.4 Functional isomers (a) propanoic acid and (b) 2-hydroxypropanal.

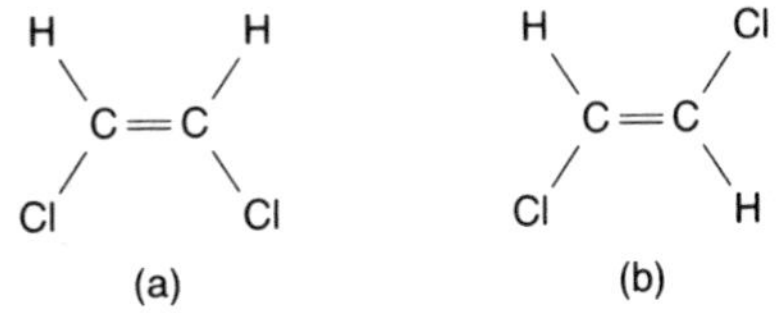
H
H
C=C
Cl
Cl
H
Cl
C=C
Cl
H
(a)
(b)

Figure 7.5 Geometric isomers (a) *cis*-1,2-dichloroethene, (b) *trans*-1,2-dichloroethene.

Geometric isomers

Geometric isomers result from the restriction that double and triple bonds as well as ring systems place on the rotation of atoms. Rotation causes these bonds to break. Atoms are effectively locked into a particular spatial position which therefore confers a fixed shape in that region (Figure 8.12). EXAMPLE: Helical molecules such as those formed from the partial double bond formed between the carbon and nitrogen in peptide bonds (Figure 7.5). The helices associated with proteins (30.3 and Figure 30.3) and the hereditary molecule DNA (Figure 24.9) are fundamental to life.

Geometric or stereoisomers are identified by prefixes. In Figure 7.5 a the prefix **cis** is used to indicate that the two structures with the same groups are located on the **same** side of the double bond. The prefix **trans** is used to indicate the location of the groups on opposite sides (Figure 7.5b). NOTE: Geometric isomers cannot occur where two identical groups are attached to the same atom as only one structure is possible.

Optical isomers

Optical isomers occur when at least one carbon atom in a molecule has four different groups attached to it. Such carbon atoms are called **asymmetric carbon atoms**. In an optical isomer the same molecular formula exists but the structures are mirror images of each other. If a model of a structure is placed in front of a mirror the reflected structure represents the arrangement of the other optical isomer. These molecules are in fact different as they cannot be superimposed on each other. EXAMPLE: Glucose and galactose are optical isomers of $C_6H_{12}O_6$ (Figure 5.9).

Optical isomers rotate polarized light in different directions with + or **d** prefix indicating that polarized light is rotated clockwise and/or **l** indicating an anti-clockwise rotation. Another prefix system of **D** and **L** is used by convention to describe the relative arrangement of atoms about an asymmetric carbon atom (Figure 7.6). NOTE: The D and L refers only to structure and not to the direction of the rotation of light.

Application: Optical activity and body function

Enzymes primarily will only act on one particular optical isomer. The body mainly uses the D series of carbohydrates and the L series of proteins. Parkinson's disease is treated with the L-dopa form of dopa as the D form is ineffective. The body uses the L form of Vitamin C(1-ascorbic acid) since the D series is inactive.

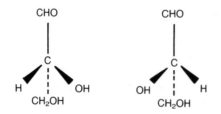

Figure 7.6 Optical isomers of gluteraldehyde. The wedges represent projections towards you while the dotted lines project away from you. (a) D-gluteraldehyde contains the OH on the right-hand side whereas (b) L-gluteraldehyde contains the OH on the left-hand side.

Table 7.1 Names and molecular formulae for the first ten alkanes

Name	Molecular formula
Methane	CH_4
Ethane	C_2H_6
Propane	C_3H_8
Butane	C_4H_{10}
Pentane	C_5H_{12}
Hexane	C_6H_{14}
Heptane	C_7H_{16}
Octane	C_8H_{18}
Nonane	C_9H_{20}
Decane	$C_{10}H_{22}$

7.5 Straight chain hydrocarbons

Hydrocarbons are compounds that consist solely of carbon and hydrogen. These compounds form the basis of oil and its derivatives such as methane and propane.

Alkanes

Alkanes are a large group of saturated hydrocarbons that exist in straight chains. All alkane compounds are named in the following manner. Each alkane's name can be split into two parts. The first part indicates the number of carbon atoms in the chain. EXAMPLES: pent- for five, oct- for eight. The second part of the molecular name is -ane. Any substance that contains an -ane at the end of a word is an alkane. The common alkanes are listed in Table 7.1. The structural formula of the alkane propane is shown in Figure 7.7a. Note that the structural difference between successive alkanes is

constant — CH_2. In a **homologous series** of compounds, each member differs from the member of next higher weight by a **methylene group** (CH_2).

The following are the IUPAC rules for naming an alkane.

1. The general name of a saturated hydrocarbon is alkane.
2. Determine the longest possible continuous chain of carbon atoms which, in branched alkanes, may include two side chains. Assign a parent name from Table 7.1 that corresponds to the number of carbon atoms in the chain. EXAMPLE: The structure in Figure 7.7e is heptane, not hexane, as the longest continuous chain contains seven atoms.
3. Locate and identify any groups or side chains that are not part of the longest chain. Satuated side chains are called **alkyl groups**. The name of any attached group is derived from the alkane of the same number of carbons by changing the **ane** to **yl**. In Figure 7.7e a methyl group occurs at carbon atom three and an ethyl group at carbon atom four.
4. When only one group or side chain is attached to the parent chain, the carbon

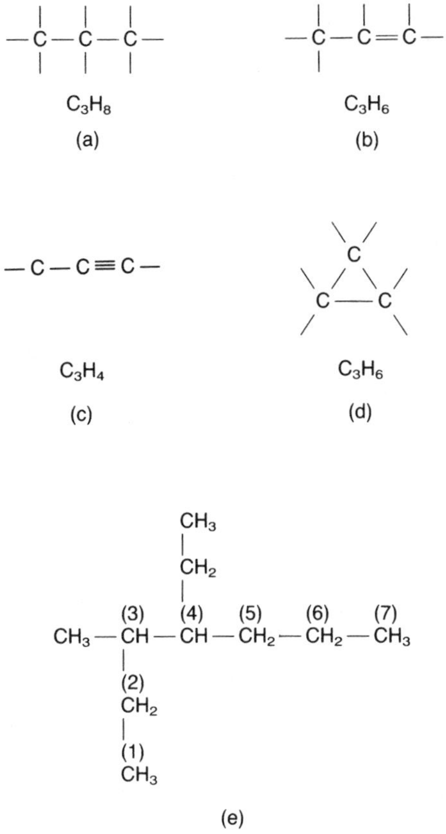

$$-\overset{|}{\underset{|}{C}}-\overset{|}{\underset{|}{C}}-\overset{|}{\underset{|}{C}}-$$

C_3H_8

(a)

$$-\overset{|}{\underset{|}{C}}-\overset{|}{\underset{|}{C}}=\overset{|}{\underset{}{C}}-$$

C_3H_6

(b)

$$-C-C\equiv C-$$

C_3H_4

(c)

C_3H_6

(d)

$$\begin{array}{c} CH_3 \\ | \\ CH_2 \\ | \\ \underset{CH_3}{\overset{(3)}{CH}}\overset{(4)}{-}\overset{(5)}{CH}\overset{(6)}{-}CH_2\overset{(7)}{-}CH_2-CH_3 \\ | \\ CH_2 \\ (2) \\ | \\ (1) \\ CH_3 \end{array}$$

(e)

Figure 7.7 Structural and molecular formulae of the hydrocarbons: (a) propane, (b) propene, (c) propyne, (d) cyclopropane and (e) 4-ethyl-3methylheptane.

atoms with side groups are numbers three and four. This adds up to seven, whereas numbering the carbon atoms from the opposite end would give a higher total. (The carbon atoms would be numbers four and five resulting in a total of nine).

5. Write the name by commencing with the location and name of each attached group. If the same group occurs more than once, the number of each carbon atom is given. In addition, the number of times each group occurs is indicated by the prefixes di, tri, etc. If several different groups occur, list them in alphabetical order and place before the parent name. EXAMPLE: Figure 8.8. NOTE: Use commas between numbers and hyphens between numbers on names of side groups.

Alkenes

An **alkene** is an unsaturated hydrocarbon with one or more carbon–carbon double bonds. All alkenes are distinguished by a numerical prefix which is identical to the alkanes, and the letters **-ene** at the end of the word. EXAMPLES: Propene for a three carbon alkene and octene for an eight carbon alkene. The structural formula of the alkene propene is shown in Figure 7.7b.

Alkynes

An **alkyne** is an unsaturated hydrocarbon that contains one or more carbon–carbon triple bonds. These compounds are distinguished from alkanes and alkenes by the use of **-yne** at the end of a molecular name. EXAMPLES: Propyne contains three carbon atoms and octyne contains eight carbon atoms. Propyne's structure is shown in Figure 7.7c. The location of triple bonds is determined by the same process as that used for alkenes.

atoms in the parent chain are numbered so that the carbon with the attached group has the lowest possible number. When two or more groups are present always begin numbering from the end of the parent chain that gives you the smallest total of numbers for the groups. EXAMPLE: In Figure 7.7e the carbon

Naming alkenes and alkynes

The location of double and triple bonds along a carbon chain can vary for the same molecular formula. The longer a carbon chain, the greater the number of positions where a double or triple bond can be located, that is, the greater the number of possible isomers. Remember that isomers have the same molecular formula but different structural formulae.

The location of double and triple bonds is described in the IUPAC system by numbering the carbon atoms in a chain from the end that will give the double and triple bonded carbon atoms the lowest possible number. EXAMPLE: 2-hexene indicates that a double bond is located between the second and third carbon atoms from the end of the chain (Figure 7.3a), 3-hexene indicates that a double bond exists between the third and fourth carbon atoms (Figure 7.3b).

7.6   Cyclic hydrocarbons

Cyclic hydrocarbons contain a ring of carbon atoms. These compounds are named by combining the prefix cyclo- to the corresponding alkane, alkene or alkyne name. EXAMPLES: Cyclopropane contains three carbon atoms linked into a ring whereas cyclohexane contains six carbon atoms in a ring. The structural and molecular formulae of cyclopropane are shown in Figure 7.7d. Note that cyclopropane contains two less hydrogens than propane. Cyclopropane has different properties from propane. Cyclopropane (trimethylene) can be used as a general anaesthetic whereas propane is a natural gas — used in conjunction with butane as a fuel.

7.7   Aromatic hydrocarbons

Alkanes, alkenes and alkynes (including cyclic ones) are collectively called **aliphatic hydrocarbons**. The aromatic hydrocarbons have a different form and different properties from the aliphatic hydrocarbons.

Aromatic hydrocarbons were originally named because many of them have a spicy or sweet smelling odour. This generalization is misleading as not all aromatic compounds are odorous and not all sweet smelling compounds are aromatic compounds. The name is now used to denote a particular form of six carbon ring. **Aromatic hydrocarbons** contain six carbon atoms joined together in an alternating sequence of single and double bonds (Figure 7.8). This structure consists of two isomers that are continually changing into each other. An abbreviated symbol is used to indicate the structure of these compounds (Figure 7.9).

The simplest aromatic compound is benzene. This compound is represented in Figure 7.8 and it has the molecular formula C_6H_6. Benzene is toxic when ingested and can cause a decrease in red blood cell and

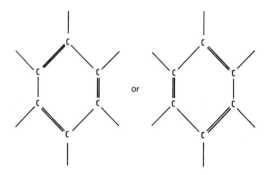

Figure 7.8   Two structural forms of an aromatic compound and the frequently depicted abbreviated symbol.

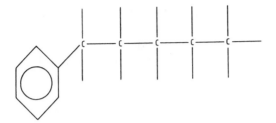

Figure 7.9   The combination of a hydrocarbon chain with a benzene molecule can lead to an infinite number of aromatic compounds.

white blood cell counts on continued inhalation of its vapour.

Benzene can have straight hydrocarbon chains, cyclic chains or other benzene molecules attached to the ring by simply replacing a hydrogen in the benzene molecule with a carbon atom in a hydrocarbon chain (Figure 7.9). The addition of these chains leads to an infinite number of aromatic compounds with an infinite number of properties. A large proportion of biologically important organic compounds exhibit both aliphatic and aromatic features. These compounds are named as follows:

1. When a single hydrogen has been substituted by a group, the group's name usually precedes the word benzene. EXAMPLES: A single chlorine substitution forms chlorobenzene whereas the substitution of a single NO_2 ion forms nitrobenzene. Some single substitutions always give a compound with a common name. EXAMPLES: A substitution involving an amine group ($-NH_2$) forms an aniline, a hydroxyl group (OH) substitution forms phenol (Figure 8.1b) and a methyl group (CH_3) forms toluene.
2. Substitution of two hydrogens results in the possible formation of three isomers. A common method of identifying or describing these isomers uses the prefixes **ortho**,

meta and **para**, which designate the position of the second substitution relative to the first (Figure 8.1b). An alternative system is the use of carbon numbers (Figure 8.1c).
3. When three or more hydrogens have been substituted it is necessary to use carbon numbers to name the compound (Figure 8.1c).
4. When naming more complex molecules the benzene ring is often regarded as the substituted entity, in which case it has had an H atom substituted and is called a phenyl group (Figure 8.1d).

Some hormones are benzene compounds with substituted H atoms. EXAMPLE: Steroids. The benzene compound toluene is used as a urine preservative while other benzene compounds are used as drugs. EXAMPLE: Benzodiazepines such as valium, librium and serepax. Some of the multibenzene ringed compounds can cause cancer. EXAMPLE: 1,2 benzpyrene which is found in cigarette smoke and automobile exhaust gases.

7.8   Environmental health and safety

Hydrocarbons present hazards to both staff and patients. Organic compounds are generally more reactive than inorganic chemicals. It is important that the correct procedures are followed for the storage, handling and disposal of organic chemicals. A common method of storing organic chemicals is to store them in small quantities. Precautions must be made to ensure that all the appropriate fire prevention equipment is readily accessible wherever organic chemicals are used. Petrol provides an example of how flammable hydrocarbons can be. Hydrocarbons are non-polar and are therefore readily absorbed through the skin and lungs.

Summary

Organic compounds contain carbon whereas inorganic compounds generally do not. Organic compounds are covalent and are usually incapable of dissolving in water.

When atoms of carbon are linked by single bonds, the molecule is saturated. An unsaturated compound contains some carbon atoms linked by either double or triple bonds.

Organic compounds can vary in shape as a result of rotation about a single carbon bond. These variations are called conformations, and are fundamental to biological processes.

Organic compounds form isomers. The four categories of isomerism are: structural, functional, geometric and optical. Stereoisomerism refers to either geometric or optical isomers. The body usually selects only one isomer for a particular process.

Organic compounds are usually more reactive than inorganic chemicals and therefore require great care in their use and storage.

Hydrocarbons or compounds consisting of carbon and hydrogen can be arranged in straight chains, cyclic configurations or a combination of both. The IUPAC system is used to identify and describe organic compounds. Many organic compounds are arranged in a homologous series in which each member differs from the one of next higher molecular weight by a methylene group (CH_2). Straight chained hydrocarbons are termed alkanes, alkenes and alkynes according to the presence of single, double or triple bonds linking respective carbon atoms. When six carbon atoms form a ring by linking the carbon atoms in an alternating sequence of single and double bonds, an aromatic hydrocarbon is formed.

Chapter 8

Important biological functional groups

Objectives

At the completion of this chapter the students should be able to:

1. describe the functional groups identified in this chapter;
2. define organic radical, hydrophobic, hydrophilic, heterocyclic compound, catecholamine, antiseptic and disinfectant;
3. draw the general structure of amino acids and a peptide bond;
4. explain the hazards associated with using organic compounds.

8.1 The biological role of functional groups

The range of different organic substances is increased by the inclusion of other groups of atoms to a hydrocarbon chain or ring.

A **functional group** is an arrangement of atoms that will have very similar chemical and physical properties whenever it is found in an organic molecule. The addition of these functional groups to a hydrocarbon chain alters the properties of the chain. Functional groups are the sites of chemical reactions. In the case of chemicals in the body, this means that these groups are the main sites at which the chemical processes that determine body function are located.

For simplicity the hydrocarbon chain is often replaced by R when referring to the properties of a functional group. The R represents an **organic radical** which refers to the chemically inactive part of a molecule, that is, the molecular part that is not the functional group. EXAMPLE: Alcohols have the general formula ROH. The OH determines the chemical properties of an alcohol and thus R represents hydrocarbon chains such as propane and pentane.

It is important to understand the structure and relative location of a functional group as these features determine the function of that compound in the body. The influence on the body of functional groups is shown by the use of drugs to alter body function or microorganisms that have invaded the body. The action of drugs results from a particular functional group or groups being located in a specific position within a molecule. The location of the position influences the final shape of a molecule. The shape of a molecule is an important factor in the biologically selective action of a molecule (5.11). The chemical and physical properties of a functional group together with its location combine to determine the biological effects of a drug within the body.

Table 8.1 Important functional groups, their structure and examples of their use

Name of functional group	Functional group structure (attached to a carbon chain)	Use
Alcohol and phenol	R—OH	Alcohol depresses nervous system while phenol is corrosive to tissue; both used as antiseptics and disinfectants
Aldehyde	$$R-C\underset{\diagdown H}{\overset{\diagup\!\!\!\!/ \; O}{}}$$	Glucose used to produce energy for cell function
Amine	$$R-\overset{\displaystyle H}{\underset{\displaystyle H}{\vert\;N\;\vert}}$$	Stimulant chemicals of the body, nervous function, inflammatory response, protein structure, hereditary molecules; many drugs contain amine groups
Carboxylic acid	$$R-C\underset{\diagdown OH}{\overset{\diagup\!\!\!\!/ \; O}{}}$$	Fatty acids are a major component of body structure; lactic acid is a by-product of energy production; many drugs contain acid groups
Ester	$$\underset{\overset{\Vert}{O}}{R-C}-O-R$$	Body fat stores energy and the ester ATP transfers energy
Halide	R—halide	Anaesthetics, disinfectants and plastics
Ketone	$$\underset{\overset{\Vert}{O}}{R-C}-R$$	Organic solvent, sugar fructose is converted into energy, by-product of fat and protein breakdown
Amide	$$\underset{\overset{\Vert}{O}}{R-C}-NR$$	Form peptide bonds in polypeptides, hormones, proteins; urea; barbiturates

Application: Differences in drug action

Adding or altering the location of a functional group is used by pharmaceutical companies to modify the actions of a drug on the body. EXAMPLE: The penicillin ampicillin has been altered to improve absorption across the wall of the gastrointestinal tract. The modified drug has an OH⁻ added and is called Amoxicillin. The addition of this structure results in a more predictable absorption and consequently a greater amount is available for use within the body. This results in an increased concentration in the blood compared with ampicillin.

A diverse range of functional groups exist. The more relevant groups involved in body function and their alteration of body function are listed in Table 8.1.

The addition of polar molecules or ions

to a hydrocarbon chain alters the previously non-polar properties of the chain. Generally, small organic molecules containing charged functional groups such as alcohols and organic acids are capable of dissolving in water. In the larger-chained molecules, the non-polar hydrocarbon chain exerts a greater influence over the charged region, and therefore the longer the hydrocarbon chain the less able is the molecule to dissolve in water. EXAMPLE: Small-chained alcohols such as ethanol dissolve in water whereas larger-chained alcohols such as octanol have difficulty dissolving in water. The non-polar region is 'water hating', and is called the **hydrophobic** region while the water attracting polar region is called the **hydrophilic** region.

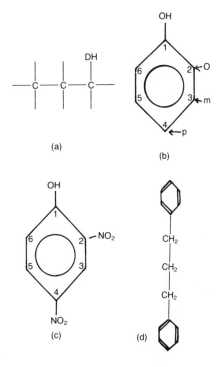

(a)

(b)

(c)

(d)

Figure 8.1 The structural formulae of (a) alcohol, (b) phenol, (c) a phenol derivative, 2,4-dinitrophenol and (d) 1,3-diphenylpropane. The ortho (o), meta (m) and para (p) positions are related to the OH group.

8.2 Alcohols and phenols

The addition of a hydroxyl ion OH^- to a hydrocarbon chain results in the formation of an **alcohol**, whereas if the OH^- is added to a benzene ring it forms a **phenol**.

Alcohols are named by replacing the 'e' at the end of hydrocarbon chains with an **-ol**. EXAMPLE: A three carbon alcohol is named propanol from the three carbon hydrocarbon propane (Figure 8.1a). All alcohols can be identified by the letters -ol at the end of the name. Phenols are usually referred to by their common names. EXAMPLE: Cresol.

Alcohols and phenols have different properties. Phenols are more acidic than alcohols and can be corrosive to tissue. Phenols are unable to dissolve in water whereas the common alcohols dissolve easily in water. The term alcohol is often used when referring to ethanol or ethyl alcohol which has the effect of depressing the nervous system resulting in the removal of a person's inhibitions. Methanol is also a commonly used alcohol which is the main constituent of methylated spirits (industrial alcohol or surgical spirit). This alcohol should never be ingested since the intake of small amounts can lead to blindness and paralysis. Both alcohol and phenol have the property of being able to kill germs.

Application: Antiseptics and disinfectants

A disinfectant is an agent that destroys most germs or renders them inert when applied to any surface (36.5).

An antiseptic is an agent that inhibits growth and multiplication of microbes without necessarily destroying them. Many useful chemical disinfectants are too irritating to the skin and mucous membranes and thus are unable to be used as antiseptics. Some alcohols and phenols are used as disinfectants and antiseptics.

Alcohols such as ethanol and propanol have anti-germ activity in the presence of water. When using alcohol as a distinfectant it is important to consider the presence of moisture on a surface. Since alcohol dissolves in water, a wet surface will dilute the amount of alcohol present, leading to a diminished action.

Oils are non-polar and are unable to dissolve in water whereas they can dissolve in alcohol. This property enables alcohols to be used to cleanse and disinfect skin surfaces by removing oils, cell debris and germs.

When other disinfectant compounds are dissolved in alcohol a tincture is formed. EXAMPLES: Tincture of iodine and tincture of zephiran. Tinctures have better disinfectant properties than either of the constituents along with better removal of oils.

Alcohols and tinctures are usually used on normal skin surfaces as alcohol may have a deleterious effect on traumatized tissue. The use of alcohols as disinfectants is restricted to small areas because of their possible irritating effect on skin.

Phenols are more corrosive than alcohols. The phenol's harmful properties are altered when it combines with soaps or detergents. The derivatives of phenol are used as disinfectants, with the less toxic compounds also being used as antiseptics. Cresol (lysol and sudol) is a phenol derivative which is frequently used for the preparation of theatre and dressing trolleys before use and for disinfecting basins and baths after use. Hexachlorophane is another phenol compound which, when combined with soap or detergents, forms relatively non-toxic antiseptics such as phisohex and dialsoap. Phisohex is used for surgical 'scrubs' and hand washing. It can also be used to disinfect and clean walls, floors and surfaces of dressing trolleys and operating tables.

8.3   Ketones

Ketones are organic substances whose structure is based on an oxygen atom being attached by a double bond to a carbon atom. This carbon atom must not be at the end of a hydrocarbon chain (Figure 8.2). Ketones are named by using the ending **-one**. Organic substances readily dissolve in ketones such as propanone which is frequently referred

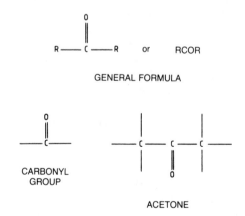

Figure 8.2   The carbonyl group and the structure of ketones.

to as acetone (Figure 8.2). This substance is used as nail polish remover and to dissolve the parts of adhesives that adhere to the skin when a dressing is being removed.

Ketones are formed from alcohols that have lost the hydrogen from the hydroxyl group. The removal of a hydrogen atom means that an electron has been removed from the alcohol group. Oxidation is the process of removing hydrogen. Oxidation can also mean the combination of oxygen with a substance (6.6). The process of oxidation is important in the production of most of the body's energy since very little energy is produced if the cells lack oxygen (33.9).

GENERAL FORMULA

FORMALDEHYDE

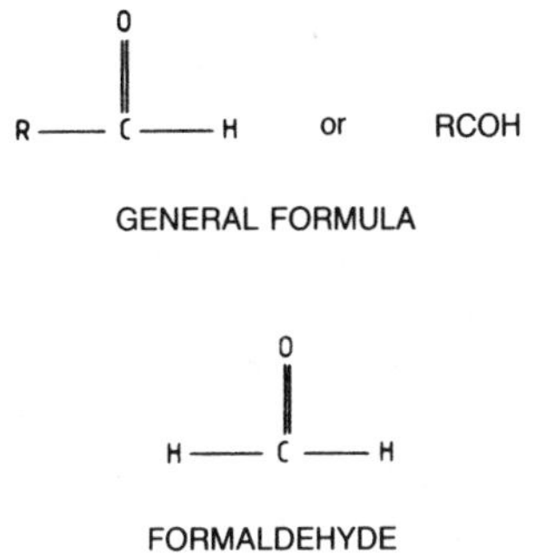

Figure 8.3   The structure of aldehydes.

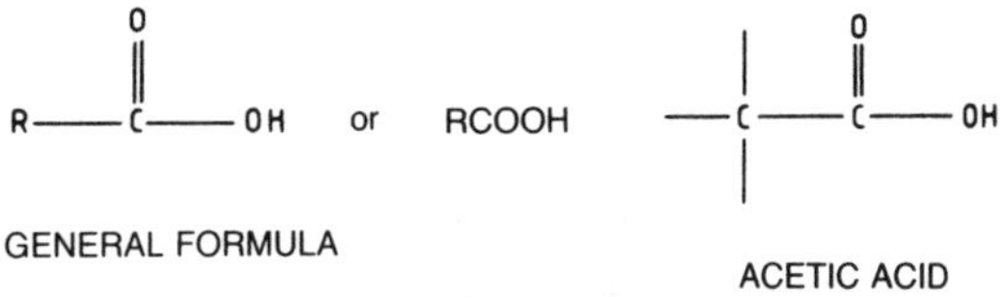

GENERAL FORMULA

ACETIC ACID

Figure 8.4   The structure of organic acids.

Application: Body ketones

Ketones are used by the body to form energy. EXAMPLE: The fruit sugar, fructose, is an important ketone that is digested and converted into energy. The breakdown of fats and protein results in the formation of ketones that are termed ketone bodies. EXAMPLES: Acetone and acetoacetic acid.

In diabetes mellitus, excessive breakdown of fat and proteins results in an excess of ketone bodies in the blood which is referred to as ketosis. The sweet smell of acetone can often be detected in the breath of people with ketosis. The onset of ketosis is associated with malaise and rapid breathing, which if not treated will be followed by vomiting, dehydration, abdominal pain and finally coma.

8.4   Aldehydes

An **aldehyde** is a compound with the general formula RCHO (Figure 8.3). Aldehydes are

formed from the oxidation of alcohols which contain the hydroxyl group at the end of the hydrocarbon chain. In naming an aldehyde, add **-al** to the end of the prefix used for the longest hydrocarbon chain which includes the C of the aldehyde group. Aldehydes and ketones are collectively called **carbonyl compounds** because they both contain the carbonyl group (Figure 8.4).

A common aldehyde used in hospitals is methanal which has the common name of formaldehyde. This substance readily dissolves in water. Formalin is a mixture of formaldehyde and water. It is used as a disinfectant and as a tissue preservative.

Glucose is an aldehyde which is used by the body, particularly the brain, to produce energy for cell function. The body's supply of glucose comes either from the ingestion of food or from the manufacture of glucose within the body.

8.5   Organic acids

An **acid** is a substance that releases hydrogen
ions (H^+) into water. The greater the number
of hydrogen ions released into water, the
greater is the acidity of the liquid (16.1). An
organic acid is a compound with the general
formula RCOOH (Figure 8.4). Most organic
acids are weak acids and are formed from the
oxidation (6.6) of an aldehyde, that is, oxygen
is added to the aldehyde functional group.
The COOH group is called the carboxyl
group, and substances with this group
are termed **carboxylic acids**. Many of the
carboxylic acids are known by their common
names in preference to their IUPAC name.

The IUPAC name for each acid is derived
by taking the longest hydrocarbon chain
that includes the C of the COOH group
and replacing the 'e' with the suffix **-oic**.
The word acid follows the -oic. EXAMPLE:
Acetic acid consists of ethane that has been
oxidized to form the carboxyl group and
is thus named ethanoic acid (Figure 8.4).
Aromatic compounds can form carboxylic
acids by combining a carboxyl group to
the aromatic compound. EXAMPLE: The
anti-fungal agent benzoic acid consists of a
carboxyl group attached to a benzene ring
(Figure 8.5).

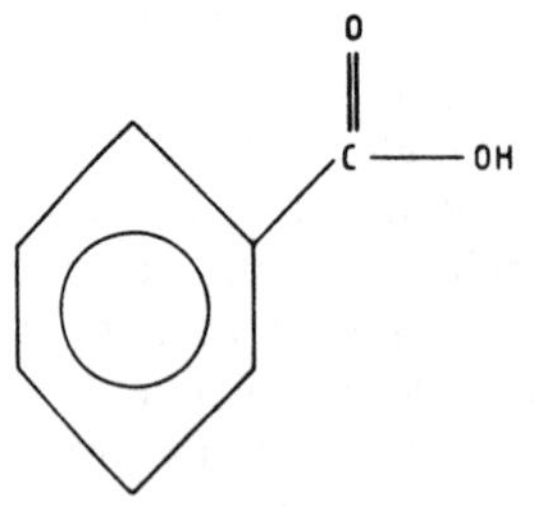

Organic acids perform a variety of important roles in body function. Fatty acids are
a major component of body structure and
function. These organic acids are essential for
the formation of all body fat (29.1). Another
important body chemical is lactic acid. This
organic acid is formed in tissue when a relative lack of oxygen exists (33.8).

Organic acids are also important constituents of many drugs and can be chemically
altered to form a wide variety of drugs.

Application: Salicylic acid

Salicylic acid is an aromatic compound
that contains both a carboxyl and an
alcohol group (Figure 8.6). This acid
exerts remarkable analgesic, antipyretic,
anti-inflammatory and anti-rheumatic
effects in humans. Compounds formed
from salicylic acid act either by conversion to this acid or by a similar
mechanism to its mode of action. These
salicylic acid preparations are termed
salicylates. EXAMPLES: Aspirin and
sodium salicylate.

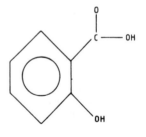

SALICYLIC ACID

Figure 8.6   The structure of salicylic acid (2-
hydroxybenzoic acid).

BENZOIC ACID

Figure 8.5   The anti-fungal agent benzoic acid
consists of a carboxyl group attached
to a benzene ring.

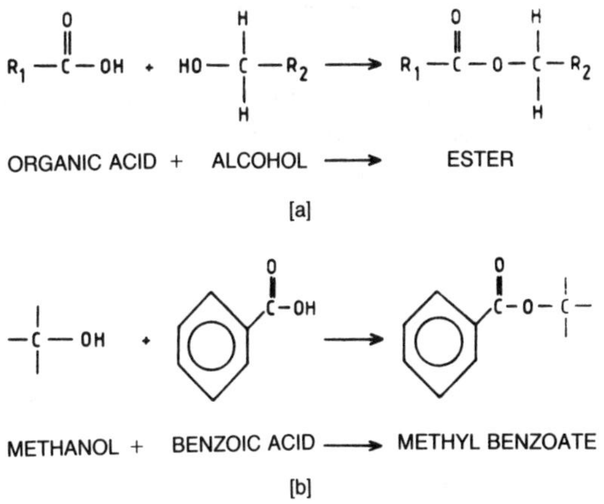

ORGANIC ACID + ALCOHOL ⟶ ESTER

[a]

METHANOL + BENZOIC ACID ⟶ METHYL BENZOATE

[b]

Figure 8.7 (a) The formation of an ester from an alcohol and organic acid. (b) Methyl benzoate is formed by combining methanol and benzoic acid.

8.6 Esters

Esters are substances produced by combining an organic acid with an alcohol (Figure 8.7a). An important example of an ester is body fat. All body fat is formed by combining an organic acid with an alcohol. In the case of fat, the acid is a fatty acid and the alcohol is glycerol.

The general formula for an ester is R_1COOR_2 where R_1 and R_2 can be either the same hydrocarbon chain or different chains.

An ester is identified by two words. The first word is derived from the alcohol by replacing the -ol with a **-yl**. The second word is derived by replacing the acid -oic with an **-ate**. EXAMPLE: Methanol is combined with benzoic acid to form methyl benzoate (Figure 8.7b).

The importance of body esters is shown in the formation and breakdown of fat. Briefly, fat is the major source of stored energy for the body. An understanding of these processes is important for gaining an insight into the utilization of fat by the body. These processes will be discussed in detail in 33.11.

Esters are used as local anaesthetics (benzocaine), preanaesthetic medications (scopolamine), and blood vessel dilators (nitroglycerin).

8.7 Halogenated hydrocarbons

Halogenated hydrocarbons or **organohalogen** compounds consist of a hydrocarbon chain where some of the hydrogens have been substituted by halogens. Halogens are the elements fluorine (F), chlorine (Cl), bromine (Br) and iodine (I). In naming these compounds the halogen is specified as **fluoro-, chloro-, bromo-** or **iodo-** which are used as prefixes with the hydrocarbon chain. The location of the halogens is determined by the carbon atom numbers where they are attached to the chain. EXAMPLE: The inhalation anaesthetic halothane has the IUPAC name of 2-bromo-2-chloro-1,1,1-trifluoroethane. This long name indicates the specific structure of the anaesthetic (Figure 8.8) but is a cumbersome term and thus the common name is often preferred.

Halogenated hydrocarbons have a variety of uses in hospital ranging from anaesthetics such as halothane and ethyl chloride to disinfectants such as hexachlorophene.

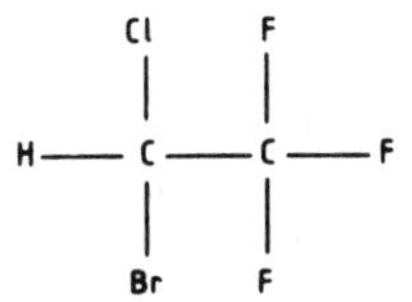

Figure 8.8 Halothane or 2-bromo-2-chloro-1,1,1-trifluoroethane.

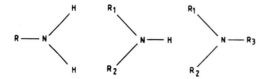

Figure 8.9   General formula of the three forms of amines. R₁, R₂, and R₃ can be different or identical.

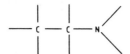

Figure 8.10   Ethylamine.

8.8   Amines

Amines are a group of compounds that are identified by the functional group —NH₂. They are derived from ammonia (NH₃). The nitrogen can combine with one, two or three hydrocarbon chains depending on the number of hydrogens that have been displaced (Figure 8.9). An amine is named by adding the suffix **-amine** to the hydrocarbon name. EXAMPLE: Ethylamine is a two carbon amine (Figure 8.10).

Amines play a vital role in both normal body function and patient care. Amines are used as cardio-vascular stimulants (epinephrine), central nervous system stimulants (amphetamines), antihistamines, antiseptics and anaesthetics.

Application: Body amines

A variety of functions are performed by body amines. The catecholamines are the amines of the nervous system. The main catecholamines are norepinephrine (noradrenaline), epineph-rine (adrenalin) and dopamine. The catecholamines are the stimulant chemicals of the body. EXAMPLE: Epinephrine stimulates the cardiovascular system and norepinephrine stimulates parts of the nervous system.

Nitrogen compounds are removed from the body mainly in the form of urea.

Amino acids

These are small organic acids that contain an amine group (Figure 8.11). Amino acids are the building blocks of proteins. They are also the source of other body nitrogen compounds such as the catecholamines, hormones and the molecules of genetic information. Amino acids will be described in greater detail in 30.1.

8.9   Amides

Amides are compounds in which a carboxyl group has had the hydroxy component replaced by the NH₂ group (Figure 8.12a). The two remaining nitrogen bonds can be attached to organic radicals (Figure 8.12). Amides result from the combination of an organic acid with an amine group. In the IUPAC system (7.7) amides are named by removing the ic or oic suffix of the carboxylic

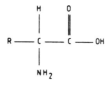

Figure 8.11   General formula for an amino acid.

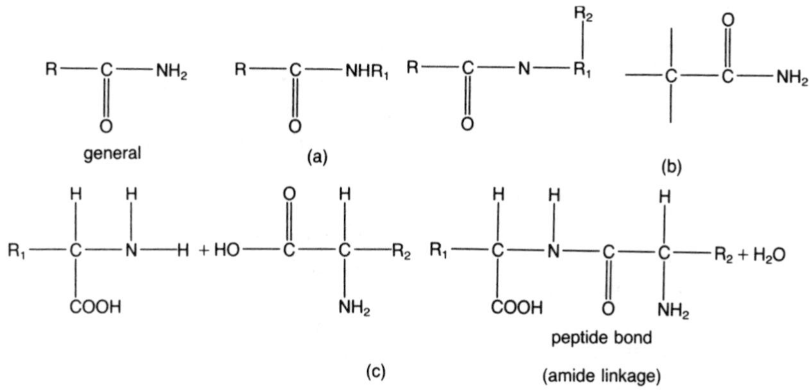

R—C—NH$_2$ R—C—NHR$_1$ R—C—N—R$_1$ —C—C—NH$_2$

general   (a)   (b)

R$_1$—C—N—H + HO—C—C—R$_2$ R$_1$—C—N—C—C—R$_2$ + H$_2$O

COOH   NH$_2$ COOH   NH$_2$

peptide bond

(c)   (amide linkage)

Figure 8.12 (a) General structure of amides. (b) Acetamide. (c) Two amino acids linked by a peptide bond. (R = organic radical.)

acid and adding the suffix amide. EXAMPLE: Acetic acid forms acetamide. An amide bond links the amine group of one amino acid to the carboxyl group of another. This is called a peptide bond and is the mechanism of linking amino acids to form polypeptides (Figure 8.12c). Amide linkages are used in the formation of synthetic materials such as nylon.

8.10 Heterocyclic compounds

Heterocyclic compounds are cyclic organic compounds that contain another element within the ring structure. The elements are usually nitrogen, oxygen or sulphur. These compounds comprise a large segment of organic chemistry. The nitrogen based heterocyclic compounds called **nucleotides** are essential for life. They are formed from the aromatic amines, purine and pyrimidine (Figure 8.13). The nucleotides are discussed in Chapter 31. EXAMPLE: The molecules deoxyribonucleic acid (DNA) and ribonucleic acid (RNA) are the key to hereditary information and the maintenance of life (24.7 and 24.8). Other important molecules that contain a heterocyclic compound are haemoglobin, vitamin B$_{12}$ and the brain chemical, serotonin.

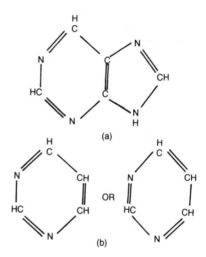

Figure 8.13 General formula for (a) purine and (b) pyrimidine.

Application: Heterocyclic drugs

Heterocyclic compounds form the basis of a group of drugs used in altering brain function.

Opiates such as morphine, codeine

and heroin depress brain function. Codeine is used to depress the cough centre of the brain.

Barbiturates are a group of drugs that have a sedative and sleep-inducing effect when administered in therapeutic doses. Nembutal and seconal are the trade names of two barbiturates that are used as sleeping pills and pre-anaesthetic sedatives.

Psychedelic drugs or hallucinogens alter sensory perception so that the boundary between real and unreal is lost. LSD appears to act by mimicking the action of the brain chemical serotonin. STP and mescaline are structurally similar to epinephrine and norepinephrine which suggests a possible link between these drugs and body chemicals.

Some heterocyclic drugs have a diverse action on the body. Caffeine stimulates brain nervous activity and acts as a diuretic. Guanethidine acts on norepinephrine and is used as a sedative and in the treatment of hypertension.

8.11   Environmental health and safety

Organic compounds formed from the inclusion of functional groups provide a wide range of potential health risks. Some of these substances are among the most toxic substances known. EXAMPLE: Dioxins and PCBs (polychlorinated biphenyls). Many common organic substances cause cancer and are referred to as **carcinogens**. Potentially carcinogenic organic substances can be taken into the body through the mouth. EXAMPLE: Substances in cigarette tar; through the skin. EXAMPLE: Some organic solvents or through breathing vapours. EXAMPLE: Vapours from some adhesive solvents. Care must be taken at all times to minimize exposure to potential carcinogenic substances.

The excessive intake of alcohol over an extended period of time leads to liver and brain damage. The intake of alcohol during pregnancy may result in the abnormal development of the foetus which is referred to as Foetal Alcohol Syndrome.

Organic substances present a fire risk due to their low flash point.

Summary

Hydrocarbon chains can have various functional groups, attached to them. Each functional group has its own chemical and physical properties which will alter the properties of a hydrocarbon chain. The hydrocarbon chain represents a hydrophobic region whereas charged functional groups attract water and form a hydrophilic region. The site of many body chemical reactions is located at the functional group and thus these groups are important for body function and the maintenance of homeostasis. The main functional groups are alcohols, phenols, aldehydes, ketones, amines, organic acids, esters, halides and amides.

Heterocyclic compounds are cyclic compounds that contain another element such as nitrogen within the ring structure. These compounds play an important role in body function and its alteration.

Care must be taken in using organic chemicals as they provide a range of toxic effects and can be highly flammable.

Unit Five
Energy and the Physical Properties of Matter

This unit integrates the physical properties of matter and applies these properties to health care, normal and abnormal body function, the uses and the dangers of diagnostic and therapeutic equipment. You will learn how the properties of matter are influenced by various forms of energy and how matter moves.

Chapter 9

Energy and the physical states of matter

Objectives

At the completion of this chapter the student should be able to:

1. explain the relationship between energy and matter;
2. relate kinetic energy to the different physical states of matter;
3. describe the properties of solids, liquids and fluids;
4. explain how matter changes from one physical state to another;
5. describe surface tension.

9.1 Matter and physics

In Unit Three the chemical levels of organization of matter (5.1) and their chemical properties were described. Matter can also undergo changes that do not result in the formation of new substances. These changes reflect the **physical properties** of matter and form the basis for the study of the field of science known as physics. The physical properties of matter can be broadly divided into:

1. **physical state** which refers to solids, liquids, gases and plasmas (9.4);
2. **physical form** which refers to features such as shape and colour;
3. **motion**;
4. **electromagnetism** which refers to electricity and magnetism;
5. **nuclear** which refers to the properties associated with the nucleus of an atom;
6. **gravitation** which refers to the attraction between two objects.

The above properties are determined by energy. An understanding of the properties of energy is important as it provides a basis for understanding the general principles of physics that pertain to health care and provides an awareness of the potential hazards associated with the use of energy.

9.2 Potential energy and kinetic energy

Energy is related to matter since energy either creates a potential to do work or it enables matter to do work. The close association of energy and matter was discovered by Albert Einstein who showed that in certain cases energy could be converted into mass and vice versa.

$$E = mc^2 \qquad \text{Eqn 9.1}$$

where E is energy, m is mass and c is the velocity of light.

Potential energy is energy stored in an object as a result of its position, chemical composition or stretching and compression of elastic material. This stored energy is shown by the release of energy when the restraints maintaining the object's position or chemical makeup is removed. EXAMPLES: Stored water in a dam being released by a floodgate, release of a stretched elastic band, breaking down of food to produce body energy.

When energy is in action or is performing work it is known as **kinetic energy**. EXAMPLES: Flow of blood, chemical manufacture and muscle contraction. Both potential energy and kinetic energy can be converted into the opposite kind of energy.

Application: Stretching and recoil of the aorta

Stretching of the elastic walled aorta results when blood is ejected from the heart during ventricular contraction or systole. The stretched aorta recoils to its original size during ventricular relaxation or diastole. In terms of energy the stretched aorta represents a potential to do work or potential energy. When the walls recoil, blood is squeezed along the artery thus doing work in the form of kinetic energy.

Potential energy and kinetic energy can be subdivided into various forms of energy, each of which has its own properties. The energy forms used in body function and health care are: electrical, radiant, nuclear, thermal, sonic, chemical and mechanical. These forms of energy can only occur in the presence of matter, apart from radiant energy (e.g. light and X-rays). These forms of energy are discussed in the remaining chapters in this unit.

9.3 Conservation of energy

Generally energy is neither created nor destroyed but is converted from one form to another. This principle of the interconversion of energy enables humans to obtain energy in the form of chemical energy stored in food, and to transform it into forms that can be utilized by the body for the growth and maintenance of normal body function. The ingested chemical energy is transformed by the body into the following forms:

1. chemical energy for cell growth and function;
2. electrical energy for nerve and muscle function;
3. mechanical energy for body movement and the movement of objects by the body;
4. thermal energy for body temperature homeostasis. The body also converts sound energy and radiant energy (light) into the electrical energy of nerve function.

The total energy in any system is constant. The total amount of energy taken into the body is either stored or removed from the body as chemical energy (faeces, urine, sweat, etc.), mechanical energy or thermal energy.

Application: Intravenous fluid administration sets

The principles of constant energy within a system and the ability of energy to be converted from one form to another are shown in the functioning of an intravenous set (Figure 19.8). The liquid contained in a raised one litre bottle contains 100% potential energy and zero kinetic energy. When the bottle is

67% full, the bottle will contain 67% of the initial potential energy. The potential energy of the liquid that has left the bottle was converted into kinetic energy as the liquid flowed out of the bottle and down the tube. Likewise, when the bottle is 50% empty, the bottle will contain only 50% of the initial potential energy. Of the original potential energy 50% has therefore been converted into kinetic energy of the infusing liquid. When the bottle is empty, all the potential energy of the liquid has been converted into kinetic energy.

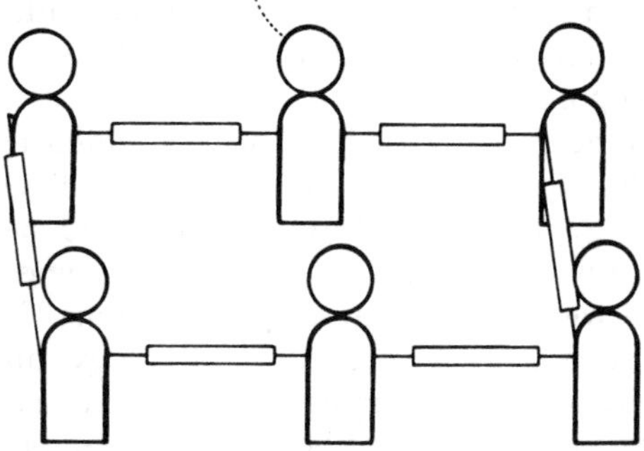

Figure 9.1   For a solid the distance between each atom is fixed and therefore a fixed shape results. People in the figure are held by bars and can therefore only be moved as a group, with no difference occurring between their relative positions.

9.4   States of matter

Matter can exist in four states or phases which are referred to as solids, liquids, gases and plasma. The amount of relative movements of atoms or groups of atoms determines the atom's state. Atoms with the lowest kinetic energy are solids whereas those with the greatest amount of kinetic energy are plasmas. Solids, liquids and gases each contain various properties which can be either similar or different to the other states. These properties are determined by the amount of kinetic energy that is contained within an atom or group of atoms.

Plasmas contain the greatest amount of kinetic energy as they exist at very high temperatures. When a very high amount of energy is imparted into a gas the atoms become ionized (form ions — 4.3). Plasma flames can be produced at high temperature nozzles to coat objects with corrosion resistant materials. The three common physical states of matter will now be discussed.

9.5   Solids

In solids, the atoms are maintained in a relatively fixed position close to adjacent atoms. These atoms are held in position by attractive forces operating between adjacent atoms. EXAMPLE: Ions are held close together by the force of attraction of opposite charges that exists between cations (positive charge) and anions (negative charge). The distance between atoms in solids is minimal, thereby preventing individual atoms from being compressed or pushed closer to adjacent atoms. Solids are therefore incompressible.

In solids, the attractive forces between atoms or groups of atoms are greater than the kinetic energy of these atoms. This difference results in atoms being unable to move with respect to other adjacent atoms, thus resulting in a well-defined shape for a solid (Figure 9.1).

The degree of attraction between different

atoms or groups of atoms varies according to each element. Distinctive structures, such as crystals, result from the particular attractive forces of the elements of which they are composed.

When energy such as heat is added to a solid, the energy is converted into kinetic energy. A liquid is formed when the kinetic energy of atoms is greater than some of the weaker forces that link the atoms. This process of imparting sufficient energy into a solid to form a liquid is known as **melting**. The rapid addition of large amounts of energy can result in a solid forming a gas. This process is called **sublimation**. EXAMPLE: When solid carbon dioxide (dry ice) is exposed to the relatively high room temperature this solid is converted directly into gas.

The loss of heat from a liquid will result in the **freezing** of a substance. The freezing point is the temperature at which freezing occurs and is unique for each substance.

9.6 Liquids

The atoms of a liquid contain enough kinetic energy to enable limited movement. The available kinetic energy is insufficient to allow all atoms complete freedom of movement. The quantity of kinetic energy is able to break the weakest attractive forces so that limited movement can occur (Figure 9.2). The variation in position of atoms results in liquids having no characteristic shape. The prevention of atoms escaping from their neighbours causes liquids to maintain a constant volume. The restricted flexibility of a liquid enables it to take the shape of the container in which it is placed.

The close proximity of atoms in a liquid results in a low compressibility, that is, a liquid is relatively incompressible when compared with gases.

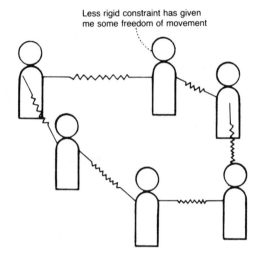

Figure 9.2 In a liquid the distance between each atom may vary in a manner similar to people being joined or linked by large elastic bands (these elastic bands can be broken and reformed).

Surface tension

Surface tension is the pull of the surface particles of a liquid into the body of the liquid. Atoms within a liquid are surrounded by a balance of attractive forces. Atoms on the surface of a liquid do not have these attractive forces surrounding them. This results in the greater attractive forces pulling these atoms towards the body of the liquid than those forces between the liquid and gas.

Liquids attempt to contract to the smallest possible area. This can be seen when drops form as liquids come in contact with solids. EXAMPLE: Rain on a windscreen. In gases, a liquid will either form bubbles or droplets. EXAMPLE: In air soap forms bubbles and droplets form from a dropper.

The strong attractive forces of solids causes liquids to adhere to a solid's surface, since the attractive forces of solids is greater than the attraction of other liquid atoms. In a narrow piece of tubing this results in an indentation

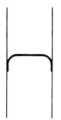

Figure 9.3   A meniscus is formed by the wall's strong attractive forces for the liquid.

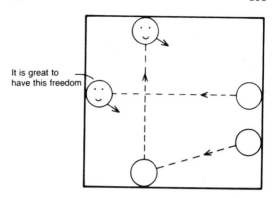

It is great to have this freedom

Figure 9.4   In a gas the distance between atoms is random, as is the location of any particular atom in a container. The high kinetic energy of gas atoms enables them to completely occupy the container by deflecting off the walls.

being formed on the surface of the liquid (Figure 9.3). This indentation is known as a **meniscus** and results from the surface of the liquid being pulled along the walls of the tubing. This movement of a liquid along the walls is often referred to as capillarity.

Application: Surfactant

A surfactant is any substance that reduces the surface tension of a liquid. In the lungs, a pulmonary surfactant is released to reduce the surface tension of the pulmonary liquids, thereby contributing to the elastic properties of lung tissue. A deficiency of pulmonary surfactant results in a collapse of the sacs within a lung.

In premature infants the amount of surfactant present in the lungs may not be sufficient to enable correct lung function. Lack of pulmonary surfactant in newborn babies is referred to as respiratory distress syndrome or hyaline membrane disease.

9.7   Gases

Gases are formed by imparting more energy into a liquid by a process termed **evaporation**.

The kinetic energy of atoms is now at a level where the attractive forces between atoms or groups of atoms are broken. The high kinetic energy results in the independent movement of atoms or groups of atoms in a random motion (Figure 9.4). **Boiling** is a special form of evaporation where liquid is converted into a gas via the formation of bubbles within the liquid. The temperature at which boiling occurs is unique for each substance and is known as the boiling point.

Gases thus have neither a defined volume nor shape and occupy the entire space available in a container. Particles continue to move within the container by deflecting off the walls of the container (Figure 9.4).

The collision of gas particles with the wall of a container results in pressure being exerted on the walls of the container. Pressure is also exerted as a result of gas particles trying to escape from a container. If the number of particles in a given volume, or the kinetic energy of particles is increased, the frequency with which these particles collide with the walls of the container will be increased thus exerting a greater pressure.

Table 9.1 Comparison of physical properties of
solids, liquids and gases

Property	Solid	Liquid	Gas
Fixed volume	Yes	Yes	No
Compressibility	No	No	Yes
Rigidity	Yes	No	No
Characteristic shape	Yes	No	No
Takes the shape of its container	Sometimes	Yes	Yes
Completely fills the container	No	No	Yes
Flows along tubes	Sometimes	Yes	Yes
Can be poured	Sometimes	Yes	Yes

lose kinetic energy they change from a gas
into a liquid, a gas into a solid or a liquid into
a solid.

A change of state is usually reversible so
that no chemical alteration occurs with a
substance when it changes from one state to
another, that is, the amount of kinetic energy
is the only variable. EXAMPLE: Heating ice
causes water to be formed whereas cooling
water results in the formation of ice. Sometimes a change of state is irreversible since
the chemical structure of a substance is
altered. EXAMPLE: Heating wood can result
in burning, with formation of ash and gas
or smoke. Cooling smoke and ash will not
reform wood.

9.8 Comparison of the physical properties of solids, liquids and gases

The main differences and similarities between
solids, liquids and gases are summarized in
Table 9.1. Note that gases and liquids contain
many similar properties. The large number of
similar properties require a collective term for
liquids and gases. A **fluid** is a substance that
takes the shape of its container and can be a
liquid or a gas.

9.9 Changes of state

A substance can change from one state to
another by gaining or losing kinetic energy.
The energy required to change a state is
referred to as the **latent heat** (13.1). The gaining of kinetic energy by atoms results in a
change from a solid to a liquid, from a solid to
a gas or from a liquid to a gas. When atoms

9.10 Humidity

The change of phase from water to a gas
occurs over a range of temperatures with the
transition being complete at the boiling point.
As the temperature increases towards boiling
point an ever increasing number of water
molecules escape from the surface of the
water into the air. If the change occurs in a
sealed container, a balance will occur between
water molecules becoming vaporized and
vapour molecules hitting the surface of the
liquid. At this point, for a given temperature,
the vapour is saturated as the rate of vapour
formation equals its rate of removal. The
mass of water per unit of volume at saturation is referred to as the **saturation vapour
density**. In air the amount of water vapour
at a given temperature is usually less than
the saturated vapour density. A convenient
reference term called the **relative humidity** is
used to reflect the relative amount of water
vapour compared to the closed system. That
is, it indicates the percentage of water vapour
in air compared with the maximum quantity
of air that can be held at that temperature.

EXAMPLE: A relative humidity of 75% at a given temperature indicates that the actual vapour density is three-quarters the saturation vapour density for that temperature. The higher the temperature, the greater is the saturation vapour density. The higher the humidity the greater is the likelihood of water condensing on cool surfaces and the more difficult it is to remove water from the skin through perspiration.

9.11 Environmental health and safety

Caution is required when working in environments where steam is being produced as the heat contained within this gas is sufficient to cause serious burns. Steam is more dangerous than hot water or boiling water burns as steam is only formed when additional energy is added to boiling water. This additional energy is referred to as the **latent heat of vaporization**. EXAMPLE: Steam at 100°C contains more heat than water at 100°C. An additional hazard associated with steam is the potential for a person to receive serious burns without being in direct contact with the source of boiling water. Care should be taken at all times to avoid direct contact with steam. Continued exposure to steam or boiling water will lead to an increase in the severity of a burn.

Application: Classification of burns

The depth of tissue damage and destruction in a burn is indicated by the degree of the burn. A **first-degree burn** involves destruction to the outer layers of the epidermis. The presence of blisters indicates a **second-degree burn**. This burn involves the destruc-

---

tion of several layers of skin. Skin regeneration can occur as sufficient tissue in the dermis still exists. A **third-degree burn** or a **full thickness burn** indicates damage to the full thickness of the skin. In addition underlying tissue may be damaged. Normal skin regeneration fails to occur thus resulting in the slow formation of scars and usually the need for skin grafts.

Summary

Matter is anything that occupies space and has some mass. The physical properties of matter are those characteristics that represent changes in the properties of matter apart from the formation of new substances. EXAMPLE: Solids, liquids, gases and plasma are called the physical states of matter and all can exist in the one substance.

To move matter requires energy. Potential energy is energy stored in an object as a result of its position, chemical composition or stretching and compression of elastic material. Kinetic energy is energy of action. These two kinds of energy can be converted into each other, and be manifested in different forms. The common forms involved in health care are electrical energy, radiant energy, nuclear energy, thermal energy, sonic energy, chemical energy and mechanical energy.

A substance can change from one state to another by gaining or losing kinetic energy. That is, these states of matter differ by the amount of movement of atoms or group of atoms

1. In solids the atoms contain small amounts of kinetic energy and thus they remain in a relatively fixed position close to adjacent atoms.

2. In liquids the atoms contain a greater amount of kinetic energy which enables the atoms to have a limited movement with respect to adjacent atoms. This movement results in liquids being able to pour and flow, that is, exhibit properties of a fluid.

3. Gases contain the greatest amount of kinetic energy. The high kinetic energy results in the independent movement of atoms or groups of atoms. Gases are also fluids since they can flow and be poured.

The difference in the attractive forces of solids with liquids and gases with liquids, that is, surface tension, results in the liquid attempting to contract to the smallest possible area.

Chapter 10

Electricity and magnetism

Objectives

At the completion of this chapter the student should be able to:

1. describe the properties of electricity and magnetism;
2. relate the properties of electrical energy to health care, normal and abnormal body function and the uses and dangers of diagnostic and therapeutic equipment;
3. describe how an action potential is formed;
4. describe the requirements for a flow of current;
5. describe the safety procedures required for using electrical equipment;
6. explain the terms electrolysis, emf, resistance, conduction, current, electromagnets, electromagnetic induction; capacitance.

10.1 Electrical energy and health care

Electrical energy results from a flow of charged particles. In the body, information is conducted along nerves in the form of electrical energy and is then converted into muscular movements (mechanical energy) or other energy forms. Electrical energy is easily converted into radiant energy as occurs in light bulbs, X-rays and short-wave radiation. Since the body relies on electrical energy for a major part of its internal communication and for muscular function, these processes can be monitored by machines which measure electrical activity in various body tissues. EXAMPLES: The electrocardiograph (ECG) for the heart, the electroencephalograph (EEG) for the brain and the electromyograph (EMG) for peripheral nerve injuries and muscle disease (10.14). Electrotherapy applies the properties of electricity to the treatment of body conditions (10.14).

10.2 Electrolytes

When opposite charges exist in nature, the charged particles are attracted to each other in an attempt to attain a zero charge.

Remember, unlike charges attract and like charges repel (4.4).

When ions are added to a solution, they move freely throughout the liquid so that they are randomly distributed. If two rods of opposite charge are placed into a liquid containing ions, negatively charged ions or anions are attracted to the positive rod and repelled by the negative rod. Positive ions or cations are attracted to the negative rod and are repelled by the positive rod (Figure 10.1). These rods or electrodes are named according to their attraction of ions. Anions are thus attracted to the **anode** (positive electrode) and cations to the **cathode** (negative electrode). Note that these ions are no longer randomly distributed in the liquid. Substances that move to oppositely charged electrodes when placed in a liquid or when molten are called **electrolytes**.

As most metals are cations, they will be attracted to the cathode. This results in the cathode being coated by the metal and this process is referred to as electroplating. EXAMPLE: Gold plating.

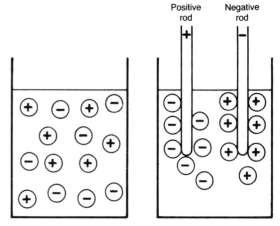

Figure 10.1   Ions are randomly distributed in solution. When two oppositely charged rods are placed in the solution there is a non-random distribution of ions, negatively-charged ions are attracted to the positive rod and positively-charged ions to the negative rod.

10.3   Potential difference

An analogy of water stored in a dam often assists in the understanding of potential difference. Water stored in a dam possesses potential energy. This water has the potential to flow down to the river below due to the influence of gravity. The potential energy is converted to kinetic energy when the dam's spillway is open, that is, the barrier that maintained the potential energy has been removed.

In a similar way to the dam, potential energy exists in a liquid between two separate regions of oppositely charged ions. This can be seen when a vessel containing a liquid is separated by a barrier into two compartments, one of which contains positively charged ions and the other contains negatively charged ions. If a positive electrode or anode is placed in the compartment with the positive ions and a negative electrode or cathode in the other, the barrier prevents the movement of ions to the oppositely charged electrode (Figure 10.2a).

The dam with a closed spillway whose water contains potential energy is analogous to oppositely charged ions being separated by a barrier. These ions possess potential energy. Removal of the barrier will cause a flow of ions and the potential energy being converted into kinetic energy (Figure 10.2b).

These differences in charge between the two regions are referred to as a difference in potential, that is, a **potential difference**. The greater the difference in charges between two

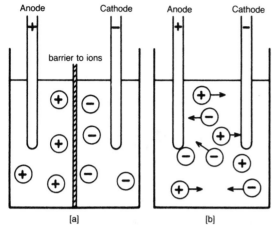

Figure 10.2 (a) A barrier separates two oppositely charged regions of a solution. The ions in these regions possess potential energy since removal of the barrier (b) results in the flow of ions and the conversion of potential energy into kinetic energy.

regions, the greater is the attraction of the oppositely charged particles to each other. Potential difference is therefore a form of potential energy, since a potential exists for the movement of charged particles.

A dam higher than another dam will possess more potential energy than the lower dam, since water from the first dam flows a greater distance. As a result, the higher dam's water is able to generate a greater amount of kinetic energy. The greater the height that water is raised the greater is the potential energy of that water. With respect to ions, the greater the difference in charges between two regions, the greater is the potential difference or voltage.

The greater the potential difference between two regions, the greater is the amount of stored energy. Potential difference is measured in **volts**. The greater the voltage, the greater is the attraction of oppositely

charged ions to each other. This potential for the movement of charges is only fulfilled if there is a medium present that allows ion movement to the differently charged regions.

The conversion of potential energy into kinetic energy results in a gradual decline in the potential difference. As the potential difference decreases, the flow of ions also decreases. A situation eventually develops whereby there is no difference in charges remaining, that is, zero potential difference and kinetic energy exist.

In the body, a potential difference exists across cell membranes. The charges are distributed so that the inside of the cell is negative and the outside is positive. The membrane acts as the barrier which maintains the potential difference. This potential difference across membranes plays an important role in muscle and nerve function, as well as in determining the distribution of electrolytes in the body. Since the potential difference is small, a unit one-thousandth of a volt is used. This SI unit is known as the millivolt and is symbolized as mV.

10.4   Static electricity

This is produced when electrons are physically transferred from one material to another and the two materials are then moved apart. The rubbing effect of walking on carpet or removing a sweater can produce high voltages. These voltages are removed when the electrons are able to jump to the positively charged region. This jumping to the oppositely charged region produces a spark. Common static sparks are rarely dangerous to the body. The danger of static electricity in hospitals is in the risk of a spark initiating an explosion in a region where flammable substances are present such as an operating theatre.

10.5   Flow of electrolytes in liquids

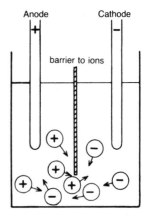

Figure 10.3   The flow of ions or current is reduced by the presence of a restriction or resistance. Complete removal of the barrier would result in a greater flow of ions as in Figure 10.2b.

Electric current

Potential difference is only converted into kinetic energy if a medium known as a **conductor** is present, which enables charged particles to move to their oppositely charged regions. In a liquid the flow of ions is referred to as an **electric current**. The passage of electric current in a liquid is called **electrolysis** and represents a chemical change as ions combine with an oppositely charged substance. The **electromotive force (emf)** represents the source which impels electricity to be conducted from a region. EXAMPLE: Battery. The unit of emf is also volts. Convention states that current flows from a positive region to a negative region. The SI unit for the measurement of current, that is, flow of charge is known as the ampere, which is symbolized as A. The ampere is often abbreviated to **amp**.

The greater the potential difference, the greater is the amount of available energy that can be converted into kinetic energy. When no restrictions to the flow of ions exist, potential difference is converted into kinetic energy in the form of an electric current. Generally, the greater the potential difference, the greater is the quantity of current that can be generated. EXAMPLE: A potential difference of 240 volts can generate more current than a potential difference of 110 volts for the same medium.

The existence of a restriction to ion flow reduces the flow of ions, that is, current (Figure 10.3). The potential difference only represents the potential for ions to flow and not the actual quantity of ions that flow.

Resistance

When considering the current that results from a given potential difference it is necessary to consider any restrictions, that is, resistance to ion flow. The amount of **resistance** present determines the quantity of current that actually flows for a given voltage. This relationship is shown by the equation

$$\text{Voltage} = \text{Current} \times \text{Resistance.}$$
$$V = I \cdot R \qquad \text{Eqn 10.1}$$

This equation represents Ohm's Law.

The greater the resistance for a given potential difference, the lower the amount of current that flows. The unit which is used to measure resistance is the **ohm**, which is symbolized as Ω. When the resistance to ion flow is absolute, a barrier occurs which results in no flow of current. In this case the potential difference is maintained until the barrier is removed.

To ensure a constant flow of ions it is necessary to maintain a constant potential difference. Without the maintenance of a constant potential difference, the flow of ions will decrease the potential difference. A decrease in the flow of current will ensue.

A constant potential difference can be maintained by the use of specific chemical reactions which replace ions that are lost as a result of current flow, and this process occurs in batteries. The quantity of current that flows is dependent upon the potential difference developed by a battery. The strength of a battery is measured by the potential difference generated by the battery and is thus measured in volts.

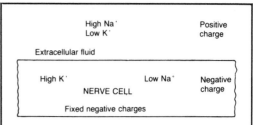

Figure 10.4 The distribution of ions inside and outside a nerve cell 'at rest'.

denoted as −70 to −90 mV. This voltage represents a nerve cell 'at rest' and is referred to as the resting potential.

The distribution of ions inside and outside a nerve cell determines the resting potential (Figure 10.4). The membrane acts as a barrier to the flow of large negatively charged proteins and the large positively charged sodium ions (Na^+). The smaller ions, potassium (K^+) and chloride (Cl^- are able to move freely across the membrane. The resting potential occurs as a result of the presence of large negative charges such as proteins and amino acids inside the cell and the high concentration of Na^+ ions outside the cell.

The large negative ions are manufactured within the cell and are incapable of passing through the nerve membrane. These negative charges are retained within the nerve cell during any nerve activity and are therefore referred to as fixed negative charges.

The negative charge within nerve cells attracts Na^+ and K^+ ions. Sodium ions are unable to move to the negative region as the membrane structure acts as a barrier to these ions. Potassium ions can move into the cells but there is an insufficient quantity of K^+ ions to

---

Application: Nerve impulses

In nerve cells, the positive ions, sodium and potassium, flow between the outside and inside of these cells. This flow of positive ions or current constitutes a nerve impulse or action potential. Nerve action potentials are extremely important in body homeostasis, since they act as units of information which are necessary for the coordination and regulation of body function. Action potentials can be divided into four stages:

1. resting potential;
2. depolarization;
3. repolarization;
4. redistribution of sodium and potassium ions.

Resting potential

The potential difference between the contents of a nerve cell and the liquid surrounding the cell is approximately 70 to 90 mV. The inside of a cell is negative with respect to the outside of a cell and therefore the potential difference is

overcome the excess negative charge and therefore the cell contents remain negative with respect to the outside of the cell.

Depolarization

A stimulus causes the nerve membrane to be momentarily altered so that the barrier to Na^+ ions is removed. The negative charge within the cell attracts a large flow of Na^+ ions into the cell and a current results. This flow of positive ions causes the inside of the cell to become more positive, that is, less negative with respect to the outside of the cell (Figure 10.5a). The decrease in potential difference is referred to as depolarization and is the first stage of a nerve impulse or action potential.

During depolarization, the rapid flow of positive ions or current results in the potential difference across the membrane firstly approaching zero and then becoming positive. This overshooting of Na^+ ions results in the potential difference attaining a voltage of approximately +45 mV. Notice that now the cellular contents are positive with respect to the outside of the cell. If this change in potential difference is measured during the depolarization stage a graph similar to Figure 10.5b would be observed.

Repolarization

At the completion of depolarization the nerve cell membrane has returned to acting as a Na^+ ion barrier. Since the inside of the cell is now positive, K^+ ions flow to the negative region outside the cell, that is, current flows to the region outside the cell.

The difference in the amount of K^+

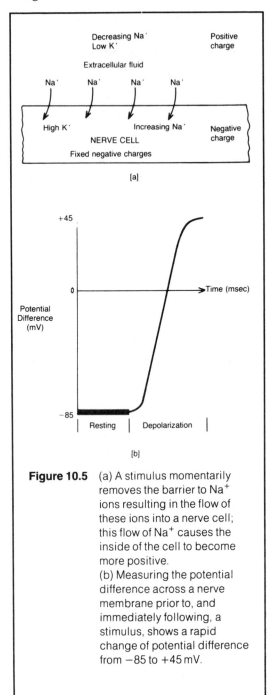

Figure 10.5 (a) A stimulus momentarily removes the barrier to Na^+ ions resulting in the flow of these ions into a nerve cell; this flow of Na^+ causes the inside of the cell to become more positive.
(b) Measuring the potential difference across a nerve membrane prior to, and immediately following, a stimulus, shows a rapid change of potential difference from −85 to +45 mV.

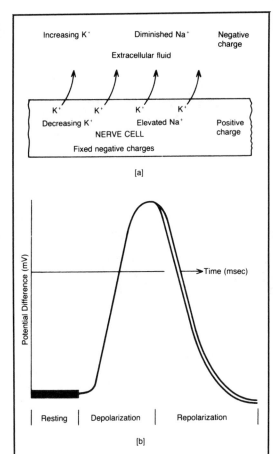

Figure 10.6 (a) K⁺ ions flow from the positively-charged nerve to the negatively-charged region outside the nerve. (b) Measuring this flow of K⁺ ions will show a changing potential difference across the membrane from +45 to −85 mV (Repolarization).

between the outside of the cell and the inside also assists the flow of K^+ from the cell (Figure 10.6a). Relatively high concentrations of K^+ ions inside the cell compared with the outside results in a flow of these ions to lower concentra-

tion by a process called diffusion. The relationship of differences in the amount of ions to ion flow is described in 23.2.

The loss of K^+ ions from the cell results in the cellular contents becoming less positive, that is, more negative with respect to the outside of the cell. The potential difference returns to zero and then decreases to the original resting potential difference. The loss of K^+ ions from the nerve, and subsequent increase in negative charge within the cell is known as repolarization. Measuring potential difference across a nerve membrane during repolarization will result in a graph similar to Figure 10.6b.

Redistribution of Na^+ and K^+ ions

At completion of repolarization, the nerve has a similar potential difference to the resting potential but the cellular contents of Na^+ and K^+ ions are different. For another action potential to occur the distribution of these ions has to return to their original resting potential distribution. The removal of Na^+ from the cell and the transport of K^+ into the cell is performed by a carrier that uses energy to carry Na^+ out of the cell and K^+ into the cell. The mechanism of this carrier is described in 23.5.

10.6 Flow of electricity through a gas

Gases are normally good insulators as most molecules in a gas are neutral. The creation of a high voltage between electrodes can cause conduction as can the ionization of a gas.

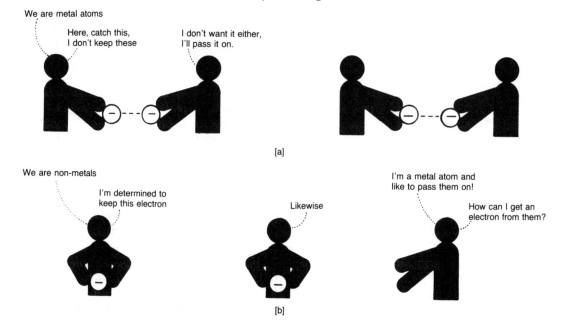

Figure 10.7   (a) The ability of metals to donate electrons enables them to pass electrons from one metal atom to the next, that is, conduct a current. (b) The inability of non-metals to donate electrons stops the flow of electrons.

Ionization of a gas can be achieved through reducing the concentration of molecules in a sealed container. This reduces the obstruction (resistance) of molecules to the movement of electrons thereby increasing the flow of electrons. EXAMPLE: Fluorescent tubes.

10.7   Flow of current through a solid

Electric current

The potential difference between two regions can be decreased by connecting a piece of metal to the two regions. Unlike ions in solution, it is very difficult to move positive or negative ions through a solid and therefore a different mechanism is used for decreasing the potential difference. The small mass of electrons enables them to flow through certain solids from a negative region to a positive region. Since the flow of negatively charged electrons decreases the potential difference between two regions, this flow is also referred to as electric current.

Conductors

Substances that carry current are known as **conductors**, whereas substances incapable of carrying current are **insulators** or non-conductors.

Conductors are generally composed of metals whereas insulators are composed of non-metals. Metals are able to conduct electricity as they are electron donors, that is, metals lose their outer orbit electrons to nearby atoms. This enables electrons to jump from one atom to another along a metal wire, from a negatively charged region to a positively charged region. The net flow of electrons is also called a current (Figure 10.7). Insulators are unable to release electrons because they require electrons to complete their outer shell (Figure 10.7). As the electrons do not move freely a current cannot occur.

Semiconductors

Conductivity is the term used to describe the relative conducting ability of a material. Some materials such as silicon(Si) increase their conductivity with increasing temperature. These materials form the basis of current electronics technology using silicon chips. A silicon chip consists of pure silicon crystal lattice (5.4) with thin layers of an insulator being etched onto the silicon thereby forming paths for electrons to flow. Adding an impurity that contains extra electrons such as arsenic provides a source of electrons if a potential is applied. Adding an impurity with less than four outer electrons such as boron(B), provides in the silicon lattice an area where 'holes' exist for electrons. If a potential difference is applied excess electrons are free to move to an electron hole. The electron hole now moves through the lattice to another position. This property of semiconduction is used in combination with other electrical components to form a complex of electrical paths which are referred to as an **integrated circuit**. Such integrated circuits are the basis of computer function.

Superconductors

In some materials, particularly special alloys, resistance rapidly decreases below a certain temperature to zero resistance. These **superconductors** can conduct current with a very high efficiency resulting in the movement of electrons with minimal loss through heat. Currently, the use of superconductors is limited as until very recently materials could only superconduct at very cold temperatures. The massive research in this area has led to the discovery of new materials that can superconduct at temperatures close to 0°C. It is expected that superconduction will play a significant role in the development of new technology used in health care in the near future. EXAMPLE: Magnetic imaging equipment.

10.8   Resistance in wires

The amount of electrons flowing along a piece of wire will depend upon certain features of the wire such as wire diameter and the type of metal, both of which alter the resistance and thus the flow of current. A thin piece of wire can only conduct a small number of electrons whereas a larger diameter wire can carry a greater number of electrons. ANALOGY: The quantity of water that can flow through a pipe is determined by the pipe's diameter. A small pipe has a greater resistance to water flow than a larger diameter pipe which results in less water being able to flow through the smaller diameter pipe at any given moment (Figure 10.8).

Metals differ in their ability to conduct electrons, with poor conducting metals carry-

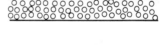

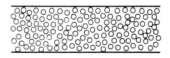

Figure 10.8   The flow of water through a smaller diameter pipe is less than that through a larger diameter pipe.

ing a smaller quantity of electrons or current than high conducting metals. The above characteristics of metal wires are used in controlling the amount of current that can flow in electrical equipment.

Application: Fuses

A fuse is a device that can be put into an electrical circuit and which breaks when an unduly high current passes through it. A fuse consists of a short length of wire which is selected according to its particular resistance to current. The greater the resistance, the less is the quantity of current that can be carried before the fuse wire overheats and breaks. The breakage of the fuse wire prevents excessive current overloading and damaging electrical components.

10.9   DC and AC electricity

Direct current (DC) always flows in the same direction from a negatively charged terminal to a positively charged terminal. Batteries are a source of DC electricity. Power stations rapidly alternate the terminal voltages between negative and positive. This rapid switching of a terminal between negative and positive charges results in an **alternating current** (AC), that is, one flowing first in one direction then in the opposite for brief periods of time. The rate of switching or alternating the direction of electron flow is called frequency. The SI unit for frequency is the **Hertz** (one cycle per second). AC is the preferred form of electricity for domestic and industrial use. Only AC can be transported from power stations at high voltages for long

distances and then be transformed to smaller domestic voltages by transformers.

AC can be produced by the relative motion of a magnet within a coil of wire. The electric current produced by this electromagnetic induction is called an induced electric current.

10.10   Magnetism and electricity

Magnetism

Magnetism is a property of certain metals called **magnets** where metals such as iron, steel and certain alloys are attracted to the magnet. A magnet consists of two poles called the **north pole** and **south pole**. A magnet creates a **magnetic field** which is a region between the poles where magnetic lines of force exists (Figure 10.9a). The earth has a magnetic field with the north magnetic pole being located near the south geographic pole. Unlike poles attract each other and like poles repel. EXAMPLE: The north pole of one magnet is attracted to the south pole of another magnet (Figure 10.9b). Magnets always have two poles as is shown by cutting a magnet in half. Two magnets are formed each with two poles. The above magnets always retain their magnetic properties and are referred to as **permanent magnets**.

Moving charges and magnetism

When an electric current moves through a wire a magnetic field is established which is perpendicular to the direction of current flow (Figure 10.9c). Electricity and magnetism represent a common physical property of matter which is referred to as **electromagnetism**. A magnetic field associated with the movement of an electric current is not permanent and

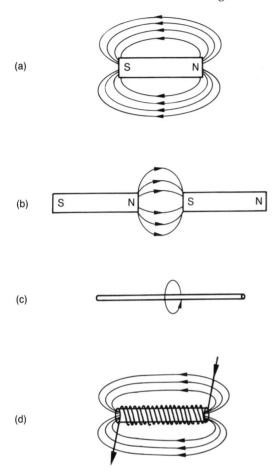

Figure 10.9 (a) Magnetic field of a permanent magnet, (b) magnetic attraction of opposite poles, (c) electric current and magnetism and (d) solenoid.

Application: Magnetic resonance imaging

Magnetic resonance imaging (MRI) or **Nuclear Magnetic Resonance** (NMR) focuses on the responses of a single element in a tissue to magnetism. The part of the body to be studied is placed in a magnetic scanner thereby exposing the tissue to a uniform magnetic field. The hydrogen nuclei are usually studied to identify any abnormalities. MRI can perform non-invasive studies of tumours, investigate biochemical differences and metabolic processes, measure blood flow and monitor the progress of a disease. The procedure takes about 30 minutes and produces results in the form of three dimensional colour images.

so can be switched off by simply stopping the flow of current. Such magnets are called **electromagnets** and are used in health care to remove metal from an eye.

The current flowing in wire wound around a piece of soft iron generates a magnetic field similar to that of permanent magnets (Figure 10.9d). Such electromagnets are called **solenoids** and are often used as switches.

Electromagnetic induction

Faraday discovered that electricity can be generated in a loop of wire by a changing magnetic field. That is, **electromagnetic induction** has occurred which is the basis of electricity supply via the use of **transformers**. A transformer uses the principle that varying an electric field will vary the surrounding magnetic field. Passing a current through a coil of wire produces a magnetic field. If a second coil of wire is located in the magnetic field of the first, an induced current will result. The amount of induced current is dependent on the number of loops forming the secondary coil of wire. Transformers can therefore be designed to generate a different current to that supplied in the primary coil. This property of transformers plays an important role in the transmission of electricity at high voltages and its subsequent reduction to lower domestic voltages.

10.11   Electric circuits

Completing electric circuits

Electrons only flow through metal when it connects two oppositely charged regions. If a wire is broken, electrons are unable to jump across the non-metal gap as this region acts as an insulator. A complete piece of metal wire is required for current to flow from one region to another, that is, a completed electrical circuit is required.

Series and parallel circuits

Electrical circuits can be arranged with the resistors or other electrical appliances such as light bulbs connected end on end (Figure 10.10a) which is referred to as a **series** arrangement. The total resistance of resistors in series is the sum of the individual resistors. If an electrical component fails an incomplete connection occurs which results in a breakdown of the entire circuit.

Circuits may also consist of resistors arranged in a **parallel** arrangement (Figure 10.10b). In parallel circuits most current will

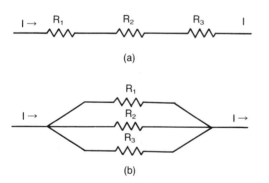

(a)

(b)

Figure 10.10   (a) Series arrangement of resistors (R) and (b) parallel circuit arrangement.

flow down the path with the least resistance and little through the high resistance paths. The total current has now been distributed among all of paths. This property of parallel circuits is used to earth electrical equipment which is further discussed in this section. Failure of one path in a parallel circuit does not result in the general failure of the circuit as the current is redistributed over the remaining parallel paths.

Short circuits

When oppositely charged regions are connected by several pathways, most electrons will flow along the path which offers the least resistance.

An active wire carries current from the power source to the electrical components of a piece of equipment. Contact between an active wire and another wire or a conducting medium can result in most current flowing along the latter path especially if the latter offers less resistance to the flow of electrons. When the current flows via an unintended, alternative pathway a short circuit occurs.

Short circuits can occur when a loose wire comes in contact with the metal casing of a piece of equipment or with a frayed electrical cord. This casing is now 'live' and contact with it can cause an electric shock.

The presence of a large quantity of electrolytes within the body enables it to conduct electricity. Metals conduct electricity better than the human body and this property is used in preventing or decreasing the intensity of an electric shock by a process called earthing.

Earthing

Earthing is the process whereby a wire connects the metal casing and other areas of equipment to the earth (Figure 10.11).

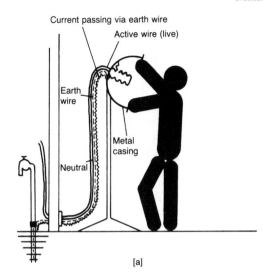

Current passing via earth wire

Active wire (live)

Earth wire

Metal casing

Neutral

[a]

Neutral

Active wire (live)

Current passes through body to earth

To earth

[b]

Figure 10.11   (a) A normally earthed lamp.
(b) A faulty lamp can lead to the active wire connecting with the outer casing.

A large potential difference exists between live wires and the earth. This potential difference enables electrons to flow to the earth whenever a short circuit occurs.

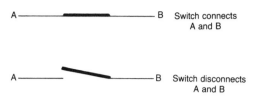

A————————————B   Switch connects A and B

A————   ————B   Switch disconnects A and B

Figure 10.12   A closed switch allows current to flow between A and B, whereas an open switch prevents current flow.

Switches

A switch is a device which closes or opens a circuit and therefore either allows current flow or stops current flow respectively (Figure 10.12). Switches are designed to regulate the flow of electricity and thus the function of electrical equipment. Solenoids (10.10) are often used as switches.

10.12   Mains wire

Electrical circuits involving hospital equipment originate from power stations which cause the flow of electrons and create a potential difference between the power station and the hospital power points. The power station usually maintains a potential difference of 260 to 250 V with electrical equipment.

A completed electrical circuit between a power station and a piece of equipment consists of:

1. a live or active wire carrying current from the power station; the wire is covered by brown or sometimes red insulating material;
2. a neutral or return wire from the equipment; the wire is covered by blue or sometimes black insulating material;

3. an earth wire which usually connects the equipment case to the earth; the wire is insulated with a green/yellow or sometimes green material.

10.13 Capacitance

A set of parallel plates of opposite charge has the capacity to store electricity. The oppositely charged plates are called capacitors and the charge which can be stored per volt of electric potential is called **capacitance**. When the circuit between the two plates is connected the electrons surge towards the positively charged plate. EXAMPLE: The two plates of a defibrillator can act as a capacitor when the body is placed between them. Defibrillators are used to shock the heart into normal rhythms of contraction (25.4 Application: Cardiac arrythmias). WARNING: Equipment containing capacitors can still produce electric shocks even when the lead has been removed from the power point.

10.14 Diagnostic and therapeutic uses

Recording body electrical events

Electrical currents and potential differences exist throughout the body and are essential for body function. The electrical activity of the heart, brain and muscle can be measured by placing external electrodes on the body's surface. Detection of various electrical events associated with the functioning of these organs can assist in determining a patient's condition.

Application: Electrocardiograph

During contraction of the heart, potential differences develop between different regions of the heart. The resultant electrical currents spread into tissues surrounding the heart, and a small proportion of these spread to the surface of the body. By placing leads at different points on the body's surface, a comparison can be made as to whether the current is flowing towards or away from a particular lead. There are various arrangements of electrocardiograph leads, each of which produces a different shaped wave of electrical activity known as electrocardiograms or ECGs. Figure 10.13 shows the most common ECG which is composed of:

1. a P wave — due to atrial electrical events;
2. a QRS complex — due to ventricular electrical events;
3. a T wave — due to ventricles returning to the resting potentials.

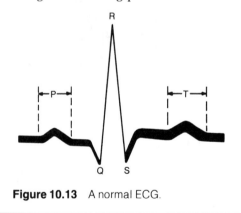

Figure 10.13 A normal ECG.

Electrotherapy

Electrotherapy refers to the range of therapeutic applications of electricity that are used in the treatment of pain, nerve damage, muscle injuries and soft tissue injuries. **Transcutaneous Electrical Nerve Stimulation (TENS)** is an electrical stimulus introduced across the skin and into the tissues where it influences the nervous system to block pain signals travelling up nerves. TENS is successful against both chronic and acute pain. Low frequency electric currents are alternating currents with a frequency of waves ranging from 1 Hz to 2000 Hz. This current stimulates nerves and muscles but has difficulty passing through the skin which results in discomfort. Medium frequency currents range from 3900 Hz to 5000 Hz and are used for the relief of pain and swelling and produce relatively little discomfort compared to low frequency currents. **Short wave diathermy** involves the use of a high frequency current to create an electrical field in the tissue. The movement of ions in the tissue results in the generation of heat to increase circulation, increase metabolism and reduce inflammation, pain and muscle spasm.

10.15 Environmental health and safety

The body can conduct electricity and its electrical activities such as nerve and muscle function are altered when exposed to the cycles associated with AC current (10.9). Electrocution is a major cause of injury and death. The body is particularly susceptible to electrocution when an area of skin is wet as the electrical resistance is substantially less than dry skin. The following steps should be taken to minimize the risk of electrocution.

1. Try to use three pin plugs.
2. Never pull a plug out of a socket by the wire.
3. Never pull a plug out of a socket with the power still on.

4. If any equipment gives a tingle turn the power off, disconnect and get the equipment serviced.
5. Additional precautions should always be taken when using electrical equipment in a wet surface area as the risk of electrocution is considerably increased due to the ability of electric current to be conducted through impure water and the substantially lower protection of resistance of wet skin.
6. Never touch a person who is electrocuted until the source of electrocution has been disconnected from them.

Application: Electric shock

A person touching a piece of earthed equipment will receive only a minor shock as most of the current will flow through the low resistance earth wire (Figure 10.11a). A short circuit in equipment that is not earthed results in a person conducting the entire current as no alternative pathway exists (Figure 10.11b). He or she therefore receives an electrical shock.

Electric shock can also be minimized by breaking the conduction path between the body and the earth by wearing non-conducting or insulating material such as rubber gloves or rubber shoes. A person receiving an electric shock, must be isolated from the main power supply by turning it off or by dragging the person away from the source of supply. The rescuer involved in moving a person that is receiving an electric shock needs to avoid receiving a shock by using insulated materials such as thick rubber gloves or rope.

Summary

Electrical energy involves the flow of charges as an electric current. The relative flow of current is influenced by the potential difference and the resistance to flow according to Ohm's Law of $V = IR$ where V is in volts, I in amperes and R is in ohms. The charges representing electricity can be electrolytes in liquids or electrons in solids. Conductors are materials that have a relatively low resistance whereas insulators are incapable of carrying a current. Semiconductors increase their conductivity with increasing temperature and they form the basis of the silicon chip and computer function. Superconductors are capable of conducting electricity with close to zero resistance. The amount of current flowing through a wire is influenced by the nature of the material and the diameter of the wire.

Magnetism results in the generation of magnetic fields containing a north and south pole. Electromagnetism is the physical property of nature involving electricity and magnetism. Current flowing in a wire produces a magnetic field while magnetic fields in turn can produce electric currents in the process of electromagnetic induction.

A completed electrical circuit arranged in series or parallel is required for a current to flow. Fuses are arranged in series to prevent the flow of damaging currents to equipment such as occurs with a short circuit. Capacitors have the capacity to store electricity.

The body uses electricity in the form of action potentials to conduct and process information. An action potential usually involves the flow of Na^+ into a nerve and K^+ out and the subsequent replenishment of the original concentrations by a membrane pump. The body's dependence on electricity is used to advantage with electrodiagnostic equipment and in the use of electrotherapy to treat a range of body conditions. The body is also susceptible to electric shock especially when the skin is wet as the resistance of the skin is substantially lowered. Safety procedures must be followed at all times to minimize the risk of electrocution to the health professional and the patient.

Chapter 11

Radiant energy or electromagnetic radiation

Objectives

At the completion of this chapter the student should be able to:

1. describe the different forms of radiant energy and their properties;
2. relate the properties of radiant energy to health care, normal and abnormal body function and the uses and dangers of diagnostic and therapeutic equipment;
3. describe how light interacts with objects;
4. explain the terms concave, convex, endoscope, reflection, refraction and scattering.

11.1 Electromagnetic radiation and body function

The sun is the major source of electromagnetic radiation in this solar system. Without this source of energy life could not exist on earth. Energy from the sun is converted into other forms of energy such as chemical energy in plants. Humans rely on the intake of this energy for maintaining body function (Figure 11.1).

11.2 Properties of electromagnetic radiation

When the electrons of atoms gain energy from sources such as heat, they jump briefly to a higher energy level (4.2). On return to their original level they emit energy in the form of waves or rays which are referred to as electromagnetic radiation. Microwaves, heat (infra-red rays), light, ultraviolet light, X-rays and gamma rays are examples of electromagnetic radiation.

The different properties of various forms of radiation are due to differences in the nature of their energy waves. Wave characteristics are determined by the degree of energy that has been absorbed and released by electrons. The electromagnetic spectrum demonstrates the range of wavelengths and thus the properties of the various forms of radiation (Figure 11.2).

Radiation exists in the form of short discontinuous bundles of waves known as photons, and not in the form of a continuous wave. A **wavelength** is composed of one complete wave or one cycle, for example, the distance between the highest point of one wave and the same point on a following

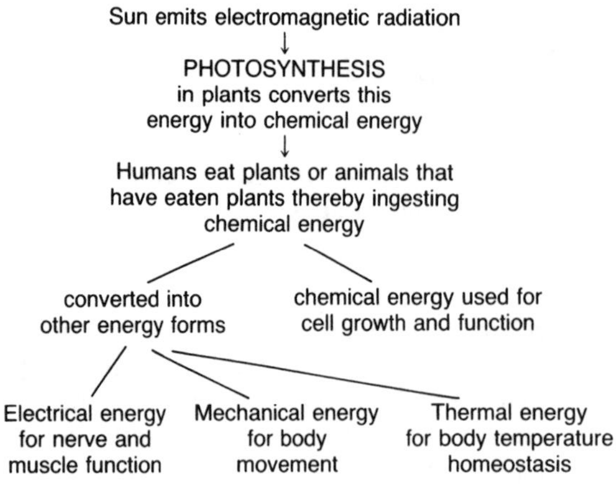

Sun emits electromagnetic radiation
↓
PHOTOSYNTHESIS
in plants converts this
energy into chemical energy
↓
Humans eat plants or animals that
have eaten plants thereby ingesting
chemical energy

converted into
other energy forms

chemical energy used for
cell growth and function

Electrical energy
for nerve and
muscle function

Mechanical energy
for body
movement

Thermal energy
for body temperature
homeostasis

Figure 11.1   Interrelationship of body function to
the sun's emission of
electromagnetic radiation.

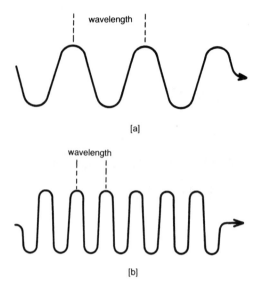

[a]

[b]

Figure 11.3   The nature of a photon. The
wavelength of the photon in (a) is
larger than in (b) but (b) has a
greater frequency than (a).

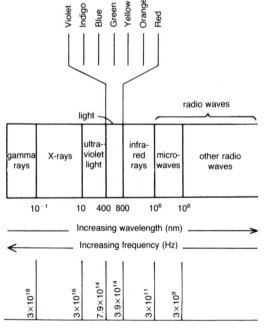

Figure 11.2   The electromagnetic spectrum.

wave (Figure 11.3a). The **frequency** of a wave
is the number of waves passing through a
point in one second.

The speed for all electromagnetic waves
is constant at about 300 000 kilometres per
second in a vacuum. The shorter wavelength
wave requires more waves to travel the same
distance, at the same speed as a wave with
a longer wavelength. Shorter wavelengths
thus have a higher frequency than longer
wavelengths (Figure 11.3b). The shorter the
wavelength, the greater is the amount of
energy of those waves. The wavelength and
energy of photons is therefore directly related
to the frequency of a wave.

Electromagnetic rays produce their effects
at the point at which the rays are absorbed.
This is achieved by changing from radiant
energy into another form. EXAMPLE: Heat
can be converted to chemical energy.

The intensity of electromagnetic radiation
at any given point from a source follows the
inverse square law.

$$\text{Intensity} = \frac{1}{(\text{Distance from source})^2}$$

Eqn 11.1

This equation indicates that a small increase in distance results in a large decrease in intensity. This rapid fall off of intensity with distance is used to minimize exposure to harmful electromagnetic radiation. During treatment using electromagnetic radiation the distance between source and patient is critical. If the source is too near the patient, or the patient moves during treatment, he or she may be exposed to a higher dose of electromagnetic radiation than intended, and burns may result.

11.3 Microwaves

Microwaves are the shortest wavelength group of a range of rays that are known as wireless or radio rays. Wireless rays have wavelengths that are greater than infra-red rays. Microwaves cause water molecules to rotate and ions to vibrate. These movements result in the generation of heat. The different electrical properties of different tissues determine the amount of heat generated. In health care, microwaves are used for the treatment for a range of conditions with the waves being generated by a **magnetron**.

Application: Microwave therapy

The application of therapeutic application of microwaves is referred to as **microwave diathermy**. The non-polar nature of fat (5.5) and the low fluid content of bone result in the poor absorption of microwaves and provide a basis for the selective heating of a

---

specific area. This form of treatment is used for the treatment of superficial conditions as microwaves can only penetrate the superficial layers of tissue (3–5 cm). The main uses of microwave diathermy are the localized treatment of: pain from superficial muscles, joints and ligaments; muscle spasm; inflammation; delayed areas of healing; chronically infected areas and fibrosis.

Care must be taken to prevent burns.

11.4 Infra-red rays

These rays have a relatively long wavelength and are emitted by hot bodies. As the temperature of an object increases the wavelength of the emitted rays will become shorter and contain more energy. The absorption of these rays by matter produces heat or thermal energy as a result of molecular vibration.

Application: Infra-red therapy

The low energy content of infra-red rays restricts the penetration of these rays to the outer regions of skin tissue. The effect of infra-red irradiation is a local rise in tissue temperature. A mild increase in temperature appears to have a sedative effect on sensory nerves, thus enabling infra-red irradiation to be a useful method of relieving pain. This heat will also lead to an increase in the diameter of superficial blood vessels which allows an improved blood supply that assists in the healing of wounds and superficial infections.

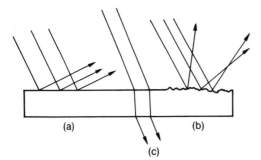

Figure 11.4 Interaction of light with matter (a) reflected light from a polished surface, (b) scattering and (c) refraction.

11.5 Light

What is light?

Everything that is seen by the human eye results from the eye detecting light waves. Light is electromagnetic rays that stimulate the retina of the human eye to produce images in the brain. Light consists of electromagnetic waves that are smaller in wavelength than infra-red rays but greater in wavelength than ultraviolet rays.

Differences in the colour of light are due to distinctive wavelengths within the range of visible light. The sequence of these distinctive wavelengths forms the pattern of a rainbow which is known as the visual spectrum. The spectrum consists of seven colours arranged in the following order of descending wavelength size: red, orange, yellow, green, blue, indigo and violet (Figure 11.2). White light is a mixture of all of these wavelengths and black is the total absence of visible light. When a single colour exists, it represents a narrow wavelength and is referred to as monochromatic light.

Light is next in the spectrum of wavelengths to infra-red radiation (Figure 11.2). When an object that is emitting infra-red radiation absorbs more heat, the resulting electromagnetic radiation will consist of waves with a shorter wavelength. As the wavelength continues to shorten with the addition of energy the colour of the object changes from a dull red to white, emitting visible light. Light can be generated in this manner by heating material such as metal wire to a level where light is given off. EXAMPLE: Light bulbs.

Interaction of light with matter

A green object owes its colour to the ability of that piece of matter to absorb all other wavelengths apart from green. The colour of matter is due to the wavelengths of light that are reflected by individual pieces of matter. A black object does not reflect any light and therefore absorbs all light falling upon it.

The penetration of matter by light depends upon the nature of the matter. Matter can be described as: transparent, translucent and opaque according to light penetration. Firstly transparent material allows light to move freely through it, so that a clear image emerges from the material. EXAMPLE: Glass. Translucent matter alters the path of light and causes light to emerge in a diffuse non-ordered manner so that a clear image cannot be seen through it. EXAMPLE: Frosted glass. Opaque matter absorbs most light waves and therefore does not emit light. EXAMPLE: This book. Some light hitting an opaque medium is **reflected** at the surface, that is, it is bent back into the original medium (Figure 11.4c). A rough surface results in light being reflected at a variety of angles which is referred to as **scattering** (Figure 11.4c). When the surface is smooth the angle of reflection is the same as the angle at which

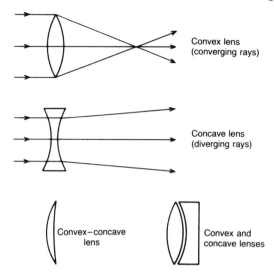

Convex lens
(converging rays)

Concave lens
(diverging rays)

Convex–concave
lens

Convex and
concave lenses

Figure 11.5 Examples of a convex and concave lens and a combination of these.

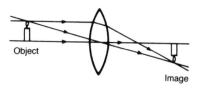
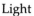

Object

Image

Figure 11.6 Formation of an image by a lens.

an object meet after passing through a lens (Figure 11.6).

A **convex** lens is able to make light rays converge to a point or focus where an image is formed. These lenses are known as converging lenses and they can be used to form an image that is smaller than the object. EXAMPLE: Camera lens. They can also be used to form images that are larger than an object. EXAMPLE: Magnifying glass. The ability of a convex lens to form a reduced or magnified image depends upon the nearness of the object to the lens. Generally, the closer the object is to the lens the larger the resultant image.

A lens that consists of a **concave** surface spreads light rays further apart, i.e. they diverge. This lens is referred to as a diverging lens and can only produce reduced images.

the light hit the object the light can reflect the original source of light. EXAMPLE: Mirrors.

When light rays enter an object at angle other than 90° it is bent. This bending or **refraction** is due to the alteration in velocity of light when it changes from one medium to another (Figure 11.4b). EXAMPLE: When light enters glass it slows down by approximately 25%.

Lenses

The size and shape of transparent matter influences the movement of light through it. This property is used in the functioning of curved transparent objects known as lenses. A **lens** consists of either a convex or a concave surface or a combination of both (Figure 11.5). They are used to form a proportionately smaller or larger visual replica of an object. This replica is called an **image**. The image occurs at the point where the light rays from

Application: The eye

The eye consists of a large convex lens which magnifies or decreases the size of an image. It forms the image on a layer of photoreceptive cells known as the retina (Figure 11.7). The retina consists of cells that convert the image into nerve impulses which are interpreted in the brain as an image. The colour characteristics of an image are determined by three types of cells that absorb either red, green or blue rays. The colour of an object is determined by the relative number and combination of these cells that are stimulated. An equal stimulation of the three cells types results in the sensation of white light. A loss of one or more types of the cell types results in colour blindness. The lack of one cell type causes an inability to distinguish some colours from others.

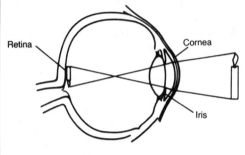

Figure 11.7   In the normal eye, light rays converge to form an inverted image on the retina.

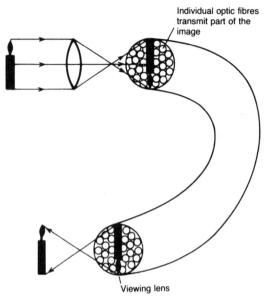

Figure 11.8   An endoscope shows the principle of fibre-optics.

11.6   Fibre optics

Fibre optics is the area of study attributed to the movement of light through optic fibres. Optic fibres are flexible glass rods that are capable of conducting light within the rod from one end to the other. The surface of each fibre is coated so that light is trapped within the core of the fibre. Since the light rays are trapped within the fibre they can only emerge from the fibre's core at the opposite end to which they have entered. A group of parallel fibres can transmit a pattern of light which is displayed at one end (image) by each fibre transmitting light from a small area of the pattern to the other end. At the viewing end the image is reassembled (Figure 11.8).

The advantage of instruments that use optic fibres over other optical systems is their

ability to reach into previously inaccessible regions.

Application: Endoscopes

Endoscopes are instruments that examine hollow organs or internal cavities such as the bladder, lung bronchi, gastrointestinal tract. These instruments consist of a long fibre of optically transparent material with a lens system at one end and a viewing head for the observer and/or camera use (Figure 11.8).

The internal examination of patients has been revolutionized by the development of various endoscopes such as the cystoscopes for bladder examination, bronchoscopes for lung bronchi, laproscope for inspection of the peritoneal cavity and the gastroscope for stomach inspection. The addition of small surgical instruments to the end of an endoscope enables biopsy material to be collected without operating on the patient.

11.7 Lasers

When light is concentrated into a beam of parallel rays consisting of the same wavelength, it is possible to focus the beam onto a tiny spot. This specific form of light is produced by a photon activating the emission of another photon which in turn activate others in a chain reaction. The result is Light Amplification by Stimulated Emission of Radiation or LASER. The ability of lasers to focus onto tiny spots results in the concentration of enormous amounts of energy. Lasers have widespread uses in health care. EXAMPLES: Removal of growths, fine cutting and cauterizing, repairing detached retinas and cleaning heart arteries.

11.8 Ultraviolet rays

These rays are of shorter wavelength and thus higher frequency and energy than light waves. Ultraviolet rays cause chemical changes. EXAMPLES: Formation of vitamin D and melanin deposition in the skin, fading of certain dyes. By removing electrons from atoms they cause the formation of ions. Ultraviolet radiation is a form of ionizing radiation. The relatively high energy of these rays can cause damage to any tissue, especially sensitive tissues such as the retina.

Most of the ultraviolet rays emitted from the sun are absorbed by ozone in the earth's atmosphere.

The higher frequency rays not absorbed by the ozone layer or a protective sun screen lotion can lead to an alteration in skin cells which may lead to the development of skin cancer. The harmful properties of ultraviolet light are used to kill bacteria and fungi. EXAMPLES: Sterilization of instruments and operating theatres.

Ultraviolet light used in therapy can be divided according to wavelength into UVA and UVB. UVA represents the long rays (290–390 nm). These rays have less energy than the short rays (180–290 nm). Ultraviolet rays from the sun are responsible for tanning and sunburn (Application: 11.10). Mercury vapour lamps generate the rays used for therapeutic purposes.

Application: Therapeutic use of ultraviolet radiation

Primarily used for conditions where a localized increase in the circulation of the skin is required. EXAMPLES: Infected wound; poor skin condition such as the area around ulcers and pressure areas and slow healing surgical incisions. The basis of UV therapy is the development of a localized inflammatory response (37.2) which is visible as a reddening of the skin which is referred to as an **erythema**.

The antibiotic property of UV is used to treat fungal and bacterial infections of the skin.

11.9 X-rays

X-rays have a shorter wavelength than ultraviolet rays and are capable of penetrating most matter including human tissue. This property is used both diagnostically and therapeutically.

Application 1: Diagnostic use

X-rays are absorbed by dense tissues such as bone; tissues such as skin absorb only minimal amounts. X-ray machines emit X-rays over a particular part of the body. Apart from dense tissue such as bone, most X-rays will penetrate the tissues and emerge on the opposite side. These emerging X-rays are recorded on a photographic plate.

Fractures in bones may therefore be detected, since X-rays can pass through the gap formed by the fracture and be recorded on a photographic plate. This X-ray film will contain a slightly different picture when compared with a normal X-ray film of the same region.

The size, shape and function of some soft tissue organs can be determined by administering a dense X-ray-absorbing metal such as barium. EXAMPLE: Barium sulphate known as barium meal is used to outline the gastrointestinal tract.

The use of a computer in conjunction with an X-ray instrument can produce an image of a slice of the body. The production of a series of cross-sectional images by an instrument is called **tomography**. A three-dimensional view of a body structure can be constructed by combining serial scans. The production of these scans is called a computerized axial tomography (CAT) scan.

Application 2: Therapeutic use

Exposure of tissue to high doses of X-rays results in chemical changes which may cause cell death or damage to cells, which may lead to tumours or genetic abnormalities in offspring. The ability of X-rays to destroy cells can be used to advantage in X-ray therapy.

High doses of X-rays are fired in a fine beam at a tumour and so kill the tumour cells and any healthy neighbouring cells. The instrument for producing these X-rays is called a linear accelerator.

11.10   Gamma rays

Gamma rays are high energy, short wavelength waves emitted from radioactive isotopes. They are similar to X-rays except that they originate from the nucleus of atoms. The energy released from nuclei is called nuclear energy and is discussed in Chapter 12.

11.11   Environmental health and safety

Exposure to high levels of electromagnetic radiation can result in injury to tissue. EXAMPLES: Burns from infra-red and ultraviolet radiation; damage to the eye from light and ultraviolet radiation and cancer from X-rays and high frequency ultraviolet rays. Increasing the distance from a source of electromagnetic radiation is an important means of minimizing exposure as intensity of electromagnetic radiation decreases rapidly with distance according to the inverse square law (11.2). Patients who are being exposed to electromagnetic radiation should be cautioned against movement as any movement can alter the amount of exposure.

Application 1: Sunburn

Excessive exposure to a specific band of ultraviolet rays called ultraviolet B produces blisters and burns on the skin which are commonly referred to as sunburn. Overexposure to ultraviolet lamps will also result in skin burns. Sunburn lotions are available which contain substances that specifically absorb the harmful portion of ultraviolet radiation. The blocking out of these rays enables the remaining rays to develop a person's suntan.

Application 2: X-ray hazards

All cells can be damaged or destroyed by X-rays, the most sensitive of which are rapidly dividing cells such as cancer and foetal cells. Pregnant women should not work in areas where a chance of X-ray exposure exists.

As a result of the hazards of X-ray exposure, it is necessary for people who work with these rays to have effective protection. High X-ray absorbing materials such as lead and concrete are used as a protective barrier in order to minimize unnecessary exposure.

Staff who work in areas where X-rays are used need to wear a photographic film which is frequently checked to determine the amount of exposure to X-ray. In the ward, mobile X-ray machines should be handled with great caution to ensure that patients or other staff are not in the line of the X-ray emission.

Summary

Radiant or electromagnetic energy consists of the movement of waves that are known as photons. The wavelength of these waves varies from very small to very large. The properties of electromagnetic radiation are dependent upon the wavelength, and it is for this reason that electromagnetic radiation has been categorized according to wavelength. Categories of waves are named in descending order of length as follows: radiowaves (includes microwaves), infra-red rays, light, ultraviolet rays, X-rays and gamma rays. The speed of electromagnetic radiation is constant for a given medium. The intensity of radiation at any given point from a source follows the inverse square law. This property is important when considering the relative risk of exposure.

The major source of electromagnetic radiation or EMR is the sun which provides the energy input into the world to support life. This energy is utilized in photosynthesis to form glucose which is used as a source of energy by animals. Visible light represents a spectrum of colours. Each colour represents a specific wavelength range. The visual features of an object are determined by the extent of reflection, scattering and refraction. This property is used by lenses to focus images. As light travels in a straight line the use of internal reflection within optic fibres is used to bend light to provide images of internal body structures. When light is concentrated in a single wavelength it is referred to as laser. The energy contained within a laser can be used to cut and weld tissues.

The properties of electromagnetic radiation can be used to treat and diagnose a range of conditions. Short wavelength (high frequency) electromagnetic radiation in the form of ultraviolet radiation, X-rays and gamma rays represent ionizing radiation. These forms have the potential to cause cancer as they can ionize the DNA molecules and therefore extreme care must be exhibited at all times when using these categories.

Chapter 12

Nuclear energy

Objectives

At the completion of this chapter the student will be able to:

1. describe the properties of nuclear energy;
2. relate the properties of nuclear energy to health care, normal and abnormal body function and the dangers of its use;
3. describe the safety requirements for working with radioactivity;
4. explain the following terms: half life, emission, becquerel, sievert, background radiation.

12.1 Nuclear energy and health care

Energy released from interactions within the nucleus of an atom is referred to as **nuclear energy**. This energy is represented as radioactivity in the form of electromagnetic radiation and particles ejected from the nucleus which are referred to as **nuclear emissions**. One of the first uses of nuclear energy were the nuclear weapons used in 1945 which heralded the start of the nuclear age. A major peaceful use of radioactivity is its use in health care where it is used extensively to save lives through diagnosis and therapy. Exposure to high levels results in an illness specific to radioactivity called radiation sickness.

Evidence that the body is able to withstand low level exposure to radioactivity is provided by the general levels of radioactivity in the environment. Radioactivity is present in the atmosphere, soil, rocks, building materials, etc. This radiation is referred to as **background radiation**. Small amounts of damage resulting from background radiation are repaired by enzymes, thereby providing the necessary protective mechanism for life to survive in a radioactive environment.

A major problem associated with the use of radioactivity is the handling and storage of radioactive waste as this often contains material that will remain contaminated for many hundreds of years. An understanding of the general properties of radioactivity and its medical applications is important for health care workers as the uses of radioactivity in health care are expanding rapidly. An understanding also provides health care professionals with the necessary knowledge to respect the potential hazards associated with working in areas where radioactivity is used yet alleviate the fear of working in such areas.

12.2   Radioisotopes

The nucleus is held together by attractive forces between protons and neutrons. For each element (4.6) an optimum number of neutrons exists that will maintain the stability of the nucleus. Any isotope of an element (4.10) that has a disproportionate number of neutrons is unstable. An unstable isotope is called a **radioisotope** or **radionuclide**.

A relatively small number of radioisotopes are naturally occurring. Most radioisotopes are artificially formed by bombarding the nucleus. Radioisotopes undergo a change in the structure of their nuclei until an optimum number of neutrons is achieved. During this period of nuclear change the nuclei release energy, called nuclear energy, in the form of gamma rays and particles. The protons and neutrons involved in the reactions within the nucleus have some of their mass converted into energy according to Einstein's equation.

$$E = mc^2 \qquad \text{Eqn 12.1}$$

where E is the energy released in the form of nuclear energy when a mass (m) is converted into energy. The other term, c, represents the speed of light which is constant during these reactions. The particles released are mainly beta and alpha particles. Nuclear change in an isotope can be shown using the changes in mass number. **Radioactive decay** involving changes in proton number results in the formation of a new element. EXAMPLE: The emission of an alpha particle results in the loss of two protons and two neutrons which can be summarized in a nuclear decay equation.

$$^{238}_{92}\text{U} \quad \rightarrow \quad ^{234}_{90}\text{Th} \quad + \quad ^{4}_{2}\text{He}$$
Uranium   Thorium   Helium

$$\text{Eqn 12.2}$$

NOTE: The total mass number and atomic number on each side of the equation are equal, that is 238 and 92 respectively.

An element may contain both stable isotopes and radioisotopes according to the mass numbers of each isotope for that element. All isotopes of an element have essentially the same chemical and physiological function regardless of their nuclear stability or instability. However the energy emitted from radioactive isotopes may be harmful to living tissue.

12.3   Radioactive emissions

Beta particles

Nuclear instability can lead to the breakdown of neutrons resulting in the formation of protons and electrons. Nuclear forces eject the electron, with its charge of −1, from the nucleus. The affected electron is called a beta particle. Since an extra unbound proton now exists in the nucleus, a new element has been formed with an atomic number that is one greater than the original element. EXAMPLE: Iodine-131 forms xenon-131

$$^{131}_{53}\text{I} \quad \rightarrow \quad ^{131}_{54}\text{Xe} \; + e$$
Iodine   Xenon + Electron

$$\text{Eqn 12.3}$$

Positrons

Nuclear instability can also lead to the breakdown of protons, resulting in the formation of positively charged particles with the same mass as electrons and with an equal but opposite charge. These 'positively charged electrons' are called positrons. When positrons encounter electrons they annihilate each other and form gamma rays.

Alpha particles

Elements that contain more than 83 protons spontaneously eject particles that consist of two protons and two neutrons. These large positively charged particles are referred to as alpha particles. The ejection of an alpha particle results in the atom changing into a new element that has an atomic number two less than before the emission (Eqn 12.2).

Gamma rays

The production of alpha and beta particles may result in the release of energy which is emitted in the form of waves of energy known as gamma rays. These rays have no mass or charge. Gamma emission does not alter the number of protons or neutrons in a nucleus and thus does not alter the atomic number.

12.4   Measurement of radioactivity

The detection of radiation is very important in medical work, particularly with respect to protecting personnel and patients from excessive exposure to radiation and for therapeutic and diagnostic purposes.

Different detecting systems are required for determining the type of nuclear emission (alpha particles, beta particles and gamma rays). The type and number of nuclear emissions can be determined for any radio-isotope and thus radioisotopes can be identified.

The physical unit of radioactivity is expressed in terms of the number of nuclear disintegrations per second from a radioactive source. The products of these disintegrations

are emitted in the form of alpha particles, beta particles, positrons or gamma rays. The SI unit (2.3) is the **becquerel** (Bq), which represents one disintegration per second. The becquerel has recently replaced the non-SI unit known as the curie. One curie equals 3.7×10^{10} Bq. For an explanation of this mathematical notation refer to 2.3.

The becquerel is used in medical work to measure the amount of radiation a person receives. It indicates the number of disintegrations per second. The SI unit that relates the amount of radiation absorbed by tissue is the **gray** (Gy). One gray equals 1 joule of energy that is absorbed by 1 kg of tissue. The gray has recently replaced the non-SI unit called the **rad**. One rad equals 0.01 Gy. The gray and rad describe irradiation of tissue regardless of whether the tissue is plant or animal. The damage to tissue by absorbing a given amount of energy varies according to the type of radiation.

A correction factor known as the relative biological effectiveness (rbe) is used to relate radiation damage to human tissue. The unit that relates specifically to the biological effect of radiation absorbed by humans is the sievert. The **sievert** replaces the non-SI unit known as the rem. One rem equals 0.01 sievert, whereas 1 sievert equals 100 rem. The relationship between the sievert-gray and the rem-rad are:

$$1 \text{ sievert} = 1 \text{ gray} \times \text{rbe}$$
$$1 \text{ rem} \quad = 1 \text{ rad} \times \text{rbe}$$

12.5   Half-life

Every radioisotope has a unique rate of nucleus decay. Some radioisotopes decay rapidly, others at a very slow rate. The rate of decay for a particular radioisotope is constant. Half-life is the time taken for half

Table 12.1 The half-life of common radioisotopes

Radioisotope	Half-life		Radioisotope	Half-life	
Caesium-137	30	year	Iridium-192	74	day
Carbon-14	5730	year	Iron-59	45.1	day
Chromium-51	27.8	day	Molybdenum-99	2.78	day
Cobalt-57	270	day	Phosphorus-32	14.3	day
Gallium-67	78	hour	Radium-226	1620	year
Gold-198	2.7	day	Thallium-201	73	hour
Iodine-125	60	day	Technetium-99	6.0	hour
Iodine-131	8.1	day	Yttrium-90	64.2	hour

Table 12.2 Half-life of ^{131}I showing its rate of decay or disintegration

Quantity ^{131}I (MB$_q$)	Time (days)
37.00	0
18.5	8
9.25	16
4.62	24
2.31	32
1.15	40

of a given number of radioactive atoms of an isotope to decay. Since the rate of decay varies for different radioisotopes, the half-life must also vary.

All isotopes have a unique half-life and thus a substance can be determined by its half-life (Table 12.1). EXAMPLE: An unknown substance has decayed from 37 MBq to 18.5 MBq in 8.1 days. Looking up the half-life table it is found that the only radioisotope with this property is the radioisotope of iodine known as ^{131}I. Furthermore, every 8.1 days half the remaining radioactive atoms will have decayed or disintegrated into a new element (Table 12.2).

The range of half-life between different radioisotopes can vary from billions of years to fractions of a second. The shorter the half-life, the greater the rate at which atoms decay

and the greater the quantity of emissions from the nucleus.

12.6 Effects of radiation on humans

The effect of radiation on humans varies according to the type of radiation emitted and the tissue that has been irradiated.

The relatively large size and mass of alpha particles (two protons and two neutrons) restricts their ability to penetrate matter. Alpha particles are relatively harmless when they strike our skin as they cannot penetrate the dead outer layer and are therefore unable to irradiate vital organs. However, when alpha particles enter the body through either inhalation or ingestion of radioactive substances, serious tissue damage can result at the site of radioactive irradiation. Alpha particles are not used in the medical field.

The small size of a beta particle (one electron) enables these particles to penetrate a few millimetres of skin which will result in an area that appears similar to a burn. They can only cause tissue damage inside the body when they have been taken in by breathing or ingestion.

Table 12.3   Recommended maximum radiation dose limits for different body structures of personnel working in radiation-related occupations

Structure	Maximum dosage (millisievert/year)
Blood-forming organs	50*
Bone marrow	50*
Eye lens	50*
Gonads	50*
Lymph	50*
Skin and thyroid	300
Arms, hands and feet	750
Other organs	150

*After age eighteen, no more than 25 mSv/3-month period.

Gamma rays have no mass and travel at the speed of light. These properties enable gamma rays to have a penetrating power about 10 000 times that of alpha particles. Gamma rays are far more harmful to the body than either alpha or beta particles, since they can penetrate further into the entire body.

The effect of radiation varies according to the type of tissue. The most sensitive tissues are bone marrow, the gonads, lymph tissue and the lens of the eye. Rapidly dividing cells, such as those in a foetus, are very sensitive to radiation, and thus exposure to radiation during pregnancy should be kept to a minimum. The International Commission of Radiological Protection (ICRP) recognizes the differences in tissue sensitivity and recommends different dose limits for different tissues (Table 12.3).

Low doses of radiation alter the structure of the chemicals involved in cell division. The alteration of hereditary information in the sex cells can result in future generations with mutations. Damage to other cells in the body can result in regions of abnormal cells which may lead to cancer. With increasing doses of radiation cell death occurs. Further increases in the amount of radiation absorbed will eventually result in rapid death of the person.

The damage to body tissue as a result of radiation exposure is similar whether the tissue has been exposed to one large dose of radiation or a series of smaller doses which equals the large dose. The effects of radiation exposure are thus cumulative. Personnel who work in areas where radiation is used are required to wear film badges that record the accumulated amount of radiation to which they have been exposed. These badges are checked at regular intervals to determine if the quantity of accumulated radiation is above the recommended safety levels.

12.7   Diagnostic use of radioisotopes

More than a hundred different radioisotopes have been used to assist in a wide variety of diagnostic tests. These radioisotopes are mainly selected according to the following criteria:

1. ability to emit gamma radiation;
2. short half-life;
3. ability to be eliminated from the body shortly after completion of the diagnostic test.

Radioisotopes administered internally should be gamma ray emitters, since these rays penetrate the tissues sufficiently to be easily detected outside the body. Also, the absorbed dose from gamma rays is much less than that from beta rays. Short half-life radioisotopes should be used and the quantity of radioactivity administered should be kept as low as possible to minimize tissue damage.

An instrument called a gamma camera produces an image of the **distribution** of radioactivity in an organ and by using this in conjunction with a computer, the functioning

Table 12.4 Some common diagnostic radioisotopes

Radioisotope	Symbol	Use
Chromium-51	^{51}Cr	Red blood cell analysis
Iodine-131	^{131}I	Testing thyroid function
Technetium-99m	^{99m}Tc	Scans of the brain, lung perfusion, bone, testing renal function, heart
Iron-59	^{59}Fe	Evaluation of body-iron concentration
Phosphorus-32	^{32}P	Detection of cancer cells
Thallium-201	^{201}Tl	Heart perfusion
Gallium-67	^{67}Ga	Inflammatory disease, detecting site of tumours

radioactive and the stable isotopes of an element. A particular isotope will provide specific information for a more precise diagnosis. Some of the important diagnostic radioisotopes are listed in Table 12.4.

Application: Thyroid function tests

To assist in the diagnosis of overactive and underactive thyroid conditions the radioisotope ^{131}I may be administered to a patient. A normal functioning thyroid gland will take up about 12% of a specific iodine dose within a few hours.

A typical thyroid uptake test scan involves a dose of 370 kBq (10 microcuries) which produces 0.002 Gy (0.2 rads — a mega Bq represents one million Bq whereas a microcurie is one millionth of a curie) to the thyroid. The neck is then viewed in the region of the thyroid gland with an appropriate detector. If the level of radioactivity over one hour is greater than 15% of the administered dose, an overactive condition may exist. When the monitored thyroid level is less than 4% an underactive condition probably exists. Note that this range of I uptake can be altered by a variety of conditions and is thus intended only as a relative guide to thyroid activity. Pinpointing the locality of areas of different function within the thyroid such as those of low accumulation in a cyst, can be done by 'scanning' with a gamma camera.

---

of an organ such as the heart or kidneys, may be determined.

Another instrument is used to measure positron emission. Positron emission tomography or PET scanning involves the detection of the two gamma rays emitted when a positron collides with an electron. EXAMPLE: Fluorine-18 is used for brain imaging.

A completely different approach is **radioimmunoassay (RIA)**. This method is used to determine minute concentrations of hormones, antibodies, drugs and many other chemicals in the body. It involves the use of a sample of blood, urine or tissue. The antigen (37.2) is combined to an isotope. The antigen competes with unlabelled antigen for the binding on the complementary body chemical such as a hormone. The sample is counted thereby identifying the level of the chemical. EXAMPLE: Early detection of pregnancy.

Elements play varying roles in body function. To evaluate a particular body function a radioisotope of an element may be used since the body cannot distinguish between the

12.8 Therapeutic use of radioisotopes

The main objective of therapeutic radio-isotope use is the selective destruction of abnormal cells such as uncontrolled rapidly dividing cancer cells. Destruction of these cells requires a highly localized intense dose of radiation. Failure to localize the radiation will result in damage of nearby healthy cells. Radioisotopes are administered to patients as either liquids (unsealed sources) or solids (sealed sources).

Firstly radioisotopes that are selectively taken up by particular tumours can be administered orally. Accumulation of the radio-isotopes by the very localized tumour cells results in a radioisotope concentration that is sufficient to destroy them. The administered dose of the radioisotopes is such that, when it is diluted throughout the body fluids, damage to general body fluids is minimal. EXAMPLE: Iodine-131 is selectively concentrated by the thyroid gland and any secondary tumours (metastases) by up to 200 times that of the rest of the body. ^{131}I administered orally at a level higher than that used for diagnosis kills the tumour cells by irradiating them with beta particles.

Secondly, sealed radioisotopes can be inserted into body cavities to irradiate adjacent tumours, e.g. in cancer of cervix, rectum. The radioisotope is encased in a biologically inert metal container such as platinum or gold. The radioisotopes radium-226 (^{226}Ra) and cobalt-60 (^{60}Co), which were used for many years, are now being widely replaced by caesium-137 (^{137}Cs). The gamma radiation from all these radioisotopes destroys the tumour cells as beta particles have difficulty penetrating the walls of the container. The long half-lives of these radio-isotopes necessitates the removal of the con-tainer when the treatment is finished so as to prevent unnecessary tissue damage.

Thirdly, radioisotopes may be implanted directly into the tumour, e.g. in cancer of the tongue. Shorter half-life radioisotopes are used, e.g. gold-198 (^{198}Au) seeds, and iridium-192 (^{192}Ir) wire. These can be used for treatment over a short period, or as a permanent implant, depending on the half-life of the isotope.

Fourthly, radioisotopes such as cobalt-60 or caesium-137 can be used externally to irradiate tumour sites within the body and destroy cancer cells. The radioactive source is housed in a heavily shielded container with an adjustable aperture, which allows the size of the radiation treatment area to be varied. The high energy gamma rays emitted from these sources are able to penetrate the body to reach the tumour. This treatment is given in small dose fractions over a 4–6 week period.

Fifthly, a recent development is the tagging of a monoclonal antibody for a specific cell (37.4) with an isotope followed by the injection of the complex into the blood. The monoclonal antibodies then bind selectively to the tumour thereby concentrating the initial low dose to a level that destroys the tumour. This method offers tremendous scope for the treatment of cancer.

Radioisotopes can also be used as a power source, by converting the emitted energy from nuclear decay into electrical energy. EXAMPLE: The radioisotope plutonium-238 (^{238}Pu) acts as a tiny nuclear battery in heart pacemakers. The pacemaker is implanted in the chest wall or in the subcutaneous tissue of the upper abdomen and is replaced about every ten years.

12.9   Environmental health and safety

Radioactivity represents a potent form of energy as it has the capacity to destroy cells and life without any physical indication of its presence. It is for this reason that anyone working in an area where radioactivity is used is required to wear a dosimetry film badge. These badges detect the extent of exposure to emissions. As emissions follow the inverse square law (Eqn 11.1), distance is a major component of protection against radiation with the further the distance from a source the better. Elongated forceps are used where possible to increase the distance when handling radioactive material. Other protection rules are the minimizing of exposure time and the use of protective shielding. When working with patients receiving internal therapy staff must organize and prepare any equipment and supplies prior to seeing the patient in order to minimize staff exposure. Any spills of contaminated material should be reported immediately to the appropriate contact person who is usually the radiation safety officer. EXAMPLES: Urine, vomit, faeces, bedlinen. Radioactive material should be disposed of in the correct containers and should never be handled with bare hands. The use of shielding further reduces the exposure to radiation. Lead is an effective shield against gamma emitting sources as its high density provides a barrier to the gamma rays. EXAMPLES: Lead aprons are often used as are lead-lined containers.

Summary

Nuclear interactions involving neutrons can result in radioactivity which represents the emission of electromagnetic radiation in the form of gamma rays plus particles. These particles can be neutrons, beta particles, alpha particles or positrons. Each particle type has its own specific properties. The disintegration of a nucleus is measured in becquerels (Bq) with one Bq representing one disintegration per second. The biological effects of radiation are measured in sieverts (Sv). Isotopes that contain a disproportionate number of neutrons in the nucleus attempt to become stable by altering the ratio of neutrons to protons by emitting particles and energy. Such isotopes of an element are called radioisotopes or radionuclides. The emissions and the rate of emissions is unique for each radioisotope. The half-life represents the time taken for half a given number of atoms to decay. Radioactive decay involving a change in atomic number results in the formation of new elements.

Radioisotopes occur naturally in the environment and are mainly responsible for background radiation. Artificial means can be used to create specific radioisotopes that are used in health care. Isotopes that predominantly emit gamma rays, have a short half-life and an ability to be eliminated shortly after completion of a test are selected for use as diagnostic radioisotopes. Therapeutic isotopes are mainly selected on their ability to destroy cells. The medical use of isotopes is based on the property that all isotopes of an element have essentially the same chemical and physiological properties.

The body can repair low level damage resulting from the ionization of molecules. Damage greater than the capacity to repair can lead to cancer so a set of maximum dose limits has been set for different body structures.

Chapter 13

Heat energy

Objectives

At the completion of this chapter the student should be able to:

1. describe the properties of heat energy;
2. relate the properties of heat energy to health care, normal and abnormal body function and the uses of diagnostic and therapeutic equipment;
3. describe the methods of measuring heat;
4. explain the terms latent heat, thermal expansion, convection, conduction, radiation, specific heat capacity.

13.1 Heat and matter

Changes of state

Heat or **thermal energy** results from the vibration of atoms and molecules. The energy imparted into the matter can originate from different forms of energy such as electrical energy and mechanical energy in the form of friction. Any increase in the vibration of atoms results in an increase in the generation of heat by these particles. Since the vibration of particles is energy of movement, the greater the thermal energy of particles the greater is the kinetic energy of these particles. As previously discussed in Chapter 9 the extent of vibration and therefore heat within matter determines the physical state of the matter with solids representing the least vibration and gases the most.

The heat involved in a change of state is referred to as the **latent heat**. This heat is not reflected in a temperature change as it is involved in the breaking apart of the particles instead of increase in vibrations. EXAMPLE: A block of ice and the forming water remains at 0°C (32°F) while heat is added until the ice has melted.

Thermal expansion

An increase in the quantity of heat in a piece of matter causes an expansion to occur as vibrations increase in size thereby increasing the distance between atoms. This expansion is referred to as **thermal expansion**. Each material has a unique response which is reported as the **coefficient of expansion**.

Application: Prosthetic devices

Prosthetic devices require similar coefficients of expansion to bone. This is required as any localized change in temperature resulting from muscle activity can create stress points at the points of contact with bone if dissimilar coefficients exist as different rates of expansion will occur.

In liquids and gases an increase in heat content results in an increase in volume. This increase can be quite large and result in a large increase in pressure within the container (19.2).

Cooling of matter generally results in a contraction in a similar rate to that of expansion. However, water expands between 4°C and 0°C. This property results in a greater quantity of water occupying a confined area which can lead to the bursting of the walls of the container. EXAMPLE: Thawing frozen blood.

13.2 Measurement of heat

Temperature

Temperature is a measure of the intensity of heat in an object, that is, the frequency of vibration of particles. Temperature indicates the degree by which particles are vibrating, it does not specify the number of particles that are vibrating. Temperature is only a measure of heat intensity and not the quantity of heat. EXAMPLE: If in a match and a log fire, all of the particles are vibrating at the same rate, then the intensity of heat will be the same in

both, although the quantity of heat will be different.

Temperature is measured in units referred to as degrees. Three scales have been devised to measure temperature: Fahrenheit, Celsius or Centigrade and Kelvin. Since temperature is a measure of particle vibration, zero degrees should indicate a temperature where no vibration occurs. The more recent Kelvin (K) scale uses this basis for determining zero degrees. Unfortunately, the older scales of Celsius (°C) and Fahrenheit (°F) base zero degrees on the zero vibration of pure water and water saturated with salt respectively. Substances such as oxygen are still vibrating at these temperatures and thus these scales do not represent the temperature at which there is no vibration of particles in all substances. The temperature at which no particles vibrate is referred to as **absolute zero** which is recorded as 0 K, −273°C and −460°F. The relationship of these scales is described in 2.2. Appendix B provides a comparative chart of the Celsius and Fahrenheit scales.

Application: Clinical thermometers

The thermal expansion (13.1) of mercury can be directly related to the temperature scales as used in a clinical thermometer. The inclusion of a constriction in the tube containing mercury prevents mercury from returning to the bulb after removing it from a patient. The design thus allows the temperature to be read away from its recording position. Shaking is required to return the mercury to the bulb and must be performed prior to its reuse.

Measuring heat quantity

The quantity of heat in an object is recorded in kilojoules (SI unit) or Calories. These units can be used to indicate the amount of heat produced or released. The major source of body heat is cellular metabolism (33.2). The rate at which heat is produced by the body reflects the rate at which foods release energy and is referred to as the metabolic rate (6.1). The amount of heat required to raise a material of a given mass will vary between different materials. This difference indicates the **specific heat capacity** of a material. The specific heat capacity is the quantity of heat required to raise the temperature of 1 kg of a substance by 1°C. The units are the Joule (J) or the non-SI unit Calorie (C). The specific heat capacity therefore represents the energy intake or loss of a given quantity of material. A comparison of the specific heat of different substances provides a guide to the relative capacity of substances to store heat. Water has a high specific heat as 1 kg of water requires 4.2 kilojoules of thermal energy to raise its temperature by 1°C. The high water content of body results in a similarly high value. This high value indicates that the body will only slowly respond to factors causing temperature changes. EXAMPLE: Holding onto a cold object results in a relatively slow cooling of the hand and not the very rapid cooling that would occur if the hand had a low specific heat such as copper.

$$\begin{array}{c} \text{Heat} \\ \text{gained} \end{array} = \text{mass} \times \begin{array}{c} \text{specific} \\ \text{heat} \\ \text{capacity} \end{array} \times \begin{array}{c} \text{temperature} \\ \text{change} \end{array}$$

Eqn 13.1

EXAMPLE: A 65 kg woman's temperature increases from 36.5°C to 38.5°C in one hour. Assuming a specific heat capacity of 4.2 kJ the heat gained is calculated as follows:

$$\text{Heat gained} = 65 \times 4.2 \times 2$$
$$= 546 \text{ kJ}$$

The approximate energy value of a food can be determined by measuring the amount of heat given off through combustion (Table 27.1).

13.3   Transfer of heat

Heat flows from matter with a higher temperature to matter with a lower temperature. Thermal energy causes particles to increase their rate of vibration, thus generating further thermal energy. The transfer of heat to other matter occurs by conduction, convection or electromagnetic radiation.

Conduction

This is the transfer of heat by particles interacting with nearby matter that contains less thermal energy. The heat spreads to the adjacent particles causing them to increase their vibrations and thus their thermal energy. EXAMPLE: Element on a stove heating pots of water.

Convection

In convection, heat is transferred by the flow of a liquid or gas with a higher thermal energy to a colder region of matter. EXAMPLE: A hot wind.

Electromagnetic radiation

Matter with high thermal energy can emit energy in the form of electromagnetic radiation. Particles that come in contact with electromagnetic rays absorb energy from these rays and this results in the particles vibrating more frequently. Heat is thus transferred from the rays to the absorbing matter. Electromagnetic radiation can transfer heat over large distances. EXAMPLE: The sun transfers heat to the earth via electromagnetic radiation.

13.4 Diagnostic use of heat

The use of thermometers has made a major contribution to the caring of patients. The properties metabolic rate, heat production and the loss of heat by radiation have been combined in the diagnostic process of thermography. The radiation given off by the surface of the body is detected by an infra-red camera and displayed on a screen or recorded photographically. An overactive area such as a cancerous region will be detected as a hot spot. In contrast, an area of poor circulation will be displayed as a cold spot.

13.5 Therapeutic use of heat

A range of therapeutic procedures based on the application or removal of heat are used in health care. The application of heat to a region is used to provide quick pain relief and alleviate muscle spasm and inflammation. Heat conduction methods include hot packs, thermal water baths, electric heating pads and wax baths. Hydrocollator packs contain a gel which has the capacity to provide heat for 30–40 minutes. The application of hot paraffin wax to the skin provides heat by conduction. The heat is trapped by the insulating properties of the wax as it cools and solidifies on the surface of the skin.

Cryosurgery is a reverse of the above as it involves the rapid loss of the relatively hot skin to a very cold probe which is filled with liquid nitrogen. This method can be used to remove cysts and warts where the region in contact with the probe attaches to the probe as a consequence of its rapid loss of heat.

The use of convection involves the transfer of heat between the skin's surface and a flow of hot fluid moving over the skin. EXAMPLES: Whirlpool baths, hot air baths and steam inhalation.

Infra-red lamps use electromagnetic radiation to apply heat (Application: 11.4).

13.6 Environmental health and safety

Heat represents a major source of injury. The burns resulting from the application of heat to the body have been previously described (9.10). The causes of burns range from the accidental spillage of boiling water to fire (6.7) and the explosion of incorrectly stored materials (6.7 — Application). It is important to treat any hot material with care and to follow the correct procedures for storing containers of volatile materials. Containers with volatile contents should not be stored in hot areas and should not be stored completely full. The treatment of burns' patients has become a specialist field with the introduction of burns units.

Another heat related occupational hazard is heat stress or hyperthermia resulting from working in a high temperature environment. Exposure to extreme cold for a period of time can lead to the condition of hypothermia. Long sleeved gloves should be used when handling very cold materials to prevent frost bite.

Summary

Heat reflects the relative vibration of particles with the greater the vibration the greater is the thermal energy of a piece of matter. The heat required to change the physical state of matter is called the latent heat. When the heat content is increased for a piece of matter an expansion occurs. In the case of solids this response is indicated by the coefficient of expansion.

Temperature is the measure of the intensity of heat in an object whereas the quantity of heat in an object is recorded in joules. Three units of measurement are used to record temperature: Celsius, Fahrenheit and Kelvin. The amount of heat required to raise the temperature of an object is referred to as the specific heat capacity.

Heat is transferred through conduction, convection and radiation. The properties of these different forms of heat transfer are used in a range of diagnostic and therapeutic processes. Care must be taken to prevent heat related accidents and to minimize excessive exposure to heat or cold.

Chapter 14

Sound

Objectives

At the completion of this chapter the student should be able to:

1. describe the different properties of sound;
2. relate the properties of sonic energy to health care, normal and abnormal body function and the diagnostic and therapeutic use of sound;
3. describe the mechanism of hearing;
4. describe the following terms: pitch, loudness, frequency, amplitude, compression, rarefaction, Doppler effect.

14.1 Properties of sound

Sonic energy or sound is the vibration of particles in the form of waves through matter. Sound cannot be transmitted through a vacuum, but only through substances in which particles are free to vibrate. Sound is transmitted when vibrating particles pass on their vibration to adjacent particles. A transfer of energy occurs without a transfer of matter. Sound travels in a similar manner to a wave that has been generated by throwing a rock into still water.

Whenever matter vibrates sound is produced. The ability to detect this sound depends upon the nature of the vibration wave. The number of vibrations per second that pass a given point is termed the frequency. The unit of frequency is the hertz which is symbolized as Hz.

Sound waves are examples of **transverse waves**. In transverse waves the particles in a wave are not permanently moved as the disturbance travels through the medium without bodily moving the medium. This is due to vibrating particles passing on their vibration to adjacent particles thereby transferring energy from one particle to the next. The speed of transfer is determined by the density of the medium. A densely packed medium contains particles close to each other which facilitates the rate of collisions while a less dense medium has a greater time interval between collisions as a result of the greater distances between particles. EXAMPLE: Densely packed solids transmit sound at 5000 metres per second compared with air where the velocity of sound is 344 metres per second.

Sound waves exhibit some of the properties of electromagnetic waves. These properties include travelling in straight lines, reflection and refraction (11.2 and 11.5). The quantity of energy in a wave is determined by the height or **amplitude** of the wave and is referred to as intensity. EXAMPLE: When the height of two waves with the same frequency

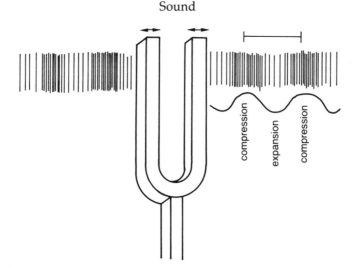

Figure 14.1 Generation of sound. The formation of repeating areas of compression and rarefaction can be represented as a sine wave.

differs, the wave with the greater amplitude contains a greater amount of energy.

14.2   Generating sound

Sound waves originate from elastic objects which vibrate back and forth. EXAMPLES: Tuning fork and drum skin. As a tuning fork is moved forwards it compresses the air molecules in front of it resulting in a region of greater density (Figure 14.1). This region is referred to as a **compression**. As the tuning fork recoils, it leaves a region containing few particles which is referred to as an area of **rarefaction** or **expansion**. The vibrations of the source of sound are therefore causing a series of alternating compressions and rarefactions to travel through air. The frequency of sound refers to the number of rarefactions or compressions that pass a given point per second. The wavelength is the distance between two rarefactions or two compressions.

14.3   Sound and hearing

Pitch and loudness

The ear is able to convert sound waves into nerve impulses in the range of 20 to 20 000 Hz. The conscious perception of any particular frequency is termed the **pitch** which may not be the true sound frequency. Pitch varies from the true frequency at very high and very low frequencies. **Loudness** is the amount of energy that is detected by the ear for a given frequency. This is a subjective term, that is, what is loud to one person may not be to another.

The ear

The ear functions by converting pressure changes resulting from the compressions and rarefactions into electrical impulses. The ear consists of three parts; outer, middle and inner ear (Figure 14.2). Sound waves hit the external outer region of the ear and are directed down a canal called the **external**

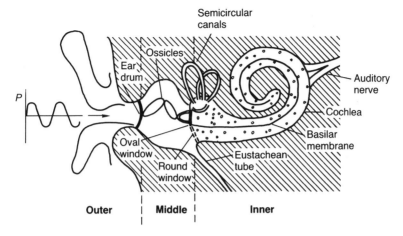

Figure 14.2 The ear.

auditory canal(meatus) to the **eardrum** or **tympanic membrane**. The extent of vibration of this thin membrane is directly related to the intensity and frequency of sound waves hitting its outer surface. ANALOGY: A drum vibrates in response to the frequency and force that the drummer hits the drum skin. The vibrations in the drum are transmitted to a small bone called the **malleus** which is in direct contact with the inner surface of the eardrum. This bone and two other very small bones, the **incus** and **stapes** are referred to as the **auditory ossicles**. The region containing these ossicles is called the middle ear. The sound is transmitted through these interconnected ossicles to the inner ear via another membrane called the **oval window**. The vibrations from this membrane are transmitted through a fluid filled spiral canal called the **cochlea**. The wide end of the cochlea responds to low frequencies and the narrow end to high frequencies. The pressure waves travelling through the cochlea vibrate a membrane called the **basilar membrane** which has attached to it the **spiral organ** or **organ of corti** which is the structure responsible for converting pressure waves into electrical impulses. Within the spiral

organ are auditory hair cells that generate an electrical impulse when moved in response to a wave. High sound intensities cause excessive movements of these hair cells. Over an extended period of time this can lead to damage of hair cells thus resulting in hearing impairment (14.6). A **round window** releases the pressure wave from the cochlea back into the middle ear thereby minimizing possible interference from waves being reflected at the end of the cochlea. The inner ear also contains three semicircular canals which are involved in balance.

Bel scale of loudness

Sound **intensity** refers to the quantity of energy in a sound wave and is measured by the amount of energy that the sound dissipates when it is absorbed at a surface. Intensity is measured in watts/square metre of surface area (Wm^{-2}). The relationship between intensity and loudness is shown in the Bel scale for loudness (Table 14.1). The **decibel** is used as the unit of loudness. This scale uses the threshold of hearing as its reference point. The scale provides a

Table 14.1 Bel scale of loudness

Noise	Decibels	W/m^2	Multiple of threshold intensity
Threshold of hearing	0	10^{-12}	1
Rustle of leaves	10	10^{-11}	10^1
Whisper	20	10^{-10}	10^2
Normal conversation at 1 m	60	10^{-6}	10^6
Busy street	70	10^{-5}	10^7
Workshop, heavy traffic at 5 m	80–100	10^{-4}–10^{-2}	10^8–10^{10}
Damage to hearing after prolonged exposure; whining power saw, siren at 30 m, workshop	100	10^{-2}	10^{10}
Threshold of pain; indoor rock concert	120	$1(10^0)$	10^{12}
Severe pain	140	10^2	10^{14}

quantitative comparison between loud and soft sounds. To achieve this comparison between large differences in intensity an exponential scale is used, that is, each increase of ten decibels represents an increase by a factor of ten. NOTE: It is important to understand that a small change in decibels represents a large change in energy being received by an ear. Also, a change of one decibel represents a different quantity of energy at different points on the scale. EXAMPLE:

10^4 dB represents an intensity of 10 000; 10^3 dB represents an intensity of 1000; 10^2 dB represents an intensity of 100

A 1 dB change from 3–2 dB is 1000–100 which represents a change of 900

A 1 dB change from 4–3 dB is 10 000–1000 which represents a change of 9000

The bel scale is an example of a **non-linear scale**. Another important example is the pH scale (16.3).

14.4 Diagnostic use of sound

Sound has a range of diagnostic uses ranging from the use of stethoscopes to the recording of blood flow with a Doppler machine. The use of high frequency sound or **ultrasound** is used as an important form of medical imaging.

The stethoscope 'bell' acts as a sound detector as it vibrates and amplifies internal body sounds such as the heart beating. The amplified sound is protected from interference from external sounds as it is conducted within tubes to the ears.

Doppler instruments use a property of waves known as the **Doppler effect**. With sound, the Doppler effect is observed whenever a moving noise passes an ear. As a siren passes, the pitch of the sound decreases as the vehicle passes. This shift in pitch represents the Doppler effect. The extent of the drop in pitch is proportional to the speed of sound of the sound source. This relationship can be used to measure the speed of sound of a moving object. The Doppler instrument involves the application of a gel to the skin

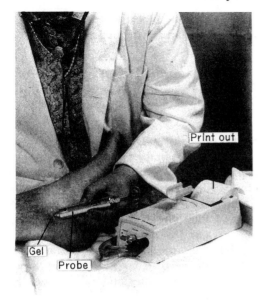

Figure 14.3 Doppler instrument measuring blood flow in the foot.

The **audiometer** is an instrument that measures the threshold of hearing at different frequencies. The sounds are applied to the ear through headphones and responses to individual frequencies are recorded. The range of maximum sensitivity is from 1000 to 4000 Hz although the ear can detect sounds from 20 to 20 000 Hz.

Ultrasound involves the use of very high frequencies ranging from 20 000 to 800 000 Hz. Ultrasound uses the property that sound travels at different speeds for different tissues. This property is used in composing pictures using sound waves that have been reflected by different tissues. These pictures are produced on television screens or can be photographed for a permanent record. Ultrasound is used in examining the heart and the brain and in determining the position of the foetus and the placenta, since it does not damage the sensitive foetal tissue.

and the use of a sound probe (Figure 14.3). The gel has similar sound conduction properties to tissue and metal and thereby provides a continuum for the sound to travel from the probe to blood and return to the probe without the interference that would occur if the waves had to pass through the less dense medium of air. The probe must be held at 45° to the skin in order to measure the difference in frequency between an emitted signal and the reflected signal from a moving red blood cell. Any factor that reduces the blood flow such as a thrombus can be located by identifying where the blood flow has slowed. The results of blood flow tests can be assessed to determine whether surgery is needed to 'clean out' the blood vessel. These tests are important in assessing the risks of strokes resulting from blockages to the carotid artery.

Audiometry is the testing for hearing loss. It represents the range of tests that are used to measure the hearing ability of a person.

14.5   Therapeutic use of sound

The main therapeutic use of sound involves the use of ultrasound. Ultrasonic beams can penetrate skin to a depth of 3–4 cm. The absorption of these waves by the skin results in a heating of the tissue, and a decrease in swelling and pain. Ultrasound causes vibrations to occur in tissue which results in the loosening of fibres and materials between cells. Vibrations soften scar tissue and cause an increased leakage of membranes which results in an increased fluid movement. Ultrasound is particularly useful for the treatment of soft tissue injuries and joint injuries.

Ultrasonic shock waves are now used to shatter kidney stones into harmless fragments.

14.6 Environmental health and safety

A major cause of hearing impairment is **noise-induced hearing loss** which mainly results from noise exposure in the work environment. Impaired hearing caused by damage to relevant nerve structures such as the hair cells can result from exposure to high sources of noise over an extended period of time as well as toxic substances and hereditary disease. This form of deafness is often called **sensorineural hearing loss** and results in the sufferer often hearing only muffled vowel sounds. The only treatment for sensorineural hearing loss is to prevent the injury by avoiding noise or by wearing suitable ear protection as hearing aids are unable to overcome the loss of discrimination between sounds.

A relationship exists between noise and stress. Repetitive background sounds can generate irritability of staff and lead to stress induced illness thereby decreasing their effectiveness as a worker.

People exposed to high levels of noise should wear appropriate protective hearing muffs. Every effort should be made to lower the noise level of a work environment through noise conservation programmes through the use of equipment containing noise suppression devices and by ensuring that equipment is maintained in good working order, as worn parts can generate high levels of sound. The understanding of the relationship between noise levels and hearing loss has led to the setting of internationally recommended maximum sound levels.

It is important when working with hearing impaired patients that health professionals speak slowly and clearly, ensuring that the deaf person can see the lips move.

Summary

Sound or sonic energy represents the vibration of particles in the form of waves through matter. Sound waves originate from elastic objects which can vibrate back and forth. The sound is transmitted when vibrating particles pass on their vibration to adjacent particles. The greater the density of the matter the greater is the contact between particles and hence the speed of transfer. Sound waves travel in straight lines and exhibit the properties of reflection and refraction. The waves represent a series of compressions and rarefactions. The higher the amplitude of the compression, the greater is the quantity of energy within a wave. The energy of a wave is referred to as sound intensity while loudness refers to the amount of energy detected by the ear for a given frequency. The relationship between sound intensity and loudness is shown in the Bel scale of loudness which uses the threshold of hearing as its reference point. The conscious perception of any given frequency is called pitch.

The ear consists of an outer ear that funnels sound to the eardrum which transmits the sound to the inner ear auditory ossicles. These three bones in turn cause the vibration of the oval window which causes hair cells in the spiral organ to move thereby generating a related electrical impulse.

The properties of sound provide a wide range of diagnostic and therapeutic uses. Overstimulation of the ear through the exposure to excessive sound can lead to temporary or even permanent hearing loss.

Chapter 15

Mechanical properties of matter

Objectives

At the completion of this chapter the student should be able to:

1. explain the terms associated with motion;
2. describe the term force and relate force to nursing and body function;
3. explain the actions of gravity;
4. explain the terms friction, coefficient of friction, mechanical advantage, work, power, inertia, momentum and elasticity;
5. perform simple vector problems.

Mechanics is a branch of science that is concerned with the motion and the maintenance of equilibrium of objects. The study of objects in equilibrium is called statics. The descriptive study of motion is called kinematics, and is used to describe the relative movement of muscles and the associated anatomical position of joints and body segments. When knowledge of the size and direction of forces is required the study is called kinetics. The human body relies upon the principles of mechanics for: body movement, balance, the movement of substances into and out of the body and the movement of substances within the body.

15.1 Terms used to describe motion

Vector

A vector has both size and direction. EXAMPLE: Velocity has a size in km/hr (mph) and a direction such as due north. Vectors are usually indicated by bold type or by an arrow over the symbol. EXAMPLE: $\vec{v}$ or **v** for velocity.

Scalar

A scalar has no direction. It can be added or subtracted mathematically. EXAMPLES: Speed, time, volume, temperature.

Velocity

Velocity is the distance that something has travelled divided by the time taken. Velocity is a measure of motion in a specified direction. **Speed** is the motion of an object without reference to any direction and is usually used when describing how fast something is moving.

Velocity is an example of a vector since it has both magnitude and direction. As speed has only magnitude, it is classified as a scalar.

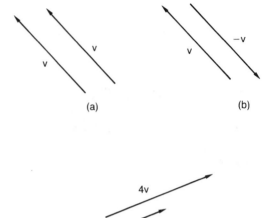

(a)   (b)

(c)

Figure 15.1   Vectors (a) equal vectors, (b) negative of a vector and (c) multiplication.

Acceleration

When velocity is altered this change is referred to as acceleration. **Acceleration** is the change of velocity divided by the time taken. A particle with an acceleration of ten metres per second per second means that the particle will alter its velocity by ten metres per second every second. Acceleration has direction and therefore requires a description of direction when referring to it. As acceleration has magnitude and direction it is a vector.

can alter the influence of the net force. Force is another example of a vector, that is, it has both direction and magnitude.

15.2   Vector analysis

Force

A **force** is any influence that either changes the position, the state of rest or the motion of an object. The SI unit of force is the **newton** (N).

Force = Mass × Acceleration   Eqn 15.1

To determine the resultant force or the relative influence of an individual force on the resultant force it is necessary to understand how vectors can be analysed. Vectors do not add or subtract in the same way as ordinary numbers. The terms used to describe vectors are described below.

Resultant force

Vector terms

The net force acting on an object is called the resultant force. It is determined by taking the sum of all of the individual forces. It is necessary to account for the direction and magnitude of each force since these factors

Two vectors are **equal** if they have the same magnitude and **point in the same direction** (Figure 15.1a).

The **negative of a vector** is a vector of equal

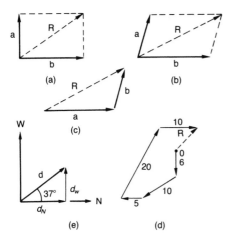

Figure 15.2 Graphical method of adding and subtracting vectors. (a) Rectangle method, (b) parallelogram method, (c) and (d) nose to tail method and (e) resolving a vector into its components.

method places the individual vectors into a 'nose tail diagram' (Figure 15.2c). The resultant is determined by joining the origin to the exposed arrow. The vector's magnitude and direction are determined by measuring the length and angle.

Application: Lifting a patient onto a bed

Lifting a patient from a bedside chair to a bed requires two main forces. Firstly, a horizontal force is required to move the patient from the chair to the bed (Figure 15.3a). A second force is required to lift the patient to the bed height (Figure 15.3b). The net force developed by the individual forces or the resultant force is determined by r̩ .acing the individual forces into a 'nose to tail' diagram (Figure 15.3c) and then joining the tail of one force to the nose of the last force (Figure 15.3d).

---

length pointing in the **opposite** direction (Figure 15.1b).

Multiplication of a vector by a simple number is that number times the original magnitude with the vector pointing in its original direction (Figure 15.1c).

Adding vectors

Addition of vectors can be achieved by either drawing the individual vectors to scale or by using trigonometry. Two individual vectors can be added using the graphical approach by forming to scale a rectangle for vectors acting at 90° or a parallelogram for vectors not at 90° (Figures 15.2a and b). In both cases the vectors, such as two forces, are drawn to scale from the one point. The rectangle or parallelogram is completed and the resulting diagonal represents the resultant vector which is measured to determine its magnitude and direction. Another graphical

Most body movements require the combined actions of many forces. The resultant of these forces can be determined graphically using the **polygon method**. The same 'nose to tail' approach is used with the vectors being added in any order. The resultant vector starts at the tail of the first vector and finishes at the head of the last vector (Figure 15.2d).

Subtracting vectors involves reversing the direction of a vector (Figure 15.1b).

Resolving vectors

Vectors can be broken down or *resolved* into individual vertical and horizontal **components**. This method is essentially the reverse of calculating the resultant. The resultant force is drawn and appropriate components are created to form a rectangle or

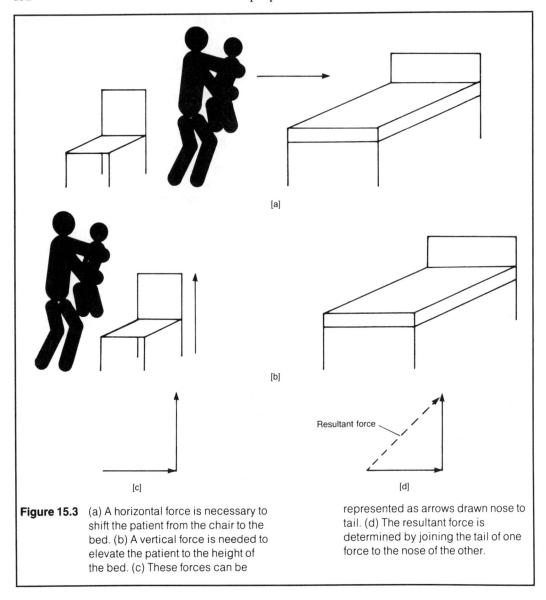

[a]

[b]

[c]

[d]

Resultant force

Figure 15.3   (a) A horizontal force is necessary to shift the patient from the chair to the bed. (b) A vertical force is needed to elevate the patient to the height of the bed. (c) These forces can be represented as arrows drawn nose to tail. (d) The resultant force is determined by joining the tail of one force to the nose of the other.

parallelogram that has a diagonal the same as the resultant (Figure 15.3d). Resolving vectors is an important process in the overall study of forces.

The alternative trigonometric method is quicker to use for resolving the components of a resultant force. This is particularly useful for analysing the forces applied to bones and joints during movement. This method requires a knowledge of trigonometry and is not discussed further in this book.

Application: Analysis of body movement

Individually, muscles are limited in the direction of the force that they can produce. However, when their actions are combined, a large number of resultant directions of muscle action are possible. A desired movement can be achieved by the body summing muscle actions; the combined action produces the desired resultant force in both magnitude and direction.

Computers are used to **resolve** the compl(x vector relationships associated with walking (**gait**) and other body movements to diagnose biomechanical abnormalities and to enhance performance in sport.

15.3   Gravity

Force of gravity

Gravity is the universal force which results in the attraction of all objects to each other. Those objects with a greater mass pull those with a lesser mass towards them. The large mass of the earth exerts a large force attracting matter to the earth's centre. The relationship between mass and its force of attraction to the earth is expressed as **weight**.

Weight = Mass × Acceleration due to gravity
W   = M   × g

$$\text{Eqn 15.2}$$

where W = $9.8\,\text{m/sec}^2$, $32\,\text{ft/sec}^2$ or $9.8\,\text{N/kg}$. The unit of mass is the kilogram which is usually also synonymous with weight. NOTE: It is important when performing calculations in physics to treat weight as a force

and not simply as an alternative expression for mass as the values are different (Eqn 15.3). EXAMPLE: For a 10 kg object the weight is

$$W = 10 \times 9.8$$
$$= 98\ \text{Newtons} \qquad \text{Eqn 15.3}$$

The movement of matter away from the earth requires a force to oppose gravity, whereas the movement of matter towards the earth will be assisted by gravity.

Application: Gravity and blood circulation

Gravity exerts a uniform effect on the blood circulation of a person lying in a horizontal position. If this person now moves to an upright position, gravity will exert different influences on the blood circulation. The regions of the body above the heart can now only receive blood from the heart if it is moved against the force of gravity. To enable blood to reach these portions of the body an increased force is developed by the heart. This force has to be of sufficient strength to overcome the effect of gravity. Failure of the heart to develop the necessary force to supply sufficient blood to the head and brain can result in fainting, and is known as postural hypotension.

Blood flows to the lower parts of the body with the assistance of gravity. Gravity, however, interferes with the return of blood from the lower extremities to the heart. This is evident by the appearance of fluid and thus swelling in the feet of people who stand for long periods of time.

The effect of gravity can be used to advantage in order to decrease bleeding. A cut hand raised above the head will receive less blood than when it is located below the heart. This is due to the heart only pumping with sufficient force to overcome the effect of gravity for the distance to the head, and not the additional distance to the raised hand.

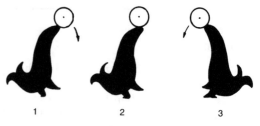

Figure 15.5 The ball is only balanced at position 2 where the force directly opposes the net force of gravity. At position 1 the ball falls to the right and at position 3 the ball falls to the left.

Centre of gravity and stability

Since gravity acts on all matter, an object will have this force acting on all its constituent particles. The resultant of the gravitational force on each individual particle is termed the **centre of gravity**. In a uniformly shaped object with a uniform mass, the centre of gravity is the centre of that object (Figure 15.4a). In objects that contain either varying amounts of particles or which are not uniform in shape, the centre of gravity will be located towards the area of greatest mass (Figure 15.4b), because more gravitational forces are acting in this region.

The position of the centre of gravity is important since it determines where forces are required to act to oppose an object falling due to the influence of gravity. The net effect of gravity on an object is exerted through a vertical line that passes from the centre of gravity to the earth (Figure 15.5). In Figure

15.5 the resultant force of gravity is exerted onto the opposing force located at position 2. This object will remain balanced or in equilibrium at this position if the magnitude of the force equals the force of gravity. **Equilibrium** exists in any object when all the forces and vectors total zero and it appears that no force is acting on the object. The position of the force at 1 results in the object falling to the right, whereas the force at position 3 results in the object falling to the left.

An object can move horizontally and not fall, as long as an opposing force acts in line with the centre of gravity. The ability of an object to move and not fall is restricted to the boundaries of action of that opposing force. EXAMPLE: A ball will not fall off a table until it moves to the boundary or edge of the table where no opposing force to gravity exists. The region of support for holding an object in a balanced position is known as the base of support.

A object has stability when it resists falling. This occurs when the base of support for that object is below or through the centre of gravity (Figure 15.6). The wider the base of support the greater is the stability of an object, since a small base of support can only support an object that has a small degree of movement.

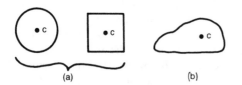

(a)   (b)

Figure 15.4 (a) In objects with uniform shape and mass the centre of gravity (C) is located at the centre of the object. (b) In non-uniform objects the centre of gravity (C) is located towards the area of greatest mass.

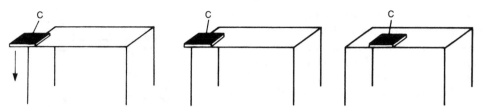

Figure 15.6 A book will remain on a table as long as the centre of gravity (C) is over the base of support.

Stability in humans

Generally, the centre of gravity in the human is located in the pelvic region near the base of the spinal column. When sitting or standing erect the centre of gravity is in line with the spinal column and in the pelvic region (Figure 15.7), its location resulting in the least strain on the body muscles. The spinal column and large thigh muscles are used to oppose the action of gravity.

Greatest stability occurs when a person has a wide base of support. Persons with their feet further apart than another person has the ability to shift their centre of gravity to a greater extent, that is, the former can have a greater variety of postural changes without falling over (Figure 15.8).

Changes of posture can alter the centre of gravity. EXAMPLE: When a person bends

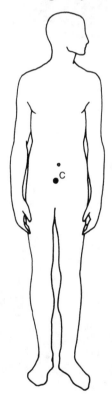

Figure 15.7 Location of the centre of gravity in humans.

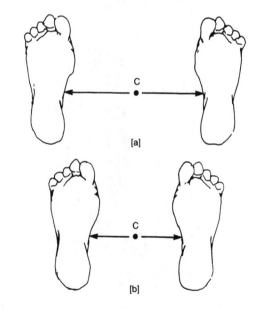

Figure 15.8 A person (a) with a wide support base can move their centre of gravity, C, a relatively large distance when compared with a person (b) with a narrow support base.

forward the centre of gravity shifts forward according to the degree of bending. Other factors that can alter the centre of gravity and require alterations in the placement of feet are pregnancy, ascites (accumulation of fluid in the abdominal cavity), loss of a limb and carrying a heavy object.

Application: Walking aids

People who have suffered a stroke or a fractured hip have decreased stability when walking. Their stability is increased if they use a walking frame (Figure 15.9), which has a wider base than a walking stick (Figure 15.10) or crutches (Figure 15.11), and hence is more stable.

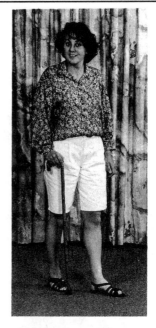

Figure 15.10   Walking stick.

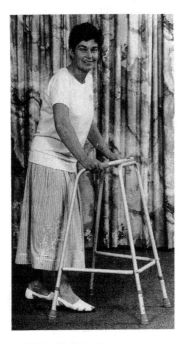

Figure 15.9   Walking frame.

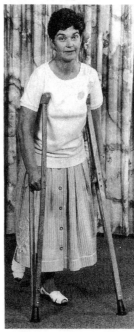

Figure 15.11   Moving with the use of crutches.

Specific gravity

Specific gravity of a substance is the weight of a certain volume of substance compared with the weight of an equal volume of water. Specific gravity can also be defined in terms of density, when density is the amount of mass in a given volume. A substance with a greater density than another substance will contain a greater amount of mass than the latter substance in the same volume. Specific gravity of a fluid is the density of a fluid compared with an equal volume of water.

Water is selected as the reference substance since the relationship between the volume and mass of water, i.e. density, is one. EXAMPLE: A volume of ten millilitres of water weighs ten grams:

$$\text{Density} = \frac{\text{Weight}}{\text{Volume}} = \frac{10}{10} = 1\,\text{g/mL} \quad \text{Eqn 15.4}$$

Specific gravity is calculated as follows:

$$\frac{\text{Specific}}{\text{gravity}} = \frac{\text{Density or mass of substance}}{\text{Density of mass of water}}$$

EXAMPLE:

$$\text{Specific gravity of urine} = \frac{1.010}{1.000} = 1.010$$

Application: Variations in urine specific gravity

Urine consists mainly of water and a few substances such as urea and sodium chloride. The normal range of the specific gravity of urine is between 1.002 to 1.040 (1002 to 1040). Note that the specific gravity of pure water is 1.000, and thus the closer the reading is to 1.000, the more diluted is the fluid. In the same way, the further that the reading is away from 1.000, the greater

---

is the amount of other substances present in the water. A reading lower than 1.002 (1002) indicates a dilute urine and may be due to diuresis. An abnormally high urine specific gravity indicates a concentrated urine. This may be due to dehydration causing excessive water retention or to the excessive excretion of a particular substance.

15.4   Newton's laws of motion

Sir Isaac Newton studied the movement of objects and determined three laws of motion. These laws explain how an object moves and what effect that object has when it collides with another object.

First law of motion

This law can be expressed as follows: matter will continue to be in a state of rest or will continue to move in a straight line with the same speed unless it is acted upon by a net external force.

When an object is at rest or is moving in a straight line at constant speed the object is in equilibrium. Most moving matter has forces such as gravity and friction acting upon it. These forces slow down the motion of matter, eventually bringing the matter to rest.

A heavy object requires a greater force to bring it to rest or change its direction than a lighter object. This relationship between mass and velocity is explained in the terms inertia and momentum.

Inertia

An object with a large mass requires a greater force to initiate motion than an object with a smaller mass. **Inertia** is the reluctance of a body to start moving after a force has been applied to it and the reluctance of the body to stop once it has begun to move. According to Newton's first law, a moving object's reluctance to move and stop moving is directly related to its mass. The greater the mass, the greater the inertia of that body and the greater the force needed to alter its motion. Mass is therefore an important factor in initiating motion and stopping motion in any matter.

Momentum

Moving objects with a large inertia require large forces to slow them down. This property is important when considering a collision between two objects and the effect that the collision has on each object's motion. The two factors of mass and velocity are important when considering the effect of a collision between two objects. In any collision it is the combined effect of the mass and the velocity of each object that determines the outcome of the collision. **Momentum** is the motion of a body as a result of the mass and velocity of the body:

$$\text{Momentum} = \text{Mass} \times \text{Velocity} \quad \text{Eqn 15.5}$$

Newton used the term momentum to explain how much force was required to alter the equilibrium of any piece of matter.

Second law of motion

Newton's second law can be expressed as follows: the net force acting on a body is equal to the rate of change of momentum of that body. A large car travelling at a low speed has the same amount of momentum as a small car travelling at a high speed. A large truck requires a greater braking force to stop it than a car when both are travelling at the same speed. When two objects collide with each other, the total momentum of the collision is the same, that is:

$$\begin{array}{cc} \text{Mass} \times \text{Velocity} = \text{Mass} \times \text{Velocity} \\ \text{object 1} \qquad \text{object 2} \end{array}$$

$$\text{Eqn 15.6}$$

This equation shows that if the mass of each object is unchanged in a collision, the velocity is the only factor that can be altered. An object with a large inertia will lose a small amount of velocity in preference to an object with small inertia. The latter has less reluctance to a change in its motion and thus tends to bounce off the object with the larger mass at a greater velocity.

Third law of motion

This law is expressed as follows: for every action there is an equal and opposite reaction exerted. EXAMPLE: A patient lying on a bed exerts a force on the bed and in turn the bed exerts an equal but opposite force on the patient.

15.5   Friction

Static and kinetic friction

Friction is a force that resists the movement of one object over another. The amount of friction depends upon the nature of the surfaces and the weight of the moving object. A relatively rough surface such as concrete will exert greater friction than a smooth surface such as ice. An object requires a greater force to move over soil than over ice, that is, a greater force is needed to overcome the friction. More friction results from heavy

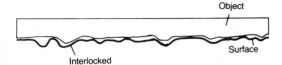

Interlocked

Figure 15.12   At rest an object settles in a
position where the surface of the
object interlocks with another
object's surface.

objects moving over a surface than lighter
objects over the same surface.

Two types of friction can be encountered
when moving a stationary object. **Static
friction** results from the rough edges of an
object interlocking with surface irregularities
of another object (Figure 15.12). Static friction
exists between most objects since very few
objects are perfectly smooth. **Kinetic friction**
is the friction exerted by a surface on an
object that is moving. This friction is less
than static friction as a greater force is
required to move an object out of an interlocked position (static friction) than to
'bounce' an object along from one minute
ridge to the next (kinetic friction).

Application: Insertion of a nasogastric
tube

In the process of inserting a nasogastric
tube, far less force is required when the
tube is inserted in a continuous motion
than when the tube is inserted in a
series of discontinuing steps. Since
less force is required for a continuous
motion, the patient will experience less
discomfort.

Coefficient of friction

Frictional force increases in direct proportion
to the force pushing two surfaces together. If
two surfaces are pushed together twice as
hard as before, the frictional force is twice its
previous value. Factors such as the nature of
the materials and the smoothness of the two
surfaces, plus the lubrication between these
surfaces, will influence the frictional force.
These factors are constant for any two particular surfaces and can be combined under
the collective constant known as the coefficient of friction (μ).

Frictional force = Coefficient of friction (μ)
                      $\times$ Applied force
                                       Eqn 15.7

The smaller the coefficient, μ, for a given
applied force the smaller the frictional force.
A smaller force is required to move an object
over a surface with a low coefficient of friction than over a surface with a high coefficient
of friction. EXAMPLES: Steel moving over
oiled steel, μ is 0.03, whereas bone moving
over bone lubricated with synovial fluid, μ
is 0.015. The coefficient of static friction is
greater than the coefficient of kinetic friction.

Lubrication lowers the friction between
two surfaces by keeping the peaks of one
surface from settling into the troughs of
another. The fluid also prevents pressure
welding at points of contact by introducing
a non-weldable point between the surfaces.
EXAMPLES: It is necessary to use lubricants
such as skin lotions and oils when rubbing
the skin, as rubbing without these lubricants
increases friction and causes pain. Baby
powder is used to decrease the friction between clothes and skin, thereby reducing
skin irritation and pain.

Friction and humans

Humans use friction to walk, as sliding
results when there is little friction. Try

walking on ice or a highly polished floor! The movement of blood through the vascular system is opposed by friction. This friction can be varied (19.4) to control blood supply to different regions of the body as the greater the friction or resistance to flow the slower the speed of blood.

Friction also has to be overcome between joint surfaces, between layers of tissue and around structures that slide on one another. EXAMPLES: A tendon and the bony prominence that it passes over. The body has several structures which are used to minimize friction:

1. Bursae. These fluid-filled sacs are frequently located at sites of wear. EXAMPLES: Between layers of muscle tissue and a tendon and beneath skin that moves across bony prominences.
2. Synovial Sheaths. These are tube-shaped structures that surround some tendons. They are lined with a synovial membrane which has a low coefficient of friction. EXAMPLES: Located on tendons passing through bony grooves.
3. Synovial Joints. These freely movable joints contain the lubricant synovial fluid enclosed within a synovial membrane. EXAMPLE: Knee joint.

Friction can also exert harmful effects on the body when the structures designed to minimize friction are altered or when the surface of the body is exposed to excessive abrasion. EXAMPLE: In bursitis excess fluid accumulates within the bursae, impairing their function and causing pain and tenderness.

15.6   Turning forces

Moments

The measure of the tendency of a force to rotate an object about a point is referred to as

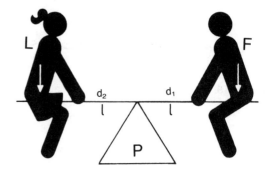

Figure 15.13   Representative diagram of a moment showing the force applied (F) to a lever (l) whereby a load (L) is moved about a pivot (P).

a **moment**. The point around which rotation occurs is called the fulcrum or pivot. The magnitude of a moment depends upon the size of the force and the distance perpendicular to its line of action from the pivot. Moments are involved in body movements to convert mechanical energy developed from muscle–bone combinations, into energy that is used to alter posture and move, or exert a force on other objects.

A **lever** is a bar which connects an object and a force. When a force is applied to the rigid bar rotation results. This force or effort is used to overcome a resistance or load on another part of the lever. The load has the tendency to rotate the lever in the opposite direction to the force (Figure 15.13). For equilibrium to occur the load or resistance must be exactly counterbalanced by the force or effort moments.

The tendency of a force to rotate an object is determined by taking the moments of that force, that is, by multiplying the magnitude of the force by the distance perpendicular to its line of action from the pivot.

There are three different ways of arranging the forces and pivot with respect to each other on a lever. Each of these types of lever is represented by bone–muscle combinations in the body.

All moments consist of a force applied to some point along a lever whereby a load is moved about a pivot (Figure 15.13).

Type 1 lever

The force and load are always located on opposite sides of the pivot. A seesaw is an example of a type 1 lever (Figure 15.13). The tendency of the boy to move the girl and vice versa is determined by multiplying the magnitude of the force, that is, their weight and their distance from the pivot. The boy and the girl will remain in a balanced state or equilibrium if the following exists:

Boy's weight × Distance from pivot =
Girl's weight × Distance from pivot
$$F \times d_1 = L \times d_2 \qquad \text{Eqn 15.8}$$

If the boy exerts a greater moment the girl is forced upwards.

A greater moment on the side of the force, rather than the side of the load, is required to move an object. When the magnitude of a force is sufficient to cause the load to rotate, the moments are known as **torque**. A clockwise rotation is a positive torque and an anti-clockwise a negative torque.

Type 2 lever

The load is located between the force and the pivot (Figure 15.14).

Type 3 lever

The force is located between the load and the pivot (Figure 15.15).

With all three types of levers, the greater the distance of the force from the load, the greater the load that can be moved. EXAMPLE: Using a crowbar (Figure 15.16).

Levers with multiple forces

In many situations involving movement and posture, several muscles may be using the

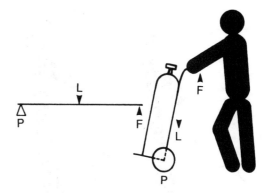

Figure 15.14 Type 2 levers have the load located between the pivot and force. When pushing a gas cylinder the wheel acts as the pivot and the gas cylinder as the load.

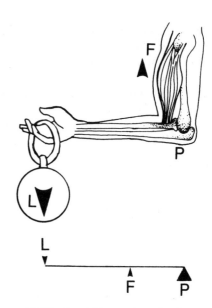

Figure 15.15 Type 3 levers have the force located between the load and the pivot. When holding a weight the biceps exert a force between the weight and the pivot or elbow.

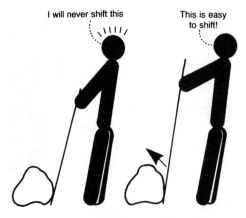

I will never shift this

This is easy to shift!

Figure 15.16   The greater the distance between load and force the greater is the effectiveness of that force.

same pivot. The resultant force is determined by calculating the moment for each individual force. Add any forces acting in the same direction and subtract any forces operating in the opposite direction to give the resultant force. The distance of the resultant force from the pivot is determined by dividing the sum of the individual moments by the resultant force.

15.7   Pulleys

A **pulley** consists of a grooved wheel on an axle, with a cord or rope passing along the groove. Pulleys are used to change the direction at which a force is acting. The body uses pulley systems to change the direction of force. EXAMPLE: The knuckles and tendons of the hands. Pulleys are also used in health care to change the direction of a force.

Application: Traction

Traction is the process in which the fractured ends of a bone are kept in position by a system of pulleys and weights (Figure 15.17). The force of gravity on the weights equals the body's opposition to the weights. This balance is important, and any adjustments should be made only after specific instructions have been given. Pulley systems are analysed by vector analysis.

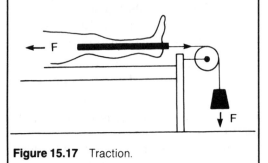

Figure 15.17   Traction.

15.8   Work

Work is the transfer of energy from one object to another. It is defined as the distance that an object is moved in the direction of a force, multiplied by the magnitude of that force.

Work = Force × Distance moved joules
Eqn 15.9

Note that time is not associated with work. A person who pushes a wheelchair from one end of a ward to another in several minutes will perform the same amount of work as a person who takes longer.

The SI unit for work is the joule (J).

The amount of energy used in performing

work does not equal the amount of work done, since some of the energy is converted into heat or other energy forms. Energy may also be used to overcome other forces such as friction. EXAMPLE: When pushing a wheelchair, additional energy is required to overcome friction. The greater the friction between the floor and the wheelchair, the greater is the extra energy required to move the wheelchair a given distance.

Efficient work is only performed when the force exerted on an object is in the same direction as the desired direction the object is to be moved. When the force is not in the desired direction an object is to be moved, some of the force that is being exerted will not contribute to the work being done. EXAMPLE: Pushing a wheelchair with a downward force (Figure 15.18).

15.9 Power

Power is the rate of doing work and is therefore different from both work and energy. The SI units for power are joules per second or watts. Since power is the rate of work being performed, the amount of work done per second determines the power. The faster a given amount of work is performed, the greater is the power.

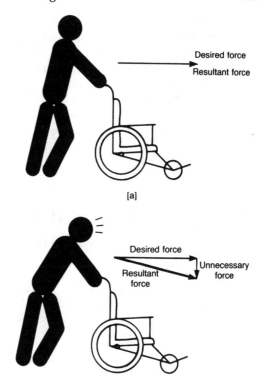

[a]

[b]

Figure 15.18 (a) The movement is in the same direction as the applied force.
(b) The pushing of the wheelchair with a downward motion results in the applied force containing a horizontal and a vertical vector. For a given distance more energy is used in (b) than in (a).

15.10 Mechanical advantage

Mechanical advantage is defined as the ratio of load to effort.

$$\text{Mechanical advantage} = \frac{\text{Size of load (L)}}{\text{Size of effort (E)}}$$
$$\text{Eqn 15.10}$$

With levers the equation is:

$$\frac{L}{E} = \frac{\text{Distance from pivot (e)}}{\text{Distance from pivot (l)}}$$
$$\text{Eqn 15.11}$$

The mechanical advantage in pulleys is equal to the number of ropes supporting the load. Mechanical advantage can be used to compare relative efficiencies of work. A large value for mechanical advantage implies that little effort is required to balance a large load or resistance. This is the principle behind the use of machines. Machines use mechanical advantage by multiplying the force so that loads can be moved with small effort. The mechanical advantage is a useful way of determining the maximum effectiveness of muscle actions. It is also useful for determining the mechanical disadvantages that occur when disabilities and incorrect posture alter correct muscle action.

thigh muscles, are now used to oppose the displaced centre of gravity. Not only are the wrong muscles used, but the relocation of the pivot substantially increases the effort required to lift a given weight, that is, using correct lifting techniques gives much greater mechanical advantage than using incorrect ones.

15.11   Environmental health and safety

Back injury is one of the major occupational injuries of health care professionals. The main cause of back injury is the incorrect lifting and moving of patients.

Application: Lifting

When lifting an object the powerful thigh muscles should be used rather than the back muscles. This is achieved by holding the object close to the body with the knees bent so that the person's centre of gravity does not shift substantially from the normal upright position. If the spine is kept straight during lifting, the large hip joints and knee joints act as the pivots, and the powerful thigh muscles provide the lifting force. When the spine is bent during lifting, the point of bending becomes the pivot, which can result in the discs between vertebrae being compressed and pressure being exerted on the spinal nerve. Moving the location of the pivot also alters the location of the centre of gravity. The relatively weak back muscles instead of the powerful

15.12   Elasticity

Elasticity is the property of matter that returns it to its original shape after a force has altered the shape. In the body, the elasticity of the lungs and arteries causes them to return to their original size after they have been stretched. There are four types of elasticity:

1. elasticity of compression — EXAMPLE: Rubber ball;
2. elasticity of extension — EXAMPLE: Rubber bands, elastic arteries, thoracic cage;
3. elasticity of torsion — EXAMPLE: The twist in a coiled spring, limited twisting of long bones;
4. elasticity of flexion — EXAMPLE: Bending a strip of steel, limited bending of long bones.

There is a limit to the elasticity of any piece of matter, and past this limit the material breaks. The limit depends on the individual elastic properties of the particular material. EXAMPLE: A piece of steel can be bent to a greater extent than an equal length of bone before it breaks.

Summary

Mechanics is the branch of science that is concerned with the motion and the maintenance of equilibrium of objects. The motion of objects in a specified direction is termed velocity. Acceleration occurs when velocity alters with time.

A force is any influence that changes the position, the state of rest or the motion of an object. Since force has direction and magnitude it is an example of a vector. Several forces may constitute a net force. The net or resultant force is determined by adding or subtracting the individual forces.

Gravity is a force of attraction between objects. The large mass of the earth pulls objects to it. Gravity exerts its net effect at the centre of gravity of an object. Equilibrium exists when an opposing force acts through the centre of gravity. The greater the boundaries of action or base of support of the opposing force, the greater is the stability of the object.

Friction is a force that resists the movement of one object over another. The amount of friction is dependent upon the coefficient of friction, that is, the nature of the materials, the smoothness of the surfaces and the lubrication between them.

The measure of the tendency of a force to rotate an object about a point is referred to as a moment. Three arrangements exist by which a force can rotate an object. These are known as type 1, type 2 and type 3 levers.

Work is the transfer of energy from one object to another. It equals the force applied by the distance moved. The rate of performing work is termed power. Mechanical advantage is the ratio of load to effort. It can be used to compare the relative efficiencies of work.

The relationship between moving objects is explained in Newton's laws of motion.

The direction in which a force is acting can be changed with the use of pulleys. This process is used in traction.

Elasticity is the property of matter that returns it to its original shape after a force has altered its shape.

Unit Six
The Composition and Properties of Fluids

In this unit the properties of fluids are integrated and applied to medications, normal and abnormal body function and safety. You will learn how these properties influence the composition of body fluids.

Chapter 16

Biological role of acids and bases

At the completion of this chapter the student should be able to:

1. describe the properties of acids and bases;
2. explain the mechanism of buffer systems;
3. describe the acid–base homeostatic mechanisms;
4. differentiate between the various acid–based imbalances;
5. explain how the body compensates for acid–base imbalance.

Various ions occur in body fluid. The properties of these ions are important in determining body function. Some of these ions can be formed in the body. In this chapter the formation and regulation of H^+ and OH^- is discussed. These ions exist in a homogeneous mixture or solution (17.2).

16.1 Acids

What is an acid?

Acids can be both useful and harmful (Table 16.1), and are continually manufactured in the body as a result of metabolism (Table 16.2). A homeostatic mechanism regulates these acids since abnormal variations in serum concentration of acids will cause a marked alteration of external respiration (breathing). The corrosive property of acids can be both beneficial and harmful. The stomach uses this property beneficially in the process of gastric digestion. The caustic nature of acids can result in harmful burns to tissue that has been exposed to an acid spillage.

An **acid** is a substance that releases H^+ ions into a solution, the greater the number of H^+ ions the more acidic is that solution. When an acid is placed in solution only a proportion of the H^+ ions are released into the solvent. **Dissociation** is the breakdown of a substance into ions when that substance is placed in a solvent. A strong acid releases most of its H^+ ions and thus mostly dissociates into H^+ ions and anions (Eqn 16.1).

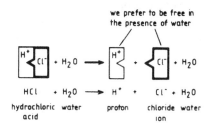

Eqn 16.1

Table 16.1 Common acids both useful and harmful to patients

Acid/medication	Effect
Acetyl salicylic	Anti-prostaglandin
Benzoic	Anti-fungal agent and germicide
Ethacrynic	Powerful diuretic effective in promoting sodium and chloride secretion
Hydrochloric	Harmful, causes burns
Hypochlorous	Disinfectant and bleaching agent, its salts are used as surgical solutions, e.g. sodium hypochlorite
Lactic	Anti-wart agent
Nitric	Harmful, causes burns
Sulphuric	Harmful, causes burns

Table 16.2 Summary of acids that are used by the body

Acid	Function
Acetoacetic	Ketone body produced during fat and protein breakdown; excessive formation results in ketoacidosis
Amino	Building blocks of protein
Ascorbic	Promotes many metabolic reactions; may combine with poisons rendering them harmless
Carbonic	Involved in the regulation of pH
Cholic	Most abundant bile acid; forms salts that assist in the digestion of lipids
Deoxyribonucleic (DNA)	Carrier of genetic information
Fatty	Important in triglyceride (neutral fat) and phospholipid structure
Folic	Vitamin that is essential for the normal production of red and white blood cells
Hyaluronic	Important interstitial chemical
Hydrochloric	Important digestive agent in gastric juice
Lactic	Waste product of anaerobic carbohydrate breakdown
Ribonucleic (RNA)	Transmits genetic information from DNA to protein-forming system of the cell
Uric	Breakdown product of nucleus metabolism and causes gout

The arrow indicates that most of the HCl has been converted into H^+ and Cl^-. A weak acid only dissociates to a limited extent, with most of the hydrogen atoms being retained by the weak acid (Eqn 16.2).

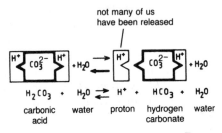

$$H_2CO_3 + H_2O \rightleftharpoons H^+ + HCO_3^- + H_2O$$

carbonic   water   proton   hydrogen   water
acid   carbonate

Eqn 16.2

The two arrows indicate that a chemical balance of fixed proportion exists between the concentration of carbonic acid and its dissociation products. The two dissociation products can also be combined to form the weak acid. Any increase in the H^+ ion and HCO_3^- ion concentrations will alter the chemical balance or equilibrium. This imbalance is returned to the correct proportions by the formation of the necessary concentration of carbonic acid.

Hydrogen consists of one proton and one electron. When an electron is removed H^+ is formed which is a single proton. Since an acid donates H^+ ions it therefore, in effect, is a proton donor (Figure 16.1). These free protons are responsible for the properties of an acid.

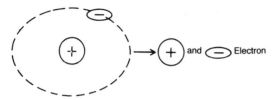

Figure 16.1 Hydrogen consists of a proton (H^+) and an electron.

General properties

Taste

An acid has a sour taste. EXAMPLE: Citric acid causes the sour taste in lemons and grapefruit.

Indicator change

Acids change the colour of substances called indicators. EXAMPLE: Blue litmus indicator changes to red in the presence of an acid.

Reaction with bases

Acids combine with bases to produce water and a salt. This process is called neutralization. EXAMPLE: Hydrochloric acid combines with sodium hydroxide to produce water and sodium chloride (Eqn 16.3).

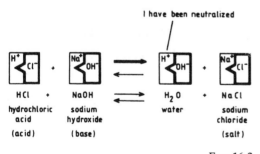

HCl	NaOH	H₂0	NaCl
hydrochloric acid	sodium hydroxide	water	sodium chloride
(acid)	(base)		(salt)

Eqn 16.3

Corrosiveness

Acids are corrosive to body tissue. The stronger the acid the greater is the corrosive effect on tissue.

Application: Gastric ulcers

Excessive production of hydrochloric acid by cells lining the stomach results in an increase in the gastric acidity. Over a period of time an elevated gastric acidity can lead to the formation of a gastric ulcer. This is a hole eaten into the stomach wall. These ulcers can also result from a localized loss of the protective mucous barrier that lines the gastric wall.

Reaction with carbonates

Acids react with carbonates to form carbon dioxide, water and salts.

Application: Gastric antacids

Sodium bicarbonate (baking powder, bicarbonate of soda) is administered to counteract excess stomach acidity. The combination of sodium bicarbonate and hydrochloric acid produces sodium chloride and carbonic acid (Eqn 16.4).

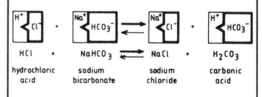

HCl	NaHCO₃	NaCl	H₂CO₃
hydrochloric acid	sodium bicarbonate	sodium chloride	carbonic acid

Eqn 16.4

Carbonic acid is a weak acid and thus it releases only a small quantity of H^+. In Eqn 16.1 a strong acid has been replaced by a weak acid. A decrease in free H^+ ions has resulted in a lower acidity. Carbonic acid breaks down to form water and carbon dioxide. (Eqn 16.5). This equation is also reversible

---

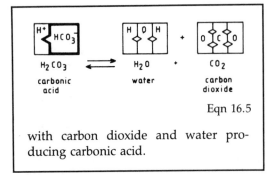

$$H_2CO_3 \rightleftharpoons H_2O + CO_2$$

carbonic   water   carbon
acid   dioxide

Eqn 16.5

with carbon dioxide and water producing carbonic acid.

16.2   Bases

What is a base?

Bases are used in the body for neutralizing
any increases in acidity. They are a component of the homeostatic mechanism that
regulates the acidity of body fluids. Water-
soluble bases are called alkalis. The terms
'basic solutions' and 'alkaline solutions' are
generally interchangeable.

A **base** is a substance that donates hydroxyl
ions (OH^-) or accepts H^+ ions from a
solution. A strong base donates relatively
large quantities of OH^- or accepts many H^+
ions. That is, the strength of a base depends
upon the degree of dissociation.

General properties

Taste

Bases have a bitter metallic taste.

Indicator change

Bases change the colour of substances called
indicators. EXAMPLE: Red litmus paper
changes to blue in the presence of a base.

Reaction with acids

Bases neutralize acids by removing protons
from solution. This is achieved by combining
the proton with an OH^- ion (Eqn 16.6) or
another anion (Eqn 16.7).

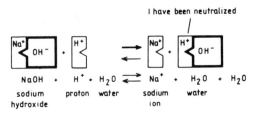

$$NaOH + H^+ + H_2O \rightleftharpoons Na^+ + H_2O + H_2O$$

sodium   proton water   sodium   water
hydroxide   ion

Eqn 16.6

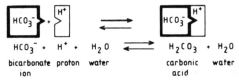

$$HCO_3^- + H^+ + H_2O \rightleftharpoons H_2CO_3 + H_2O$$

bicarbonate proton water   carbonic   water
ion   acid

Eqn 16.7

Corrosiveness

Strong bases such as sodium hydroxide
(NaOH) are corrosive to body tissue. They
can also react with fats and dissolve proteins.

16.3   Measurement of H^+ and OH^-

Whenever the number of H^+ ions and OH^-
ions is equal, a neutral solution exists. When
the H^+ ion concentration is greater than the
concentration of OH^- ions the solution is
acidic. Solutions that contain a greater concentration of OH^- ions than H^+ ions are
basic solutions.

In one litre of pure water, 10^{-7} moles of
water is dissociated into H^+ ions and OH^-
ions (Eqn 16.8).

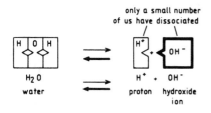

only a small number
of us have dissociated

H$_2$O
water

proton   hydroxide
ion

Eqn 16.8

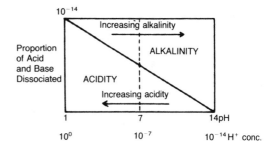

Figure 16.2 Relationship between pH and the concentration of H$^+$ and OH$^-$ ions. The total number of H$^+$ and OH$^-$ ions is constant, and at pH 7 the number of H$^+$ and OH$^-$ ions is equal.

Pure water is a neutral solution since it contains 10^{-7} moles of H$^+$ ions and 10^{-7} moles of OH$^-$ ions. In water, a balance exists between the proportion of H$^+$ ions and OH$^-$ ions for any given acid or base. The properties of water are such that the minimum concentration of H$^+$ ions and OH$^-$ ions is 10^{-14} mol/L. The maximum concentration of H$^+$ ions and OH$^-$ ions is 1 mole or 10^0, that is, the dissociation properties of water restrict the concentration of H$^+$ ions and OH$^-$ ions to the range of 10^{-14} to 10^0 mol/L.

A scale of acidity and alkalinity has been devised that uses the range of 10^{-14} to 10^0 mol/L of H$^+$ and OH$^-$ ions. The addition of H$^+$ ions to pure water results in a proportionate decrease in OH$^-$ ions from the initial concentration of 10^{-7} mol/L. A H$^+$ ion concentration of 10^{-6} mol/L results in a OH$^-$ concentration of 10^{-8} mol/L, whereas a H$^+$ ion concentration of 10^{-3} mol/L results in a OH$^-$ concentration of 10^{-11} mol/L. Note that in both these examples the combination of the powers of ten totals -14. The combination of the powers of ten for H$^+$ ions and OH$^-$ ions will always equal -14.

The pH scale represents the powers of ten of H$^+$ ions from 10^{-14} to 10^0 mol/L. For convenience, this scale uses positive numbers and expresses them as pH 14 to pH 0 (Figure 16.2). At pH 7 an equal number of H$^+$ ions and OH$^-$ ions occur. Solutions with a pH lower than 7 are acids and those with a pH greater than 7 are bases.

In blood the physiologically normal pH range is 7.35 to 7.45. A blood pH lower than 7.35 is considered acidic whereas a pH greater than 7.45 is alkaline, either of which can have a serious effect on body function.

A change of one pH unit differs in the number of H$^+$ ions gained or lost when compared with another pH unit.

EXAMPLE:
pH 8 contains 10^{-8} mol/L H$^+$ or 10 nmol
pH 7 contains 10^{-7} mol/L H$^+$ or 100 nmol
pH 6 contains 10^{-6} mol/L H$^+$ or 1000 nmol

A change from pH 7 to pH 8 represents $100 - 10 = 90$ nmol, whereas a change from pH 6 to pH 7 is $1000 - 100 = 900$ nmol.

Every change in a pH unit represents a tenfold change in H$^+$ ion concentration. An alteration of pH from pH 7.4 to 7.3 results in a doubling of the H$^+$ ion concentration. A small change in pH indicates a very significant alteration in H$^+$ ion concentration. The pH scale actually represents a logarithmic scale and not a linear scale. The H$^+$ ion concentration can also be expressed in nmol/L. This is a linear scale with pH 7 being 100 nmol/L, pH 6 = 1000 nmol/L and pH 8 = 10 nmol/L.

16.4 Buffers

Buffers are chemicals that resist changes in pH on addition of acids or bases. They act by replacing a strong acid or base with a weak one, that is, a stronger acid is replaced by a weaker acid. Since a weak acid releases only a small number of H^+ ions then the formation of a weak acid effectively removes most of the H^+ ions that were present with a strong acid (Eqn 16.9). EXAMPLE: Lactic acid (strong acid) is replaced by a carbonic acid (weak acid) thereby reducing the number of free H^+ ions in solution.

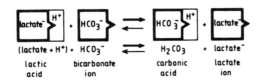

(lactate + H⁺) + HCO₃⁻ ⇌ H₂CO₃ + lactate⁻
lactic   bicarbonate   carbonic   lactate
acid   ion   acid   ion

Eqn 16.9

Application: Hydrogen carbonate/carbonic acid buffer

In the hydrogen carbonate/carbonic acid buffer system bicarbonate combines with excess H^+ ions whereas carbonic acid combines with excess OH^- ions. When excess H^+ ions are added to the blood they may combine with the hydrogen carbonate ion to form carbonic acid, which is a weak acid and thus does not release H^+ ions readily (Eqn 16.7). Removing the majority of H^+ ions results in the blood retaining its original pH. Addition of OH^- ions to the blood can cause carbonic acid to combine with it and form hydrogen carbonate ions (Eqn 16.10). The removal of excess hydroxyl ions results in the blood retaining its original pH.

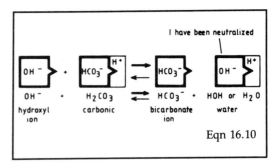

OH⁻ + HCO₃⁻ ⇌ HCO₃⁻   OH⁻

OH⁻ + H₂CO₃ ⇌ HCO₃⁻ + HOH or H₂O
hydroxyl   carbonic   bicarbonate water
ion   ion

Eqn 16.10

Buffers are used by the body to maintain very narrow pH ranges of body fluids (Table 16.3). These narrow ranges are necessary since biochemical reactions are extremely sensitive to changes in H^+ ion concentration. The pH at which biochemical regulators or enzymes function will vary for different enzymes. An enzyme that operates in the highly acidic stomach cannot function effectively in the alkaline small intestine. Also, the elimination of carbon dioxide and the transport of oxygen are dependent upon blood pH; small variations result in marked alterations in the amount of carbon dioxide

Table 16.3 The narrow pH range within fluids, and the diversity of pH between different fluids

Body fluid	Locality	pH
Cerebrospinal fluid	Associated with the central nervous system	7.4
Blood	Vascular system	7.35–7.45
Bile	Gall bladder and bile duct	7.6–8.6
Gastric juice	Stomach	1.2–3.0
Intestinal juice	Small intestine	7.6–7.8
Pancreatic juice	Pancreas	7.1–8.2
Saliva	Mouth	6.5–7.5
Semen	Vas deferens	7.35–7.50
Urine	Bladder	5.5–7.5
Vaginal fluid	Vagina	5.2

removed by the lungs. Buffers are needed to counteract the non-stop production of acids. These acids mainly result from the breakdown of carbohydrates, fats and proteins. EXAMPLES: Lactic acid and ketone bodies.

16.5 Acid–base balance

Body-fluid buffers

Carbonic acid–hydrogen carbonate buffer system

This buffer system is important in the regulation of pH changes that result from alterations in blood carbon dioxide levels. The relationship between carbon dioxide and this buffer system is shown in Eqn 16.11.

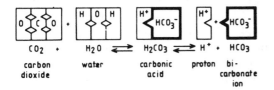

$$CO_2 + H_2O \rightleftharpoons H_2CO_3 \rightleftharpoons H^+ + HCO_3$$

carbon dioxide | water | carbonic acid | proton | bi-carbonate ion

Eqn 16.11

Carbon dioxide combines with water to produce carbonic acid. This is a weak acid and thus a small proportion of the acid is dissociated into H^+ ions and HCO_3^- ions.

The bicarbonate and carbonic acid buffer system acts in the following way. Factors that elevate the H^+ ion concentration cause a proportionate release of HCO_3^- ions. HCO_3^- combines with excess H^+ ions to produce carbonic acid (Eqn 16.7). Excess carbonic acid dissociates into carbon dioxide and water which is removed by the lungs. Production of excess OH^- ions results in carbonic acid releasing a proportionate quantity of H^+

ions to neutralize the excess OH^- ions (Eqn 16.10).

The body tends to acidify the blood and thus needs more HCO_3^- than carbonic acid. It is necessary to have a proportion of one carbonic acid molecule to twenty HCO_3^- ions (1.2 mmol/L : 24 mmol/L) if the pH of the blood is to remain in the normal range. Alterations to this ratio will result in a proportionate change in the relative concentration of carbonic acid and HCO_3^- so that the chemical equilibrium ratio is returned. Therefore, any factor that causes an increase in the ratio of carbonic acid to HCO_3^- indicates a greater acidity, since a greater amount of HCO_3^- has been used to remove the excess H^+ ions. Thus a greater proportion of carbonic acid has been formed. To overcome an increase in acidity, HCO_3^- is administered to a patient so that the proportion of carbonic acid to HCO_3^- is returned to the ratio of one to twenty.

Whenever a buffering reaction occurs, the concentration of one chemical in the buffer pair is increased while a decreased concentration results in the other. An elevated carbonic acid concentration results from a decreased HCO_3^- concentration.

In summary, HCO_3^- soaks up excess H^+ ions and carbonic acid soaks up excess OH^- so that the pH is maintained at normal levels. The excess carbonic acid can be eliminated by the lungs in the form of carbon dioxide and water vapour.

Phosphate buffer system

This buffer system consists of an acid phosphate, $H_2PO_4^-$ and an alkaline phosphate, HPO_4^{2-}. Addition of H^+ converts the alkaline phosphate into the weak acid phosphate. Likewise, addition of OH^- results in alkaline phosphate formation.

The phosphate buffer system is an important control mechanism in red blood cells, kidney tubular fluid and cellular contents. In

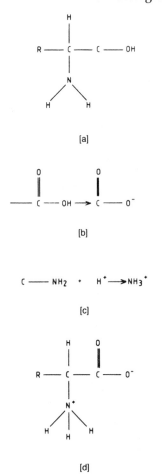

Figure 16.3 (a) General structure of an amino acid. (b) Carboxyl group acts as an acid by releasing H^+ ions. (c) Amine group acts as a base by accepting H^+ ions. (d) The net result is an internal self-neutralization and the formation of a zwitterion.

kidney tubules excess H^+ ions combine with HPO_4^{2-} to form the weak acid $H_2PO_4^-$ which is then excreted.

Protein buffer system

This is the most abundant buffer in cells and plasma. Proteins consist of chains of amino acids (30.2). The general structure of an amino acid is shown in Figure 16.3a. These acids consist of a weak acid group called the carboxyl group (Figure 16.3b) and a base structure known as the amine group (Figure 16.3c). The carboxyl group donates its proton to the amine group forming a **zwitterion**. This is a covalent compound containing positive and negative ionic regions (Figure 16.3d). When amino acids exist as zwitterions they can function as buffers. When excess H^+ ions are present the COO^- combines with the H^+ (Figure 16.4).

Addition of excess OH^- ions results in the release of H^+ from the amine group to combine with the OH^- ions to form water (Figure 16.4).

Ammonia–ammonium buffer system

This buffer system is used by the kidneys to eliminate H^+ ions from the body. Amino acids such as glutamine are broken down to form the base ammonia (NH_3). This base combines with excess H^+ ions to form the weak acid ammonium (NH_4^+) which combines with Cl^- to form ammonium chloride (NH_4Cl). Removal of ammonium chloride in the urine results in the removal of H^+ ions without the need for a high urine acidity.

Haemoglobin buffer system

In red blood cells carbon dioxide and water are converted to carbonic acid by the action of an enzyme. The H^+ ions released by this acid combine with a base known as reduced haemoglobin (Figure 16.5). When haemoglobin loses oxygen it is called reduced haemoglobin. The formation of a weaker acid than carbonic acid results in a lower concentration of H^+ ions within the red blood cells. Reduced haemoglobin soaks up most of the H^+ ions released by carbonic acid and in turn fewer H^+ ions are donated to the intracellular fluid. Hence fewer H^+ ions have been added to the intracellular fluid than

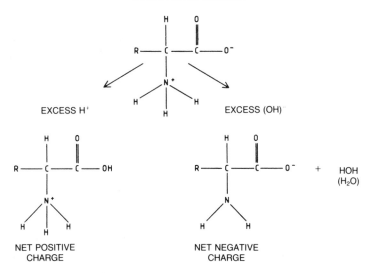

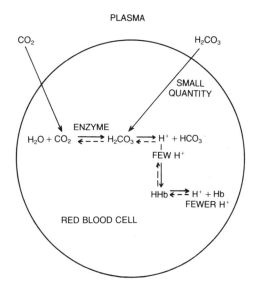

Figure 16.4 An individual zwitterion acts as either an acid buffer or a base buffer according to the relative concentration of H^+ and OH^- ions present in solution.

PLASMA

would have been added without an additional buffer.

The presence of large quantities of oxygen promotes the loss of H^+ ions from haemoglobin. In pulmonary capillaries the high oxygen concentrations convert reduced haemoglobin into oxygenated haemoglobin or oxyhaemoglobin. Since H^+ ions are released more readily with oxyhaemoglobin than with reduced haemoglobin, the former is therefore a stronger acid than reduced haemoglobin.

The H^+ ions released in the presence of high oxygen concentrations are buffered by hydrogen carbonate to form carbonic acid. This acid breaks down to carbon dioxide and water. The carbon dioxide moves into the blood and subsequently into the lungs (Figure 16.6).

In summary, the haemoglobin buffer system is important in both the regulation of blood pH as it passes through the tissues and

Figure 16.5 The buffering of carbonic acid by reduced haemoglobin (Hb) results in the addition of fewer H^+ ions to the red blood cell intracellular fluid. A small quantity of carbonic acid originates from the plasma and the removal of this acid results in a lower H^+ ion concentration in the blood.

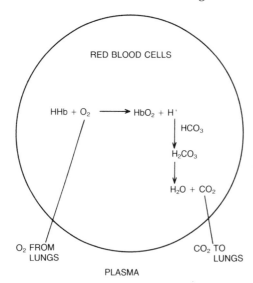

O₂ FROM LUNGS

PLASMA

CO₂ TO LUNGS

RED BLOOD CELLS

$HHb + O_2 \longrightarrow HbO_2 + H^+$

HCO_3

H_2CO_3

$H_2O + CO_2$

Figure 16.6   The influence of oxygen on reduced haemoglobin (HHb) to form the stronger acid oxyhaemoglobin (HbO₂). The subsequent release of H⁺ ions is buffered by bicarbonate to form carbonic acid. This acid is broken down to water and carbon dioxide with the carbon dioxide being released to the lungs.

the release of carbon dioxide in the pulmonary capillaries.

Respiratory regulation

An increase in cell respiration effects an elevation of serum carbon dioxide concentration which results in an increase in acidity (Eqn 16.11).

Removal of carbon dioxide by breathing results in an alteration of the chemical balance in Eqn 16.11. The net effect of breathing is that elimination of carbon dioxide results in a proportionate decrease of carbonic acid, H⁺ and hydrogen carbonate ion as these substances are converted to carbon dioxide, water and carbonic acid.

Alterations in breathing rate can greatly influence the pH of the blood since alterations in carbon dioxide elimination change serum H⁺ ion concentration. Doubling the breathing rate effects an increase in pH by 0.23 units whereas reducing the breathing rate by a quarter results in a pH decrease of 0.4. From Eqn 16.11 we see that an increase in serum carbon dioxide causes an elevation of H⁺ ions whereas a decrease in serum carbon dioxide results in a decrease in H⁺ ions.

Eqn 16.11 also shows why H⁺ ion concentration influences ventilation rates. The greater the acidity in blood the greater is the need for the body to remove these excess H⁺ ions. The more carbon dioxide that is eliminated by the lungs, the greater is the amount of H⁺ ions and hydrogen carbonate that is converted to carbonic acid. The carbonic acid is then converted to carbon dioxide and water, so that the relative concentration of each substance returns to normal proportions. Thus the effect of increased acidity is to increase the levels of carbon dioxide.

Removal of the excess carbon dioxide occurs by an increase in ventilation rates (hyperventilation). High blood acid levels stimulate an increase in ventilation rates. Likewise, a decrease in serum H⁺ concentration requires the retention of carbon dioxide by slowing the breathing rate (hypoventilation). The buildup of carbon dioxide results in a proportion of it being converted to carbonic acid, H⁺ and hydrogen carbonate.

The sensitivity of the respiratory rate to changes in pH is such that the ventilation rate is approximately doubled if the pH decreases by 0.1 units, and halved if the pH increases by 0.1 units.

In summary, hyperventilation decreases carbon dioxide and thus H⁺ ions, whereas hypoventilation increases carbon dioxide and thus H⁺ ions (Figure 16.7). The rate of respiration stabilizes the carbonic acid to hydrogen carbonate ratio by altering the rate

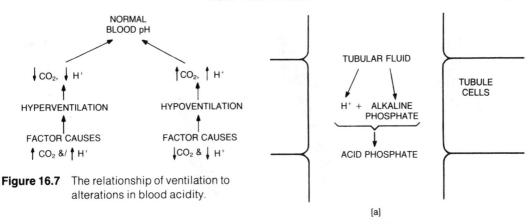

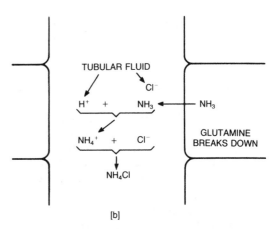

Figure 16.7 The relationship of ventilation to alterations in blood acidity.

of ventilation so that the proportion of one carbonic acid to twenty hydrogen carbonate ions is maintained.

Renal regulation

The kidneys serve two important functions in H^+ ion homeostasis:

1. They reabsorb hydrogen carbonate from the urine to the blood. This prevents the loss of hydrogen carbonate and the subsequent alteration of the carbonic acid/hydrogen carbonate buffer system.
2. They counteract a rise in serum H^+ concentration by secreting the excess H^+ ions in the form of weak acids of the phosphate and ammonium buffer systems. Acids such as sulphuric, uric and keto acids which cannot be removed by the lungs are eliminated.

Kidney cells effect both of these functions by the following mechanisms. The kidney tubule cells are sensitive to changes in blood pH. Within these cells a decrease in pH accelerates the conversion of carbon dioxide and water into H^+ and hydrogen carbonate. The hydrogen carbonate is released into the blood and assists in returning the blood pH back to normal levels.

Figure 16.8 Mechanisms involved in regulation of elevated H^+ ion concentration in tubular fluid. (a) Elevated levels of acidity are buffered by phosphate. (b) A substantial increase in H^+ ion concentration requires the ammonia buffer system.

H^+ ions are secreted into the kidney tubular fluid. This fluid contains alkaline phosphate which combines with the excess H^+ ions to form a weak acid called acid phosphate. The effective removal of most of the H^+ ions returns the urine pH to normal levels (Figure 16.8a).

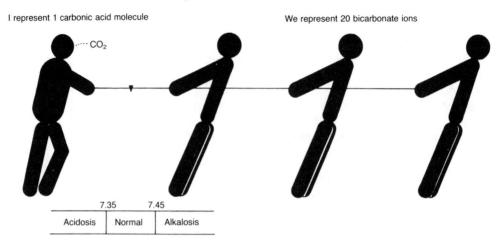

I represent 1 carbonic acid molecule

We represent 20 bicarbonate ions

CO_2

7.35	7.45
Acidosis	Normal	Alkalosis

Figure 16.9 To maintain the normal blood pH range of 7.35 to 7.45 a ratio of 1 $H_2CO_3 : 20\ HCO_3^-$ is required.

When acidity increases substantially in the tubular fluid, the tubule cells form ammonia (NH_3) by breaking down the amino acid glutamine. The ammonia is secreted into the tubular fluid where it combines with H^+ ions to form the weak acid NH_4^+. The NH_4^+ combines with Cl^- to form NH_4Cl or ammonium chloride (Figure 16.8b).

When H^+ ion concentration decreases, large quantities of bicarbonate are not reabsorbed. Thus the ratio of serum carbonic acid to bicarbonate is returned to normal since bicarbonate levels are lowered.

16.6 Acid–base imbalance

Acidosis occurs when the serum pH value falls below 7.35. There are two forms of acidosis called respiratory acidosis and metabolic acidosis. Acidosis depresses the central nervous system, and, if it remains uncorrected, will result in a decreased mental capacity, delirium, coma and death.

Alkalosis exists at serum pH levels greater than 7.45. As with acidosis, there are two forms of alkalosis called respiratory alkalosis and metabolic alkalosis. In this pH imbalance, the nervous system becomes overexcited. Failure to correct this disorder results in muscle spasm, convulsions and eventually death.

Respiratory acidosis

This results from any condition that decreases the removal of carbon dioxide by the lungs, that is, the removal of carbon dioxide does not keep pace with its production. Elevated arterial carbon dioxide concentration causes a rise in blood H^+ ion concentration. Decreased carbon dioxide removal results from chronic respiratory diseases such as pneumonia and emphysema. In addition, drug abuse such as excess morphine therapy and barbiturate poisoning can diminish respiratory function and therefore carbon dioxide removal. Arterial carbon dioxide can also increase as a result of impaired pulmonary circulation.

Elevated arterial carbon dioxide results in an increased carbonic acid and subsequently

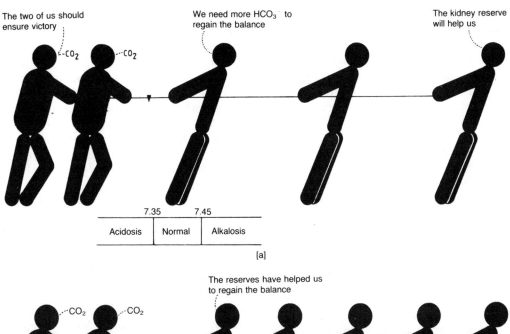

The two of us should
ensure victory

We need more HCO₃ to
regain the balance

The kidney reserve
will help us

[a]

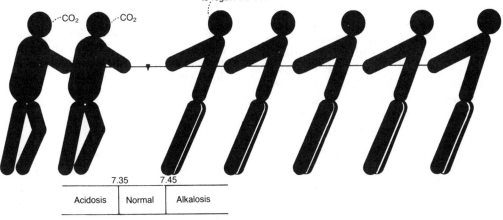

The reserves have helped us
to regain the balance

[b]

Figure 16.10 Respiratory acidosis.
(a) Uncompensated respiratory acidosis results in elevated CO_2 and H_2CO_3. The ratio of $H_2CO_3 : HCO_3^-$ is now $2:20$.
(b) Compensated respiratory acidosis results in increased CO_2, H_2CO_3 and HCO_3^-. The ratio of $H_2CO_3 : HCO_3^-$ is now $2:40$, that is $1:20$.

hydrogen carbonate level (Eqn 16.11). The hydrogen carbonate (bicarbonate) is increased so that the proportion of carbonic acid to hydrogen carbonate is returned to its normal buffering capacity of one to twenty (Figure 16.9). Thus over a period of time the body compensates for the elevated carbonic acid by stimulating the kidneys to release an increased quantity of hydrogen carbonate ion. At the onset of respiratory acidosis the ratio may have changed from one:twenty to two:twenty (Figure 16.10a). The kidneys respond to this acidosis by releasing hydrogen carbonate ions until the ratio is once again one to twenty, that is, over one to two days the hydrogen carbonate ion concentration increases so that the ratio is two to forty (Figure 16.10b). Compensation therefore effects an increased blood hydrogen carbonate level.

Metabolic acidosis

Metabolic acidosis results from an abnormal increase in acidic metabolic products other than carbon dioxide. The acidosis may be caused by:

1. an inability of the kidneys to eliminate the dietary H^+ ion load due to renal disorders;
2. elevated H^+ ion load due to diseases such as diabetes mellitus, starvation, excess lactic acid production due to insufficient oxygen supply or ingestion of salicylates;
3. excessive hydrogen carbonate loss occurring in renal tubular failure where hydrogen carbonate reabsorption is diminished, and also severe diarrhoea since large amounts of sodium bicarbonate are lost in the gastrointestinal contents.

The accumulated metabolic acids react with bicarbonate in the extracellular fluid to form carbonic acid, that is, the ratio of carbonic acid to bicarbonate is altered such that a greater proportion of carbonic acid is formed. This change in the buffering capacity results in a lower blood pH. The decreased pH stimulates hyperventilation or increased breathing rate which effects a greater removal of carbon dioxide from the lungs. Increased carbon dioxide levels, according to Eqn 16.11, lower the concentration of carbonic acid in the blood. If the carbonic acid is reduced sufficiently, the ratio of carbonic acid to hydrogen carbonate will return to normal. Figure 16.11a shows a change in the ratio during metabolic acidosis of one carbonic acid to ten hydrogen carbonate ions.

Increased breathing rates reduce the blood carbonic acid concentration to a level such that the ratio is returned to normal, that is, carbonic acid concentration is decreased so that the ratio of carbonic acid to hydrogen carbonate is 0.5:10, which is effectively 1:20. A respiratory compensation has maintained the carbonic acid/hydrogen carbonate ion buffer system, and thus near normal pH, but at the expense of decreased hydrogen carbonate (Figure 16.11b).

When the production of acid is too great for the compensatory mechanisms, the blood pH falls causing disturbances to the nervous system. In summary, compensated metabolic acidosis has low levels of blood hydrogen carbonate and carbon dioxide along with a normal pH, whereas uncompensated metabolic acidosis has a decreased blood hydrogen carbonate and pH but a normal arterial carbon dioxide level. Metabolic acidosis is treated by correcting the factors causing the imbalance, plus administration of sodium bicarbonate.

Respiratory alkalosis

Respiratory alkalosis results from hyperventilation removing excessive quantities of carbon dioxide. A decrease in blood carbon dioxide and carbonic acid levels results. The carbonic acid to hydrogen carbonate ratio is altered, with the carbonic acid decreasing with respect to the hydrogen carbonate. A ratio of 0.5:20 indicates that a relative excess of hydrogen carbonate ions exist (Figure 16.12a).

Body compensatory mechanisms or treatment may adjust the pH to normal levels by returning the carbonic acid to bicarbonate ratio to 1:20 (Figure 16.12b). This ratio can be achieved by either decreasing the concentration of hydrogen carbonate (0.5:10) or by increasing the carbonic acid concentration (1:20). Some causes of hyperventilation are

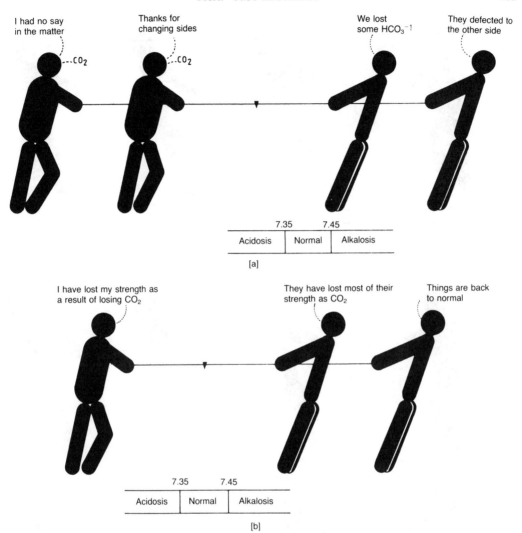

Figure 16.11 (a) Metabolic acidosis results in a decreased HCO_3^- concentration and an elevated H_2CO_3 concentration. The ratio of $H_2CO_3:HCO_3^-$ is now $1:10$. (b) Compensation occurs by removal of the excess H_2CO_3 as CO_2. The ratio of $H_2CO_3:HCO_3^-$ is $0.5:10$, that is $1:20$.

hysteria, anxiety, high fever, aspirin overdose, hypoxia, brain injury and excessive artificial ventilation.

Metabolic alkalosis

Metabolic alkalosis results from a decreased H^+ ion concentration or an elevated bicarbonate ion concentration. Two causes of this imbalance are the loss of acid due to vomiting

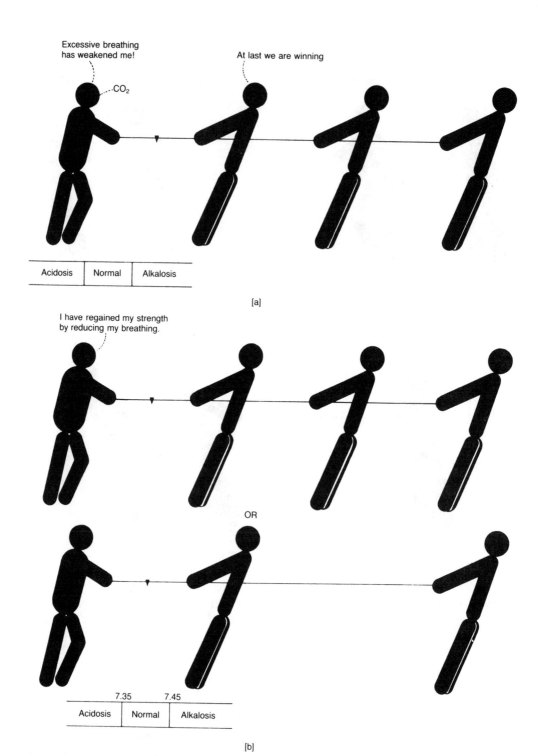

Figure 16.12 Respiratory alkalosis. (a) Hyperventilation causes decreased blood CO_2 and H_2CO_3 levels. The $H_2O_3 : HCO_3^-$ ratio is 0.5:20. (b) Compensation can occur by either returning the H_2CO_3 level to normal or by proportionally decreasing the HCO_3^- concentration.

of gastric juice and the ingestion of large amounts of antacids for indigestion relief.

The relative excess of bicarbonate may be compensated by decreasing carbon dioxide removal by the lungs and thus increasing carbonic acid in the blood. Elevating carbonic acid will alter the alkalotic state by returning the carbonic acid: hydrogen carbonate ratio from an excess of hydrogen carbonate ions (1:40) to the normal ratio of 2:40 or 1:20 (Figure 16.13). The kidneys assist this compensation by excreting excess hydrogen carbonate ions.

Metabolic alkalosis can also result from a decrease in blood K^+ concentration. EXAMPLE: A decrease in K^+ concentration can result from the use of diuretics such as frusemide (lasix, frusid) and ethacrynic acid (edecril). In these cases administration of K^+ is prescribed.

16.7   Environmental health and safety

Acids are corrosive chemicals that can damage human tissue. Acid vapours can damage the respiratory tract (16.6).

Care must be exercised when handling strong acids such as concentrated hydrochloric acid (HCl), sulphuric acid (H_2SO_4) and nitric acid (HNO_3). Acid burns require the spilt acid to be diluted with copious quantities of water. This dilution is followed by a neutralization of the acid with, for example, sodium bicarbonate.

Summary

An acid is a substance that releases H^+ into a solution. The greater the number of H^+ in a solution, the greater is the acidity of that solution. A base is a substance that donates OH^- or accepts H^+. Neutralization of an acid solution is achieved by adding a base to the solution.

The pH scale is used as a relative indicator of acidity and alkalinity. Acidic solutions have a pH range of 1 to 7 whereas alkaline solutions have a pH range from 7 to 14. At pH 7 a solution is regarded as neutral. In blood, the normal physiological pH range is 7.35 to 7.45.

Buffers are chemicals that resist changes in pH on the addition of acids or bases. They act by replacing a strong acid or base with a weak acid or base. The major buffer systems involved in acid–base balance are:

1. Carbonic acid/hydrogen carbonate ion which is important in the regulation of pH changes that result from altered blood carbon dioxide levels. To maintain normal blood pH, it is necessary to have one carbonic acid molecule to twenty hydrogen carbonate ions. Alterations to this ratio indicate changes in either acidity or alkalinity.
2. Phosphate which is important in the maintenance of pH in red blood cells, kidney tubular fluid and cellular contents.
3. Protein which is the most abundant buffer in cells and plasma. The formation of zwitterions by its constituent amino acids enables proteins to soak up either excess acid or base.
4. Ammonia/ammonium which is used by the kidneys to eliminate H^+ in the form of NH_4^+.
5. Haemoglobin which is important in the regulation of blood pH as it passes through the tissues and because it releases carbon dioxide in the pulmonary capillaries.

Elevated blood carbon dioxide concentrations result in the formation of greater carbonic acid concentrations. The net effect is an elevated acidity of the blood. Any factor

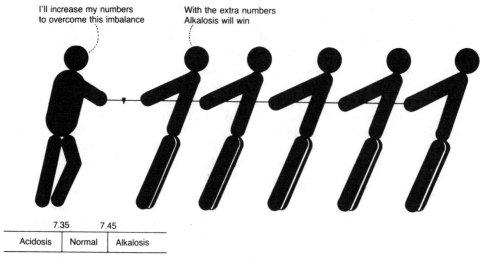

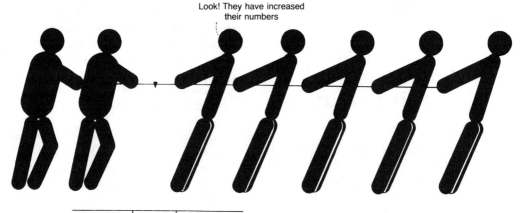

Figure 16.13 (a) Metabolic alkalosis can result from HCO_3^- excess. The $H_2CO_3 : HCO_3^-$ may alter to $1 : 40$. (b) An increase in the H_2CO_3 results in the $H_2CO_3 : HCO_3^-$ ratio returning to $1 : 20$.

that increases or decreases carbon dioxide in the blood thus influences blood pH.

Hyperventilation removes greater quantities of carbon dioxide which results in a more alkaline blood, whereas hypoventilation increases blood carbon dioxide and thus H^+.

The kidneys serve two important functions in H^+ homeostasis. They reabsorb hydrogen carbonate ions thereby preventing alterations to the carbonic acid to hydrogen carbonate ion ratio of one to twenty. They also counter-act elevated blood H^+ concentration by removing excess H^+ in the form of the weak acids in the phosphate and ammonium buffer systems.

Acidosis occurs when the serum pH value falls below 7.35. This fall can be due to a decreased removal of carbon dioxide from the lungs (respiratory acidosis). This may be compensated by the kidneys over one to two days by releasing additional quantities of hydrogen carbonate to return the ratio of carbonic acid to hydrogen carbonate to normal. Metabolic acidosis results from an abnormal increase in acidic metabolic products other than carbon dioxide. A respiratory compensation may maintain the normal pH by hyperventilation causing in-creased removal of carbon dioxide. Com-pensated metabolic acidosis has a decreased carbon dioxide and hydrogen carbonate ion whereas uncompensated metabolic acidosis has a decreased blood hydrogen carbonate ion and pH but a normal blood carbon dioxide level.

Alkalosis occurs when the serum pH levels are greater than 7.45. Respiratory alkalosis results from hyperventilation removing ex-cessive carbon dioxide. Metabolic alkalosis can result from excessive loss of acid from the stomach, the ingestion of large amounts of antacids or from a decrease in blood K^+ con-centration. The body can usually compensate by decreasing respiratory rate and increasing hydrogen carbonate secretion by the kidneys.

Chapter 17

Properties of fluid mixtures

Objectives

At the completion of this chapter the student should be able to:

1. describe the differences between solutions, suspensions and colloids;
2. explain why certain substances are soluble in water while others are insoluble;
3. relate the properties of solutions, suspensions and colloids to the administration of medications;
4. relate the properties of fluid mixtures to normal and abnormal body function;
5. describe a salt and relate its structure to the formation of electrolytes;
6. differentiate between electrolytes and non-electrolytes;
7. relate the properties of fluid mixtures to the need to follow correct protective measures.

17.1 Composition of fluids

A **fluid** is any substance that will take the shape of its container. Fluids can thus be either gases or liquids. There are various ways in which substances can be combined in a fluid. These combinations are known as solutions, suspensions and colloids.

17.2 Solutions

General properties

A **solution** is a fluid consisting of a homogeneous mixture of two or more substances. The greater quantity of substance in a solution is called the **solvent**. All other substances are **solutes**. An aqueous solution uses water as the solvent. EXAMPLE: Body fluids. Non-aqueous solutions use other liquids such as alcohol as the solvent. EXAMPLE: Iodine tincture contains iodine dissolved in alcohol.

In all solutions, solutes are loosely attached to the solvent and uniformly dispersed in

Table 17.1 Nature of solute and its ability to dissolve in a solvent

Solute	Solvent	Dissolves
Ionic	Polar	Yes
	Non-polar	No
Polar	Polar	Yes
	Non-polar	No
Non-polar	Polar	No
	Non-polar	Yes

them. This loose linking or bonding is called dissolving. When a substance dissolves in a solvent the solute cannot be distinguished from that solvent. Thus when the solution is left to stand the solute does not settle to the bottom of the container unless the solution contains excess solute.

How substances dissolve

Solvent molecules are loosely linked together. The ability of a solute to dissolve depends upon the breaking of the interactions that link solvent molecules. A solute will dissolve in a solvent if the formation of loose linkages occurs between the solute and solvent. The forces that form the solute–solvent interactions have to be great enough to break the solvent–solvent linkages. Solutes incapable of breaking solvent–solvent interactions remain undissolved. Generally, polar and ionic solutes (for example, glucose and sodium chloride) dissolve in polar solvents such as water, whereas non-polar solutes such as oil, will not (Table 17.1). A general rule is that like solvents dissolve like substances.

Polar substances contain a **dipole** which consists of one part of a molecule containing an excess of electrons and the other having a deficiency. This difference in charge results from an unequal sharing of electrons be-

tween atoms within a polar molecule (5.5). The slightly negative part is shown as δ^- and the slightly positive part as δ^+. The delta indicates that a charge exists which is less than the complete acceptance or donation of an electron. Polar molecules dissolve in water by forming **dipole–dipole interactions**. These interactions or loose-linkages between solute and solvent result from the fundamental force of oppositely charged particles attracting each other (Figure 17.1a).

Ionic substances form **ion–dipole interactions** with a polar solvent. Ions loosely link with oppositely charged solvent dipoles (Figure 17.1b). In Figure 17.1 both polar and ionic substances have water molecules attached to them. The effective size of the solute has been increased to the size of the solute–water complex. This increase in the size of the solute is an important property in determining the movement of substances through a membrane. The solute–water complex is the hydrated form of that substance. The hydrated diameter is the diameter of the solute and water molecule combination (Figure 17.1c).

Non-polar solutes have a low capacity to form linkages with polar solvents and therefore both remain in an undissolved state or only small quantities are dissolved in a polar solvent such as water. EXAMPLE: Oxygen is a non-polar molecule and thus only small quantities can dissolve in plasma. Van der Waal's forces link non-polar solutes to a non-polar solvent (5.5). This linkage results in non-polar solutes easily dissolving in non-polar solvent. EXAMPLE: Most adhesives are non-polar and can therefore be removed by being dissolved in a non-polar solvent such as acetone.

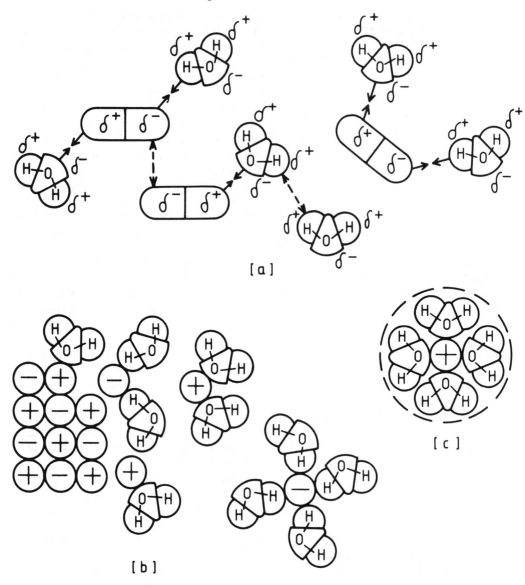

[a]

[b]

[c]

Figure 17.1 The dissolving of solutes in water. (a) Polar substances dissolve by forming dipole–dipole interactions between oppositely charged dipoles (δ^+ is slightly positive and δ^- is slightly negative). (b) Ionic compounds dissolve when polar solvent molecules pull the ions apart; the ions form loose linkages with oppositely charged solvent dipoles. (c) The hydrated diameter represents the solute–water complex diameter.

Application: Drug delivery systems

The controlled entry of drugs into the body is dependent on the dissolving properties of the drug and its coating. Non-polar drugs and polar substances with sufficient lipid solubility dissolve readily through cell membranes and therefore the skin. EXAMPLES: Topical creams and ointments. Transdermal patches (skin patch) enable the controlled release of a drug through the skin. This method of release is achieved through coating a drug with a bio-erodable organic compound that slowly releases its contents. EXAMPLES: Skin patches of glyceryl trinitrate are applied to the chest every 24 hours for the prevention and treatment of angina. Prevention of the symptoms of motion ('sea') sickness by applying a patch of Hyoscine (Scop) behind the ear five to six hours before travelling. The slow release provides protection for up to 72 hours.

A greater number of drugs are being designed to enter the body through the process of dissolving in the mucous membranes of the mouth as this method of entry is more efficient and rapid than the traditional oral method of entry through the small intestine and stomach. EXAMPLE: Sublingual glyceryl nitrate (Anginine) for angina. The use of suppositories applies the same principle to the absorption of drugs across the rectal mucosa.

Slow release can also occur through the intramuscular injection of non-polar drugs such as the sex steroid hormones. EXAMPLE: Medroxyprogesterone.

Intravascular drugs are usually polar as they readily dissolve in the blood and other fluids. Some substances com-bine the dissolving properties of both non-polar and polar molecules by containing both a polar region and a non-polar region. EXAMPLE: The amide (8.9) local anaesthetics such as lignocaine are able to be transported through the body fluids by the polar region linking to water and cross the epineural membranes by the non-polar region dissolving in the non-polar membrane.

Solubility

Solubility is a measure of the amount of solute that will dissolve in a specified volume of solvent and is thus the relative ability of a solute to form loose linkages with a solvent.

Solutes differ in their ability to dissolve in a given volume of solvent. A solute with a high solubility has a large number of solute particles that are able to combine with a given number of solvent molecules. A low-solubility solute can only dissolve a smaller number of particles in the same volume of solvent, that is, a highly-soluble solute can exist in high concentrations whereas a substance with a low solubility can exist only in low concentrations. The solubility of a solute can be increased by raising the temperature and vice versa.

Saturation of solutions

A **saturated solution** contains the maximum quantity of dissolved solute. Any additional solute remains in an undissolved state and usually settles as a precipitate. A large quantity of a solute that is highly soluble can be dissolved in a given quantity of solvent before saturation occurs. With a low-solubility solute, only a relatively low concentration can exist before saturation occurs. Any factor that decreases the ability of a solute to form loose linkages with a solvent or that decreases the number of solvent molecules may effect precipitation of that solute. This means that some of the previously dissolved solute forms a precipitate and thus a saturated solution.

An unsaturated solution has the ability to dissolve additional solute and therefore does not contain precipitate. To determine whether a solution is saturated or unsaturated add a small quantity of solute. If it dissolves, the solution is unsaturated.

Several factors can cause an unsaturated solution to change into a saturated solution. This usually results in the formation of precipitate.

Solute quantity

Increasing the quantity of the solute in a specific volume, that is, increased solute concentration, can cause precipitation. EXAMPLE: Small quantities of sugar dissolve in a cup of tea. The further addition of large quantities of sugar can result in some of the sugar remaining in its undissolved state.

Solvent pH

A substance may have a high solubility at a certain pH and a low solubility at another pH. Thus, pH changes can cause the precipitation of some substances by altering the substances' solubility. EXAMPLE: Calcium has a high solubility in acidic solutions and a low solubility in alkaline solutions.

Solvent volume

When the number of solvent molecules is decreased the remaining solvent may not be sufficient to form loose linkages with all the solute. The excess solute forms a precipitate. EXAMPLE: Evaporation of water from salt water results in the precipitation of salt crystals.

Application: Renal calculi

In the kidneys, solutes can be precipitated in one of three ways:

1. by increased quantities of serum calcium;
2. by alterations in the acidity of the kidney tubule fluid;
3. by increased reabsorption of water resulting in a decreased volume of solvent that can pass through the kidneys:

The precipitate produced by any of the above changes may result in renal calculi (kidney stones). These calculi are usually a combination of calcium and phosphate. The solubility of calcium is greater in acidic conditions than in alkaline conditions, and therefore patients suffering from renal calculi are frequently treated with acidotic diets and drugs.

17.3   Salts

A salt is an ionic compound, that is, a compound composed of cations and anions other than H^+ or OH^-. The salt is usually formed by a metal combining with a non-metal. A salt can also be formed by combining an acid with a base in the process of neutralization. Salts are important in body function and medical use (Table 17.2).

Generally, salts are soluble in water when the ions in the salt have a greater attraction for water molecules than for oppositely-charged ions within the salt. The greater attraction for water molecules by ions results in the dissociation of the salt into cations and anions in the process of ionization. The process of ionization occurs when the inter-

Table 17.2 Examples of salt use

Salt	Use
Calcium and phosphorus salts	Formation of teeth and bones
Iodine salts	Thyroid function
Sodium, potassium and chloride salts	Maintenance of cell function
Barium sulphate	X-rays of gastrointestinal tract
Calcium sulphate (plaster of Paris)	Limb casts
Magnesium sulphate (Epsom salts)	Purgative action

action between solute and solvent results in the formation of ions. (Figure 17.16).

Not all compounds that are composed of metals and non-metals are salts, as such substances can consist of covalent bonds. EXAMPLE: Aluminium chloride ($AlCl_3$). These substances are distinguished from salts by their property of not being able to conduct electricity when dissolved in water. These solutes are called non-electrolytes. Salts and their breakdown products or ions can conduct electricity when dissolved in water and are called electrolytes.

17.4 Electrolytes

Electrolytes are solutes that contain a charge in aqueous solutions. Most acids, bases and salts that are soluble in water are electrolytes, whereas most organic compounds are non-electrolytes. EXAMPLE: Na^+ and Cl^- are electrolytes and glucose is a non-electrolyte. A solution of electrolytes consists of positive and negative ions that are independent of each other. If oppositely charged regions or poles exist in an electrolyte solution the independent ions move to the oppositely charged regions, that is, the cations move to the negatively charged region. The movement of these charges represents an electric current (10.5).

The greater the difference in charge (potential difference) between two regions, the greater is the potential for ions to move to their oppositely charged regions (see 10.3). In the body there is a potential difference between the extracellular fluid and the cell's contents. Membrane barriers restrict the flow of ions from one region to another. The combination of the potential difference and the membrane properties results in the maintenance of cell electrolyte concentrations. Nerve and muscle membranes can be altered to allow the flow of ions (current) between the positive extracellular region and the negative intracellular region. This flow of ions results in nerves conducting information and muscles contracting.

17.5 Suspensions

General properties

In defining solutions, it was stated that they were homogeneous mixtures. Not all mixtures of fluids have this property. EXAMPLE: A container of blood will only be a homogeneous mixture after shaking, because the relatively large red blood cells and white blood cells settle to the bottom of the container upon standing. Such fluids are called suspensions.

Solubility

Suspended particles are insoluble in fluids.

Settling upon standing

On standing, the suspended material will settle at the bottom of the container. The heavier the particles, the faster is the settling time, and so the suspended particles will settle in order of weight.

Application 1: ESR (erythrocyte sedimentation rate)

Constant movement of blood maintains erythrocytes (red blood cells) in an even distribution. The sedimentation rate of erythrocytes is altered by various pathological states. Factors such as inflammatory conditions, myocardial infarction, menstruation, pregnancy, pulmonary tuberculosis and septicaemia elevate the ESR as a result of the erythrocytes clumping together to form large and heavy aggregates.

Application 2: Medications

Medications that are a suspension are labelled 'shake before using'. It is important that this instruction is followed immediately prior to use, since particles may settle rapidly. Failure to administer a thoroughly mixed suspension will result in the patient receiving an incorrect dosage. In most cases the patient would receive a diluted or less concentrated medication since some of the medication has settled and remained in the container. A stock suspension such as milk of magnesia requires shaking prior to each use. If the initial samples from the bottle are diluted due to an incorrect procedure, then subsequent samples will have a proportionately elevated concentration.

Relative size

Particles are relatively large. These particles do not pass through ordinary filter paper or cell membranes.

Most liquid medications are suspended in either water or an oil. EXAMPLES of water based suspensions are: milk of magnesia, calamine and benzathine penicillin Gs (LPG injection — a sterile ready-made aqueous suspension). EXAMPLES of oil based suspensions are: epinephrine s. and mandelamine.

17.6   Colloids

General properties

Particles that are too large to be solutes, and too small to form suspensions, form a colloid. The particles are dispersed or distributed throughout a medium called the dispersion medium. A colloid particle can consist of aggregates of molecules or a very large single molecule such as protein.

Solubility

Colloidal particles are insoluble in the dispersion medium.

Settling upon standing

Colloidal particles remain in suspension or settle slowly upon standing. The heavier the particle the greater is the chance that the particles will settle over an extended period of time. Colloidal medications therefore require shaking before use.

Relative size

Particles pass through filter paper but have difficulty passing through cell membranes.

Adsorption of substances

The relatively large surface area of colloid particles can attract and hold specific substances to it. The holding of a substance to a surface is called adsorption.

Most colloids selectively adsorb cations or anions (but not both) onto their surface. This results in the colloid becoming positively or negatively charged. These charged colloids attract either negatively- or positively-charged particles and other colloids. The addition of positively-charged colloid particles to negatively-charged colloid particles results in the combination of the oppositely-charged colloids. The resulting increase in size causes the colloid complex to act as a suspended particle and settle. This latter process is called coagulation and is used in the neutralization and removal of toxic substances. One form of **coagulation** is the combination of antagonistic blood antibodies and antigens which is referred to as **agglutination** (see multiple allele. 24.5).

Application: Adsorbent medications

Various medications use adsorption to selectively combine with and condense an unwanted substance. Activated charcoal is administered via a nasogastric tube to patients who have overdosed with a polar drug, e.g. barbiturates. The drug is bound to the charcoal and then the colloidal complex is removed by pumping the stomach. Non-polar substances are not adsorbed by charcoal. Diarrhoea relief is obtained from colloid medications such as aluminium silicate (kaolin, kaomagma, kaopectate) which act as an adsorbent. Aluminium silicate condenses and holds the irritating substances.

Colloid categories

Colloids are frequently categorized according to the state of matter (solid, liquid or gas) of the colloidal particles and the dispersion medium. The main categories are sols, gels, aerosols and emulsions.

Sols

Sols consist of solid particles dispersed but not dissolved in a liquid. They can be formed by combining small particles or by breaking down large particles. EXAMPLES: Proteins in plasma and intracellular fluid, aluminium silicate.

Gels

Gels consist of solids that are set in a semi-solid that has jelly-like properties. EXAMPLES: agar, gelatine, petroleum jelly, cell membranes.

Gels are semi-rigid and thus do not flow easily whereas sols are easily poured. Small substances can penetrate and move through gels at approximately the same rates as they flow through liquids. Sols can be converted into gels under certain conditions, that is, sols which can flow easily, are converted to gels which do not flow easily. The contents of a cell have been found to alter between sols and gels.

Application: Interstitial fluid

Tissue spaces consist of compartments of sols and gels. In normal conditions the amount of sol occurring in these spaces is negligible. The gel consists of various colloidal particles, the most abundant of which is hyaluronic acid. Fluid in the gel cannot flow readily from one area of tissue to another. The non-mobile properties of the gel hold the interstitial (intercellular) fluid in place and thus prevent the flow of liquid under the influence of gravity from the upper parts of the body to the lower parts. Since only small substances can readily penetrate gels, larger sized particles such as bacteria are prevented from spreading throughout the gel and thus the tissue. This gel barrier assists in restricting the spread of infection in tissues.

Aerosols

Aerosols consist of liquid or solids dispersed in a gas. They are used in inhalation therapy and also in room sterilization. The latter involves the use of the contents of aerosol cans.

Application 1: Inhalation therapy

Inhalation therapy may require the use of a device that can propel the aerosol into the trachea, bronchi and lungs. A nebulizer is a device that uses either compressed air or ultrasonic waves to disperse liquids or solids into a medium of gas, thus forming an aerosol. Drugs that can act directly on the respiratory system can be administered using this device. EXAMPLE: Salbutamol.

Application 2: Aerosol cans

On standing, the chemicals and liquid settle to the bottom of an aerosol can. When a can that contains a bacteriocidal solution is used without shaking, the resulting spray will consist of mainly the dispersing medium. The liquid containing the bacteriocidal solution will remain at the bottom of the can and not be atomized into the spray. Vigorous shaking ensures a dispersion of the colloid throughout the gas and therefore the spray.

Emulsions

These colloid particles exist as a liquid distributed in small globules or droplets throughout a second liquid, that is, the two liquids do not dissolve in each other. These two liquids are immiscible, whereas liquids that are soluble in each other are miscible.

In some emulsions, the droplets come together when left to stand and form a separate liquid layer from the solvent. Emulsions with this property are called temporary emulsions. EXAMPLE: Mixing oil and water. Other emulsions do not settle or separate into two separate layers upon standing. These are permanent emulsions which exist as homogeneous mixtures. EXAMPLE: Mineral oil emulsion (liquid petrolatum) consists mainly of mineral oil, water and alcohol.

The addition of charged particles to dispersed temporary emulsion globules results in each globule resisting recombination with other globules. The repelling of identically charged globules prevents the formation of a liquid layer and thus results in the formation of a permanent emulsion. Substances can form emulsions by the introduction of chemical agents. This process is used in the body to digest and absorb fats.

Application: Formation of body emulsions

In the gastrointestinal system, bile acts as an emulsifying agent in the small intestine. Bile breaks down the ingested fat into droplets. Most of this emulsion is then digested by enzymes and absorbed across the small intestine wall. In addition, some droplets are absorbed as a temporary emulsion in the intestinal cells. These droplets or chylomicrons are converted in these cells into a permanent emulsion by the addition of charged proteins. The identical charges on each droplet prevent the droplets from sticking to each other as like charges repel. Absence of the protein coat, due to poisons or genetic disorders, results in fat accumulating in the intestinal cells.

17.7 Separation of solutions, suspensions and colloids

Solutions, suspensions and colloids can be separated by their individually different properties. A summary of these different properties is listed in Table 17.3.

Table 17.3 Relative properties of solutions, suspensions and colloids

Particle property	Solution	Suspension	Colloid
Solubility	Potential	No	No
Settles upon standing	No	Yes	Yes
Relative size	Small	Large	Medium
Medications require shaking	No	Yes	Yes
Pass through membranes	Potential	No	With difficulty
Pass through filter paper	Yes	No	Yes
Adsorb substances	No	No	Yes

17.8 Environmental health and safety

The appropriate protective measures must be taken at all times to minimize the risk of exposure to harmful fluid mixtures that can occur at work and in the general environment. The properties of fluid mixtures determine how, where and in what concentrations substances are able to enter the human body. EXAMPLE: Exposure to non-polar substances results in widespread areas of entry into the body as these substances dissolve through the skin and other membranes. EXAMPLE: Organic solvents. The burning of sulfur-containing coal and wood leads to the formation of sulphur dioxide (SO_2) in the atmosphere. The (SO_2) reacts with water vapour to form droplets of sulphuric acid creating **acid rain**. Inhalation of these droplets can cause damage to the lungs over a period of time. The suspension of small fibres such as asbestos in air and the subsequent inhalation of the suspension can lead to the development of cancer.

Summary

A fluid is any substance that will take the shape of its container, that is gases and liquids. Fluids can exist as solutions, suspensions and colloids.

A solution consists of a homogeneous mixture of two or more substances. The lesser quantity of substance is known as the solute and it combines with solvent molecules in the process of dissolving. Generally only polar and ionic solutes dissolve in polar solvents, whereas non-polar solutes dissolve in non-polar solvents. In aqueous solutions water is the solvent, and the size of the solute/water complex is known as the hydrated diameter. A precipitate settles out of a solution when some of the solute has not combined with the solvent. A saturated solution exists when a precipitate occurs. Factors such as the quantity of solute, the solvent pH and the volume of solvent can cause an unsaturated solution to change into a saturated solution.

A salt is composed of cations and anions. Salts usually dissociate in water which results in the presence of free ions which are known as electrolytes. An electrolyte has the ability to move to oppositely charged regions in a solution. Non-electrolytes are not attracted to charged regions.

Suspensions and colloids differ from solutions in that;

1. particles settle upon standing;
2. the size of particles are larger;
3. particles are unable to pass through membranes;
4. they require shaking to form a homogeneous mixture.

In addition, colloids can selectively adsorb cations and anions. Also, colloids can combine together in the process of coagulation to form suspended particles.

Colloids are categorized according to the type of matter that is mixed with the gas or liquid dispersion medium:

1. sols — solids dispersed in a liquid;
2. gels — solids dispersed in a jelly-like liquid;
3. aerosols — solids or liquids dispersed in a gas;
4. emulsions — liquids distributed in liquids.

The properties of fluid mixtures determine the possible sites of entry of harmful substances into the body. Correct protective measures must be followed in order to minimize the risk of exposure to such substances.

Chapter 18

Composition and properties of body fluids

Objectives

At the completion of this chapter the student should be able to:

1. relate the properties of fluids to body fluid composition;
2. describe the differences in fluid composition between the different body fluid compartments;
3. relate the properties of fluids to kidney function and urine composition;
4. describe the process of dialysis.

18.1 Composition of body fluids

Body fluids consist of a combination of solutes, suspended particles and colloidal particles. Body fluid characteristics depend upon the properties of solutions, suspensions and colloids. Substances that can penetrate membranes (solutes) are dispersed throughout all body fluids. Substances that are unable to pass through membranes (suspended particles and colloidal particles) are restricted in their distribution.

The widespread distribution of solutes results in these substances being capable of performing a diverse range of functions (Table 18.1). Suspended particles and colloidal particles are restricted in their distribution since cell membranes act as a barrier to the movement of these particles. The relative distribution of substances in the various body fluid compartments is shown in Figure 18.1. The properties of solutes, suspended particles and colloidal particles along with the properties of each fluid compartment can be used to explain the composition of body fluid compartments. Body fluids can be separated into intracellular fluid and extracellular fluid, with the latter being subdivided into various compartments.

Intracellular fluid

Each cell contains an individual mixture of different substances, but the concentration of these substances is similar for all cells. Thus the fluid composition of cells is considered as one large fluid compartment known as the **intracellular fluid**. This fluid is formed from substances passing through cell membranes and by the manufacture of substances within cells.

Intracellular fluid contains mainly electrolytes, glucose, large quantities of protein (four times plasma concentration) and small quantities of lipids. (Note that most of this protein and lipid has been manufactured within the cell from solute particles.) Electrolytes such as K^+, Mg^{2+}, HPO_4^{2-}, and SO_4^{2-}

Table 18.1   A list of common body solutes. The
importance of solutes to the body is
shown by their diversity of function

Solute	Function
Amino acids	Chemical building blocks of protein
Ammonium complex	Involved in the regulation of kidney tubular fluid pH
Bicarbonate	Involved in the regulation of blood and kidney tubular fluid pH
Bilirubin	Breakdown product of haemoglobin
Carbon dioxide	Waste product of tissue metabolism
Calcium	Necessary constituent of bone and teeth; essential for hormone manufacture, blood clotting, nerve and muscle function
Chloride	Important in fluid balance
Creatinine	Produced by muscles; the rate of elimination from the kidneys is used to evaluate kidney function
Glucose	Chemical building block of stores carbohydrate (glycogen); it is the main carbohydrate used in energy production
Hydrogen ion	Released from body acids and metabolism (Chapter 16)
Iron	Essential constituent of haemoglobin and respiratory enzymes
Lactic acid (Lactate)	Waste product of metabolism formed during oxygen deficiency
Phosphate	Important regulator of pH in the kidney tubular fluid, red blood cells and other cells
Potassium	Important in nerve and muscle function
Sodium	Esssential in blood volume control, nerve and muscle function
Urea	Chief nitrogenous end product of protein metabolism

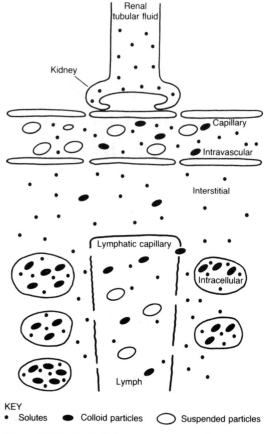

KEY
● Solutes   ⬤ Colloid particles   ◯ Suspended particles

Figure 18.1   Body fluid compartments showing
the relative distribution of solutes,
colloid particles, and suspended
particles.

Phosphate also is involved in the regulation
of cell pH. The term pH refers to the concentration of H^+ ions and is explained in
detail in 16.3.

Cells contain a predominant quantity of
negatively charged proteins and other colloid
particles. These particles confer a net negative
charge within a cell when compared with the
extracellular fluid. This potential difference
is an important factor in the functioning of
nerves and muscles (10.5).

are found in cells in relatively large quantities
compared with extracellular fluid (Figure
18.2). The large quantities of protein within
cells act as an important intracellular buffer.

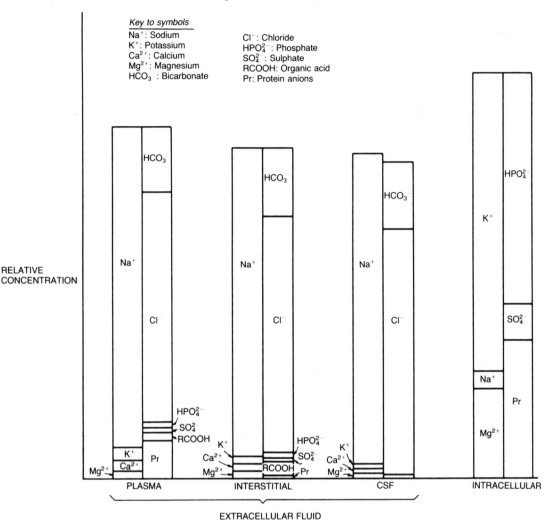

Figure 18.2 Comparison of electrolyte concentrations in plasma, interstitial fluid, cerebrospinal fluid and intracellular fluid.

Extracellular fluid

Interstitial fluid

Interstitial fluid (intercellular fluid) is formed from substances passing through either capillary walls or the cell membranes of nearby cells. Interstitial fluid contains only trace quantities of proteins and blood cells, thus indicating that these particles have difficulty in passing through membranes. The small quantity of plasma proteins in interstitial fluid is due primarily to some proteins that leak through the gaps between the cells that form the capillary walls. Damage or alteration to these cells results in a large quantity of proteins and blood cells moving into the interstitial fluid.

Large quantities of solutes, especially electrolytes, are found in this fluid since these substances can readily penetrate membranes and capillary wall gaps. Interstitial fluid contains relatively large concentrations of Na^+, Cl^- and HCO_3^- compared with intracellular fluid (Figure 18.2). The large concentrations of HCO_3^- and the low concentrations of protein and phosphate indicate that the main interstitial buffer system is the HCO_3^-/H_2CO (16.5).

Lymph

Interstitial fluid contains a small concentration of proteins and suspended particles. These particles have difficulty in passing through the capillary wall and thus they require an alternative route through which they can return to the circulatory system. A drainage system known as the lymphatic system returns interstitial fluid containing colloids and suspended particles to the blood. The **lymphatic system** is composed of channels that link the interstitial fluid with the circulatory system. Fluid enters this system via porous endings at the beginning of a drainage channel. As soon as the fluid enters the lymphatic channels it is called **lymph**.

The lymph vessels drain fluid, cellular secretions of proteins such as hormones and enzymes, suspended particles such as blood cells and cell debris. In addition to these particles, cells (lymphocytes) and proteins (antibodies) involved in the body defence mechanisms are released into the lymph from lymphoid tissue such as the lymph nodes.

Intravascular fluid (blood)

Blood consists of suspended particles or cells and a liquid referred to as plasma (26.1). **Serum** is another term used in describing the liquid component of blood, but serum differs from plasma in that serum does not contain the colloid factors involved in blood clot formation. **Plasma** is the naturally-occurring intravascular liquid whereas serum is the liquid formed when blood is allowed to clot in containers. The two terms serum and plasma are often (incorrectly) interchanged when referring to the concentration of substances in the blood.

Plasma is almost identical in solute composition to interstitial fluid (Figure 18.2). However, the concentration of protein is about three and a half times greater in plasma than in interstitial fluid. Proteins and a large quantity of cells found in the blood do not enter the vascular system by passing across membranes but pass directly into the blood stream from areas such as the bone marrow.

The high concentration of proteins and HCO_3^- indicates that these substances are the main intravascular pH regulators. The presence of red blood cells and therefore haemoglobin results in the blood also being buffered by the haemoglobin buffer system (16.5).

Cerebrospinal fluid (CSF)

This fluid originates from blood being passed through a network of capillary membranes in the brain. This network is known as the choroid plexus. The CSF functions as a protective cushion for the brain. It also acts as a carrier of nutrient and waste materials between the blood, brain and spinal cord. Fluid leaves the CSF compartment via ducts that connect with the venous system.

The composition of CSF is restricted to substances that can pass through the capillary walls of the choroid plexus. These wall cells appear to selectively secrete solutes and not colloid or suspended particles into the CSF. The composition of electrolytes in CSF is similar to interstitial fluid (Figure 18.2).

Generally any substance that has a molecular weight greater than 500 is excluded from CSF. This restriction is important in the effectiveness of drugs acting on the brain. The CSF differs from interstitial fluid in that it contains lower concentrations of phosphate ions. The CSF contains an excess of cations whereas the interstitial fluid and blood consists of a balance of cations and anions. Thus CSF has a more positive charge, and therefore a potential difference exists between CSF and these fluids such that the CSF is more positive.

The pH of CSF is 7.32 and it is maintained by the bicarbonate buffer system (16.5), since only small quantities of proteins and phosphate exist in CSF.

Application: Lumbar puncture

This process involves the insertion of a needle into the CSF in the lumbar region of the spinal cord to take CSF samples or to administer substances to the CSF. Due to the choroid plexus barrier, normally only solutes exist in the CSF. Analysis of CSF for the presence of white blood cells and blood is used for diagnostic purposes. Culturing CSF samples assists in determining the presence of bacteria. In addition, anaesthetics that are unable to penetrate the choroid plexus can be administered via a lumbar puncture.

Urine

Urine is formed from substances that can normally pass through capillary membranes. These substances pass through a membrane filter and then into kidney tubules. Some of these substances are taken up by the kidney cells and returned to the blood. EXAMPLE: Na^+ and glucose. Other substances such as urea pass through the kidney tubules and form urine. The main constituents of urine are waste products of metabolism such as urea and creatinine (Table 18.2). Note that the constituents of urine are solutes. Proteins, cells and hardened moulds of cells

Table 18.2 Normal constituents of urine

Constituent	Comment
ORGANIC	
Urea	Usually 60–90% of all nitrogen solutes; varies with dietary protein intake
Uric acid	Product of nucleic acid breakdown; low solubility results in kidney stones
Creatinine	Produced during muscle contraction from creatine
Ketone bodies	Usually found in small amounts, the result of protein and fat breakdown; high levels are found in individuals receiving low carbohydrate diets, pregnant women, untreated diabetes mellitus and acute starvation
Hippuric acid	Results from benzoic acid, a toxic substance in fruits and vegetables; diets containing a high vegetable content result in increased levels
INORGANIC	
Sodium chloride	Most abundant inorganic salt
Potassium, magnesium and calcium ions	Combine with anions, chloride, sulphate and phosphate to form salts
Sulphate, phosphate ions	Combines with sodium to form buffers; used to remove hydrogen ions in the urine
Ammonium ions	Used as a compensatory mechanism to remove high levels of acids; combines with chloride to form ammonium salt

known as casts only normally occur in trace amounts.

The inability of proteins to penetrate a membrane results in the kidneys using solutes for buffers. The main solute buffers are the phosphate and ammonium buffer systems. These buffers are used to remove acids from the body in the form of weak acids. These acids can result in a slightly acidic urine.

Damage or alteration of the kidney filtering system results in the presence of an elevated concentration of proteins and suspended particles. Calcium precipitates known as calculi may also be present. When the kidneys are unable to return a substance such as glucose to the blood the excess is eliminated in the urine. The presence of glucose in urine can be due to either high blood glucose concentrations or a decreased capacity of the kidney to return substances to the blood.

In summary, the kidney separates suspended particles and colloidal particles from solutes. The solutes are in turn separated by kidney cells so that toxic waste products are eliminated in urine and essential solutes are returned to the blood. Artificial methods have been developed that mimic the kidney filtration system. These methods are known as dialysis.

18.2 Dialysis

Haemodialysis

Dialysis is the separation of suspended particles and colloids from solutes by a membrane. Renal problems can be overcome by the use of a kidney machine (artificial kidney) in the process of **haemodialysis**. This is the removal of soluble toxic substances from the blood stream by an artificial membrane. In haemodialysis, a patient's blood is pumped

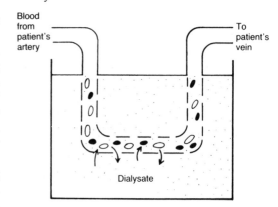

Figure 18.3 Principle of haemodialysis whereby solutes are separated from colloids and blood cells. Toxic solutes flow from a relatively high concentration in the blood to a low dialysate concentration.

through a tube of artificial membrane. This tube has both ends connected to the patient's vascular system. The plastic membrane tube is immersed in a bathing solution called the **dialysate**. It contains the required concentration of soluble substances for the patient. Soluble particles pass through a dialysing membrane from a high concentration to a lower concentration (Figure 18.3). Initially, no waste products occur in the dialysate so waste substances move from the blood to the dialysate. No net flow of other substances will occur since the concentration of these substances is the same as in the blood. Proteins and suspended particles are unable to penetrate the membrane and thus are retained by the dialysing tube.

If a patient requires substances such as glucose, the dialysate concentration is increased. The greater glucose dialysate concentration results in a flow of this substance into the blood. Also, to lower a patient's blood solute concentration, simply decrease the concentration of that substance in the dialysate to the required level.

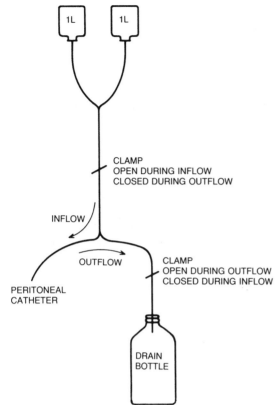

Figure 18.4   Principle of peritoneal dialysis showing the infusion of dialysate into the patient via a peritoneal catheter. Clamps control the inflow and outflow of the dialysate.

As the dialysate concentration of toxic substances increases, the efficiency of removal of these waste products from the blood decreases. Therefore it is important to change the dialysate at regular intervals.

Peritoneal dialysis

In this procedure the dialysate flows via a special catheter into the sealed peritoneal cavity (Figure 18.4). The dense capillary net-work of the peritoneal cavity is used as the dialysing membrane. This large surface area of membrane enables efficient movement of solutes from the peritoneal capillaries to the dialysate and dialysate solutes into the blood. In adults, two litres of sterile body temperature dialysate is infused over a fifteen minute period. The process of dialysis is allowed to occur for thirty to forty-five minutes. This period is called the dwell time. After dialysis the bathing solution is removed by siphonage over approximately twenty minutes. The contents of the outflow and its volume are then measured and recorded.

The infusion, dwell time and outflow are varied according to the patient's symptoms. EXAMPLE: Overhydration and oedema usually require a short dwell time. The procedure is repeated any number of times until the desired plasma concentration of solutes has been attained. Peritoneal dialysis is usually a short-term therapy since the risk of peritonitis is great.

18.3 Environmental health and safety

Prolonged physical work or exercise in a hot environment leads to hyperthermia (elevated body temperature), dehydration and hypoglycaemia (13.6) and a sodium and potassium electrolyte imbalance resulting in acidosis (16.6). During such activities such as marathon running or working near furnaces it is therefore important to maintain an adequate intake of water, glucose and electrolytes.

Summary

Body fluid compartments consist of varying mixtures of solutes, suspended particles and colloidal particles.

The distribution of colloids and suspended particles is restricted by their difficulty in penetrating membranes, whereas solutes are widely distributed throughout the body.

Intracellular fluid, lymph and blood contain relatively large quantities of colloids compared with interstitial fluid, CSF and urine.

Lymph and blood contain large quantities of cells.

Body fluid buffers are determined by the distribution of proteins. Blood and intracellular fluid rely on proteins as a major source of buffers, whereas interstitial fluid, CSF and urine rely entirely on solutes such as bicarbonate.

The kidneys separate solutes from suspended particles and colloidal particles. Kidney cells separate the toxic waste products of the body from the essential solutes and eliminate the waste solutes in urine.

Dialysis is a method by which an artificial membrane separates suspended particles and colloidal particles from solutes. The solutes contain toxic waste substances that flow into the dialysate. Removal of the dialysate at intervals results in the effective elimination of toxic solutes from the patient.

Unit Seven
Pressure

This unit integrates the properties of pressure and applies these properties to normal and abnormal body function. You will learn how pressure influences the supply, movement and removal of nutrients and waste products in the body.

Chapter 19

Properties of pressure

Objectives

At the completion of this chapter the student should be able to:

1. define pressure and apply this definition to the laws relating to pressure;
2. explain the laws of pressure using either physiological, nursing or clinical examples;
3. explain how respirators can artificially control or assist external respiration;
4. describe the principle of hydrostatic pressure;
5. describe how hydrostatic pressure may be altered by either normal or abnormal body function;
6. explain the term blood pressure;
7. explain the role of pressure in environmental health and safety.

19.1 Principle of pressure

Pressure is the force exerted by particles on an area of matter. Pressure can be developed by all forms of matter. The properties of pressure have many applications in body function and patient care. Throughout the body, pressure is used to move liquids and maintain a fluid balance. In the process of breathing (ventilation), pressure is required to move oxygen and carbon dioxide into and out of the lungs.

With liquids and gases, the degree of pressure on an object is determined by the number of molecules colliding with that object. To determine the amount of pressure imposed on an object the following equation is used:

$$\text{Pressure} = \frac{\text{Force applied}}{\text{Area of application}} \quad \text{Eqn 19.1}$$

This equation implies that the greater the area upon which a given force is applied, the less the pressure.

This principle is shown when pressure sores develop in long-term, bed-ridden patients. EXAMPLE: Spinal injuries. When lying on a firm mattress a large proportion of body weight is born by projections of the skeleton such as the scapula, coccyx and elbows. These small areas of contact bear the body weight and thus a large amount of pressure is exerted on these protrusions, resulting in bed sores (Figure 19.1a). It is therefore advisable to spread the pressure of

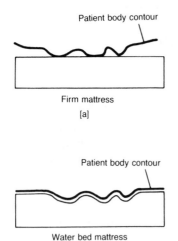

Figure 19.1 Pressure between patient and bed surface. (a) With a firm bed a small area of contact occurs between the patient and the bed resulting in the weight of the patient (force) being born by several small body projections. The flesh between the bones and the bed therefore develops sores. (b) With a flexible bed, a large area of contact occurs between the patient and the bed. Low pressure between the patient and the bed minimizes the development of pressure sores.

increases, one of the following effects will occur:

1. If the surface on which the pressure is exerted is elastic it will stretch.
2. If the surface is incapable of withstanding this increased pressure it will break. EXAMPLES: In fluids the rupture of blood vessels and subsequent haemorrhaging, in solids the fracturing of bones due to excessive pressure upon the bone.
3. Material that can resist changes in pressure will increase the potential of the matter within the container to exert pressure. EXAMPLE: Compressed gas in a cylinder.
4. Inelastic material that is capable of resisting an increase in pressure exerted by a solid will effect an increase in resistance, i.e. friction between the solid and the surface that is in contact with it. EXAMPLE: Bed sores develop on areas where an increase in pressure occurs between the patient's body and regions of contact with a bed.

Pressure can be increased by accelerating the number of particles that collide with the walls of a container at any given moment, i.e. exerting an increased force on a given area. Thus any body function that increases the number of collisions of particles will increase pressure. EXAMPLES: Expiration, changes in blood pressure and osmotic pressure.

the body protrusions over a wider area. This is achieved by using materials that will mould with the body contours such as water beds or an individually moulded cast (or bed). Decreased pressure results from increasing the area over which a force is applied (Figure 19.1b).

The force applied for a given pressure is always opposed by an opposite or resistance force. The effect of this opposite force is to resist the further movement of particles (15.5). When the pressure exerted on the walls of a container or the surface of solids

19.2   The gaseous state

Several physical laws assist in the understanding of pressure and how pressure may be altered in gases.

Charles' law

Charles' law states that if pressure is constant, then the volume of gas is directly proportional to its absolute temperature. That is, an increase in temperature results in an increase in the movement of particles resulting in an increase in the area that these particles can occupy. When the container walls are inelastic, raised temperature will cause an increased pressure due to the increased frequency with which particles collide with the wall.

Application: Compressed gas cylinders

Compressed gas containers (aerosol cans, gas cylinders) will explode if the temperature inside the container is increased to a level where the gas pressure becomes too great for the container walls to withstand this pressure.

Boyle's law

Boyle's law. The volume of a gas varies inversely with pressure when the temperature is constant:

$$\text{Volume} \propto \frac{1}{\text{Pressure}} \text{ or Pressure} \propto \frac{1}{\text{Volume}}$$

$$\text{Eqn. 19.2}$$

This means that if the volume is doubled the pressure is halved since a given number of gas molecules now occupy a greater volume. This results in less molecules colliding with the wall of a container at any particular moment. Conversely if the volume is halved the pressure is doubled. In effect the density of gas has been altered. Thus the number of particles colliding with the walls of the container has been altered.

Application: Ventilation

See Figure 19.2.

Standard temperature and pressure

Because of the relationships between pressure and temperature, a reference standard is used called the standard temperature and pressure or STP. The STP is used in calculations involving gases. The standard temperature is absolute zero $0\,K$ ($-273.15°C$). The standard pressure is one atmosphere $1.013 \times 10^5\,Pa$ (760 mm Hg).

Positive and negative pressure

Pressure that is greater than standard atmospheric pressure (101 kPa or 760 mm Hg) is often referred to as positive pressure, and pressure that is less than 101 kPa is referred to as negative pressure. Positive and negative pressure are used in respiration. Both of these pressures are also used by machines to mechanically assist respiration (respirators). The elimination of air and blood following thoracotomy also uses differences in positive and negative pressure.

Application 1: Ventilation

Inspiration occurs when a difference in pressure exists between the atmosphere and the lungs, with the pressure in the lungs being negative. Expiration occurs when the pressure in the lungs is positive. In the latter the greater pressure within the lungs forces air to move to the atmosphere. To understand the process of breathing it is necessary to know how pressure changes occur within the lungs, since prior to inspiration pressure in the lungs is approximately equal to atmospheric pressure.

The lungs are surrounded by a sealed thoracic cavity (Figure 19.2). According to Boyle's law, an expansion of this

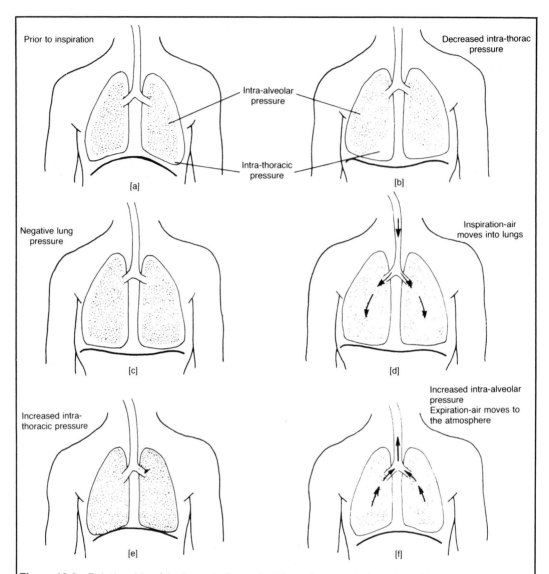

Figure 19.2 Relationship of the lungs to the sealed thoracic cage during a breathing cycle.
(a) Lungs and thoracic cage prior to inspiration, pressure in the lungs equals atmospheric pressure.
(b) Contraction of the diaphragm and intercostal muscles effects an increased volume within the thoracic cage, expansion of this sealed cage decreases the intra-thoracic pressure compared with the intra-alveolar pressure.
(c) The lungs expand until the intra-alveolar pressure has decreased sufficiently to regain the original balance in pressure with the intra-thoracic region. There is now a lower pressure in the lungs compared with the atmospheric pressure.
(d) Air moves from the atmosphere to the lungs until the intra-alveolar pressure equals the atmospheric pressure, that is, inspiration occurs.
(e) Relaxation of the intercostal muscles and diaphragm results in a decreased intra-thoracic volume, and an increased intra-thoracic pressure.
(f) Lungs recoil as a result of this alteration between the intra-alveolar and intra-thoracic pressures, the decreased lung volume develops a positive pressure. Air moves from the lungs in the process of expiration.

sealed area (volume increase) will result in a decrease in the intra-thoracic pressure. This event occurs when the diaphragm and intercostal muscles contract. This contraction effects an increase in the size of the thoracic cavity (Figure 19.2b). A decreased intra-thoracic (intra-pleural) pressure results in less particles colliding with the walls of the lung that line the intra-thoracic cavity. A relative difference in the number of particles colliding with the two surfaces of the lung (intra-thoracic and intra-alveoli) develops with a greater number of particles colliding with the intra-alveoli wall. Since lung tissue exhibits elastic properties an expansion of the lung occurs until the forces are once again balanced. This expansion of the lung results in a decreased density of air and air pressure within the lung (Figure 19.2c). This decreased pressure (negative) allows particles to flow from the atmosphere into the lungs in an attempt to equalize the lung pressure with that of the atmosphere (Figure 19.2d).

At a certain point in the expansion of the intra-thoracic cavity, stretch receptors are activated, resulting in the inhibition of diaphragm and inter-costal-muscular contraction. These muscles relax, effecting a decrease in intra-thoracic volume. This allows the stretched elastic tissue in the thoracic cage to recoil to its original unstretched length. Now a greater density has developed within the intra-thoracic cavity, since a decreased volume for a given number of particles exists. This increased density results in a greater number of particles from the intra-thoracic cavity colliding with the wall of the lung (Figure 19.2e). The balance of

forces between the intra-thoracic and intra-alveolar walls of the lung has been altered, with the elastic tissue of the lungs being forced to recoil. A decrease in lung volume results, causing an increased density and thus pressure of the intra-alveolar air. The pressure within the lungs becomes positive, thus forcing air to move to the atmosphere (Figure 19.2f).

It should be noted that expiration is regarded as a passive process since little muscular contraction occurs. Contraction of the internal intercostal muscles assists expiration to a limited extent.

Application 2: Respirators

Breathing can be assisted, and if necessary controlled, by the use of respirators. These machines mechanically alter the pressure difference between the atmosphere and the lungs. Various forms of respirators are available, each designed to overcome specific breathing problems: EXAMPLES: Iron lungs, intermittent positive-pressure respirators (IPPR), positive expiratory end pressure (PEEP) and continuous positive airways pressure (CPAP) respirators. All of these respirators effect a negative or positive pressure in the lungs.

Negative pressure respirators

These machines indirectly develop a negative pressure within the lungs to initiate inspiration. The respirators are called iron lungs. They are large, with the machine enclosing the entire body apart from the neck and head (Figure 19.3).

A pump creates a negative pressure between the patient and the machine's

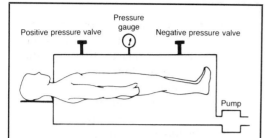

Figure 19.3   Patient in an iron lung.

wall. This negative pressure effects an expansion of the thoracic cavity. The expansion results in air flowing from the atmosphere to the lower pressure that has developed within the lungs. This expansion is similar to the normal process of inspiration. Expiration occurs when the thoracic cavity recoils to its original size. This step is aided by the use of a positive pressure developed within the machine. Iron lungs can be used with patients suffering from respiratory muscle paralysis and are continually used with patients who have poliomyelitis.

Positive pressure respirators

Positive pressure respirators force gas into the lungs at greater than atmospheric pressure. The intermittent positive pressure respirators (IPPR) force air into the lungs. This forced intake of air results in an expansion of the lungs and inspiration. The elastic recoil of the stretched tissue effects a passive expiration. These machines can be used to regulate breathing rates in unconscious patients or to improve lung expansion in patients suffering from obstructive or restrictive lung disease. Gas mixtures can be altered to regulate blood oxygen levels and pH of the blood.

Often it is necessary to retain a small positive pressure within the lungs throughout breathing. In premature babies immature alveoli may collapse preventing gaseous exchange. Therefore continuous positive pressure must be maintained. This is usually done by continuous positive airways pressure (CPAP) in which the neonate relies on its own respiratory mechanisms but a small constant pressure is retained within the lungs at the end of expiration. This positive pressure prevents the collapse of the alveoli. With IPPR respirators a small positive pressure can be retained at the end of expiration. This pressure allows a longer period for gaseous exchange and is referred to as positive end expiratory pressure (PEEP).

Application 3: Underwater drainage apparatus

Underwater drainage is used to remove plasma, blood and air from the thorax following thoracotomy. The underwater drainage apparatus is shown in Figure 19.4. The tube is inserted at the time of operation and it is essential that it has air-tight fittings. The leakage of air from the atmosphere into the tube will cause collapse of the lung, therefore care must be taken at all times to ensure that the apparatus is not accidentally knocked.

A positive pressure is created in the thoracic cavity by coughing or sneezing. This positive pressure forces air and blood to flow via the tube to the water. The air then passes through the water to the atmosphere. On inspiration, expansion of the intra-thoracic cavity creates a greater negative pressure in the thoracic cavity. Atmospheric

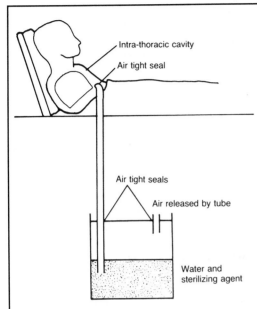

Figure 19.4 Underwater drainage apparatus consisting of a sealed tube connecting the intra-thoracic cavity to a solution of water and sterilizing agent about 1 m below the patient's chest.

pressure forces water into the tube. Deep inspiration results in water rising approximately 40 cm in the tube, thus to prevent fluid entering the thoracic cavity the underwater drainage bottle is placed 1 m below the patient's chest.

Dalton's law

Each gas in a mixture of gases exerts its own pressure as if all other gases were not present. That is, each gas exerts a **partial pressure**. The total pressure exerted by a mixture of gases is the sum of the partial pressures of the constituent gases. This is not the case with gases that combine (react) within the mixture. When gas molecules combine a decrease in the total number of random moving molecules occurs.

In one atmosphere of pressure (101 kPa or 760 mm Hg), the pressure consists of a summation of individual gas components within the atmosphere:

$$101 \text{ kPa or}$$
$$760 \text{ mm Hg} = PO_2 + PCO_2 + PN_2$$
$$+ PH_2O \text{ (water vapour)}.$$
$$\text{Eqn 19.3}$$

To determine the partial pressure of a gas, multiply the percentage of the component gas present within the total amount of gas by the total gas pressure of the mixture. Oxygen represents approximately 21% of total air content, and thus:

$$\text{atmospheric } PO_2 = 21/100 \times 101 \text{ kPa}$$
$$\text{or } 760 \text{ mm Hg}$$
$$= 21.2 \text{ kPa or } 160 \text{ mm Hg}$$
$$\text{Eqn 19.4}$$

Partial pressure is important in determining the relative pressure differences of individual gases, such as oxygen and carbon dioxide, between the lungs and blood and the blood and body cells. Pressure differences indicate the likelihood of gas movement between two regions and thus our ability to exchange gases such as oxygen and carbon dioxide.

Application: Exchange of alveolar and blood gases

Oxygen has an alveolar PO_2 of 13.3 kPa (100 mm Hg) and a venous PO_2 of 5.3 kPa (40 mm Hg). The wall separating these two regions allows oxygen to pass through it and thus a net movement of oxygen molecules will occur from the region of higher pressure (concentration) to the region of lower pressure in the blood. A decrease in the difference of partial pressure between these two regions would result in less oxygen moving to the blood thus resulting in dizziness. For example, at high altitudes the PO_2 of the atmosphere, and therefore the alveoli, decreases. The lower amount of oxygen moving from the alveoli to the blood results in altitude sickness.

Carbon dioxide has a greater partial pressure in the blood (PCO_2 6.0 kPa or 45 mm Hg) returning to the lungs than in the alveoli (PCO_2 5.3 kPa or 40 mm Hg). Thus, carbon dioxide moves from the blood to the alveoli, as the lung wall allows carbon dioxide to pass through it.

where the previous oxygen levels were too low for the effective movement of oxygen to the damaged area of tissue.

Gas flow in tubes

The flow of gas molecules through a tube is influenced by the diameter of the tube. The greater the diameter the less chance a molecule has of colliding frequently with the tube wall and losing kinetic energy. Excessive collisions of molecules with the wall result in the slowing down of gas molecules. This slowing down occurs when the tube diameter has been decreased or an obstruction blocks part of the tube, that is, an increase in resistance to gas flow has occurred.

Henry's law

The amount of gas dissolved in a liquid varies proportionately with the partial pressure of the gas, when the temperature remains constant. Thus the greater the PO_2 in the alveoli the greater is the amount of oxygen that can dissolve in blood.

Application: Hyperbaric chambers

Hyperbaric chambers are used to increase the PO_2 of the alveoli. A hyperbaric chamber contains oxygen at approximately two to three times the atmospheric pressure. Thus the level of dissolved oxygen in the blood is increased proportionately. The increased PO_2 of blood results in a greater ability for oxygen to move to the tissues. This principle is used in the treatment of anaerobic infections, spinal injuries, etc.

Application: Obstructive airways disease

A decrease in the effective diameter of the airways occurs by obstruction or constriction of vessels. Resistance to air flow increases, resulting in a need to overcome this resistance. Use of respirators can assist patients by forcing air into the lungs with a positive pressure. This greater than atmospheric pressure overcomes the airway resistance, enabling patients to receive the correct volume of gas into their lungs. In asthma patients, bronchodilators such as salbutamol dilate the air passage thus reducing the resistance to air flow.

19.3   The liquid state

The properties of liquids under pressure are important for body function. EXAMPLES: Movement of blood and lymph, fluid movement across membranes, bladder function.

Pascal's law

Pressure exerted on a confined liquid is transmitted equally in all directions. A change in pressure at any point will result in the pressure change being transmitted equally throughout the liquid.

Hydrostatic pressure

Hydrostatic pressure refers to the force that pushes a liquid against the walls of its container. This pressure is developed by the heart and bladder. The pressure developed will depend upon the ability of the container wall to compress the fluid within it. Since liquids consist of molecules that are loosely held together (9.6), the distance that molecules can be pushed towards each other (compressed) by a given force is minimal, when compared with the freely-moving gas molecules. Thus a relatively large force is required to compress liquids. Small changes in the volume of a confined liquid result in a large increase in hydrostatic pressure. This increased pressure will be applied, according to Pascal's law to all regions of the container. If a region of the wall is unable to withstand this pressure increase, then that region will collapse and fluid will be pushed through it. This principle is used by valves in the heart and sphincters in the bladder wall to release fluid into vessels. The amount of fluid moving from the bladder or heart into vessels will depend upon the resistance of the vessels to fluid.

Application 1: Micturition

Micturition, also known as urination or voiding, refers to the process of expelling urine from the bladder. As the bladder fills, it expands due to the relaxation of muscles. This expansion, with the resulting increase in volume, enables fluid to be stored with only slight increases in pressure. When full, the bladder exerts an equal pressure on the surrounding tissue which results in pain if the pressure is not relieved.

When the volume reaches 300 to 400 ml, stretch receptors are activated causing a contraction of muscles in the bladder wall and a relaxation of the internal sphincter located at the entrance to the urethra. Contraction of the muscles effects an increase in pressure on the fluid. Since the internal sphincter is the region of lowest resistance and is not strong enough to oppose the increase in pressure, fluid from the bladder will flow through it in order to reduce the pressure within the bladder. Urine then flows to the external sphincter (consciously controlled) and urethra resulting in urination.

Application 2: Cardiac cycle

The pressure developed by the heart is dependent upon the size of the chambers and the volume of blood within a chamber. When blood flowing into the atria creates a hydrostatic pressure greater than in the ventricles, the resistance to blood flow through the atrio-ventricular valves is diminished. This region of low resistance allows blood to flow through it from the atria to the ventricles. At the point where intra-ventricular pressure is greater than the intra-atrial pressure, a backflow of blood closes the atrio-ventricular valves. The ventricles contract and develop a greater hydrostatic pressure. The semilunar valves (between ventricles and arteries) are forced open since the pressure in the aorta and pulmonary arteries is lower than the intra-ventricular pressure. That is, the resistance to the flow of blood from the ventricle has been overcome by an increased ventricular pressure, resulting in blood entering the arteries. The blood (hydrostatic) pressure in the arteries increases as the ventricle contracts. This increased pressure is referred to as systolic blood pressure.

The loss of blood from the ventricle decreases intra-ventricular pressure to a point where a greater arterial hydrostatic pressure exists. The semilunar valves are forced to close and the arterial pressure is now called the diastolic pressure. This pressure decreases until the intra-ventricular pressure is again greater than the arterial pressure, at which point the above cycle is repeated. Throughout the cardiac cycle, blood has moved from an area of high pressure to an area of low pressure by the assistance of valves.

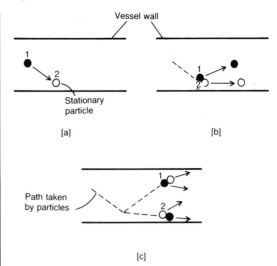

Figure 19.5 The collision of particles in a liquid results in a flow of the liquid. (a) Particle 1 is pushed towards particle 2. (b) Particle 1 collides with particle 2. (c) Particle 1 continues moving forward but in a different direction. Particle 2 moves forward as a result of the collision and collides with other particles in its path forcing these particles to move forward.

19.4 Flow of liquids through tubes

The volume of fluid passing a point in a given time period (mL/hr, L/min, drops/min) is called flow rate. If a pressure difference exists between the two regions of a tube, fluid will flow between the two regions.

A force that increases the movement of particles in a specific direction will cause these particles to collide with any other particles in their path. These collisions result in the forward movement of other particles in the liquid (Figure 19.5).

The greater the force imposed on these particles the greater is the kinetic energy gained by them, and this results in more frequent collisions. This increased frequency of collisions results in an increased flow of particles and thus a greater number of particles collide with the vessel wall per unit time. The pressure on the walls due to these collisions is called hydrostatic pressure.

The net movement of liquids through a vessel can be influenced by several factors.

Viscosity

The greater the thickness of a liquid, the greater is the force required to move that liquid. Viscosity of a fluid increases with an increase in the tendency to resist flow and bind to each other. The unit of measurement is the **poise**. A thick fluid with a high viscosity such as grease pours more slowly than a less dense liquid such as water.

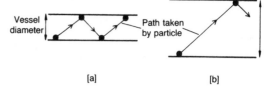

[a]   [b]

Figure 19.6 Effect of vessel diameter on the flow of a liquid. Particles collide more frequently with the wall of vessel (a) compared with (b). Each collision results in the loss of some kinetic energy, and so the greater number of collisions in vessel (a) results in a slower movement of the particle than in vessel (b). That is, the resistance to particle movement is greater in vessel (a) than in vessel (b).

Application: Blood viscosity

Normal human blood is from two to five times more viscous than water, due to plasma proteins and red blood cells within the blood. A condition that increases the number of red blood cells results in the heart having to use more force to overcome this liquid resistance. The increased work load placed upon the heart may result in cardiac failure if the viscosity remains elevated for a long period of time. An elevated viscosity results in an increased blood pressure.

Vessel diameter

The smaller the diameter of a vessel the greater is the resistance to the movement of particles. An increased resistance results from a greater probability of particles colliding with the vessel wall (Figure 19.6). When a particle collides with the wall some of the particle's kinetic energy is lost on impact, resulting in a slowing of the particle. In a smaller diameter vessel, excessive collisions of particles with the vessel wall will result in a marked decrease in the speed of particles moving through the vessel. This results in a decrease in hydrostatic pressure at regions further away from the constriction.

Application: Atherosclerosis

In this disease an accumulation of fat occurs in an arterial wall. This mass of fat is called an atheroma. As atheromas grow the build-up of fat decreases the vessel diameter resulting in the flow of blood being impeded. The change in blood flow can be detected using a Dopler instrument (Figure 14.3). Damage to tissues supplied by the blood vessel will depend upon the location and degree of atheroma development.

Vessel length

The longer a vessel, the greater is the resistance to the flow of liquid through it. A longer vessel will require a greater pressure to force a given volume of liquid through it than a shorter vessel. An increased pressure is required to overcome the resistance developed from the greater number of collisions of particles with the wall of the longer vessel.

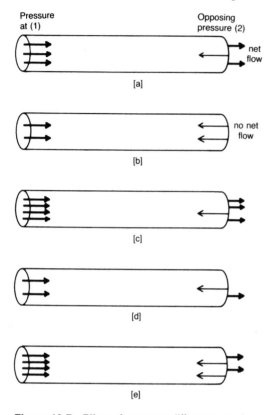

Pressure at (1)

Opposing pressure (2)

[a] net flow

[b] no net flow

[c]

[d]

[e]

Figure 19.7 Effect of pressure difference on the flow of liquids. (a) Pressure at (1) is greater than an opposing pressure at (2) which results in a flow of liquid. (b) There is no net movement of liquid, since equal but opposite pressures exist. (c) An increased difference in pressure between (1) and (2) results in an elevated flow of liquid. (d) A decreased pressure difference reduces the net flow of a liquid. (e) To overcome an increased opposing pressure that reduces net flow, an increased pressure is required at (1). Regions (1) and (2) can be compared with the heart (1) and peripheral vessels (2).

Difference in pressure between two regions

The net flow of a liquid depends upon the difference in pressure existing between two regions. A flow of liquid will occur from a region of high pressure to a region of low pressure (Figure 19.7a). If no pressure difference occurs between the two regions no net flow of liquid occurs (Figure 19.7b). An increased pressure difference results in an increase in the flow of liquid (Figure 19.7c). A decreased pressure difference between the regions reduces the flow of liquid (Figure 19.7d).

Application: Influence of blood pressure on blood flow

Blood flows throughout the body from regions of high pressure to regions of low pressure. Increasing the pressure difference between the large arteries and veins results in a greater flow of blood to the veins. That is, an increased flow of blood, containing oxygen and nutrients, occurs to the tissues. In exercise, muscles require a large increase in oxygen and glucose. These chemicals are supplied by increasing the arterial pressure and decreasing the peripheral pressure. That is, increasing the difference in pressure between the heart and tissues.

An increase in the pressure that opposes blood flow results from an increase in the resistance to blood flow. Increases in peripheral resistance cause a decrease in the pressure difference between the heart and tissues. This decrease results in a diminished flow of blood. An increase in the arterial pressure is required to maintain normal blood flow levels (Figure 19.7e). A sustained elevation of resistance, due to constriction of vessels by atherosclerosis and arteriole constriction results in chronic hypertension. As a result, an increased workload is placed on the heart. This increase may lead to cardiac failure if hypertension is not corrected.

Poiseuille's law

The above factors can be related by **Poiseuille's equation**.

$$\text{Flow Rate} = (P_1 - P_2)\frac{\pi r^4}{8\,nL} \quad \text{Eqn 19.5}$$

where $(P_1 - P_2)$ is the difference in pressure, $\pi = 3.14$, η is the viscosity of the liquid, L is the length of the tube and r is the inside radius of the tube. NOTE: This equation is limited to smooth-flowing liquids or **laminar flow**.

From the equation it can be seen that the driving force for the liquid is the pressure difference. Diameter, viscosity and length all contribute to the resistance to flow. The determining factor that controls flow is the tube radius since doubling the radius results in a substantial increase in flow. EXAMPLE: A change in the radius from 1 to 2 results in a change from 1^4 to 2^4 that is, 1 to 16. A doubling of the radius has resulted in a 16-fold increase in flow rate. Conversely a halving of the radius would reduce the flow rate by 1/16. **A small decrease in diameter causes a large increase in resistance and a large decrease in blood flow**.

The body uses this principle in the homeostatic mechanism for blood pressure. Arterioles alter their diameter in response to nerve stimulation. This property of arterioles controls the flow of blood to the capillaries and the resistance that results from the **constriction** of capillaries is referred to as **peripheral resistance**.

Application: Peripheral vascular resistance

Peripheral resistance refers to the resistance of small diameter blood vessels (arterioles, capillaries) to blood flow. The small diameter arteriole blood vessels can vary their diameter by vasoconstriction and vasodilation. These alterations in diameter are a result of muscular contraction and relaxation. The resistance to blood flow developed by the arterioles accounts for approximately half of the total systemic circulation resistance.

The greater the general resistance of the peripheral vessels to blood flow the greater is the amount of blood left in the arteries. A sustained increase in arterial pressure is referred to as hypertension. The greater the peripheral resistance, the greater is the force required by the heart to move blood through the body. This increased work load by the heart may lead to cardiac failure.

Turbulent flow

Turbulent flow results from an irregular surface inside the tube such as fatty deposits. In turbulent flow, eddies occur resulting in the backward and forward motion of blood. These opposing directions of flow result in a lower flow rate than laminar flow for the same conditions. The noise from the collisions between blood flowing in an eddie and blood flowing in a forward direction can be detected at times by a stethoscope (Application: Atherosclerosis).

Blood pressure

Blood pressure consists of two separate pressures due to the pulsatile pumping action of the heart. The greater pressure is developed by the left ventricle which pumps blood into the aorta. This is called the **systolic** pressure. The lesser pressure develops when the left ventricle is closed and being filled. This is called the **diastolic** pressure. The latter pressure is created by the recoiling of large elastic arteries.

These two pressures are recorded as follows:

16.0 kPa (120 mm Hg)   systolic pressure
10.6 kPa (80 mm Hg)   diastolic pressure

These values are for an average person at rest. Factors such as exercise, age, weight and stress will alter these values. Pressures that are considered normal are: systolic — 12.0 to 18.6 kPa (90 to 140 mm Hg) and diastolic — 6.6 to 12.0 kPa (50 to 90 mm Hg).

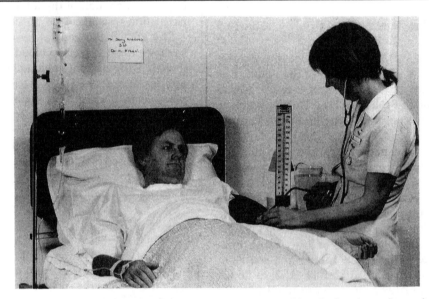

Figure 19.8 Measuring blood pressure and pulse rate and administering fluid through an intravenous fluid administration set.

Application: Measuring blood pressure and pulse rate

Blood pressure is usually measured by a sphygmomanometer (Figure 19.8). Compression of the upper arm by the cuff of the sphygmomanometer prevents blood flowing through the brachial artery. A gradual release of pressure allows the higher blood pressure (systolic) to flow through the arm, and is detected by a stethoscope placed over the artery. When the first sounds are heard on releasing the cuff pressure, the pressure on the sphygmomanometer should be noted. At the same time the mercury in the sphygmomanometer moves up and down in pulses. This is the systolic pressure. Further release of the cuff pressure allows the diastolic pressure to move blood through the arm. Since this pressure creates a continuous flow and not a pulse, the sounds due to the systolic pressure become muffled and will eventually disappear. Diastolic pressure occurs at the point where the regular beating sound becomes muffled. The pulsatile movement in the mercury column also ceases near the diastolic pressure.

The pulsatile property of systolic pressure can be used to determine heart beat, since every systolic pulse indicates another ventricular contraction. Systolic blood pressure and thus heart beats, can be felt wherever an artery occurs near the skin's surface. A firm background is required so that the artery can be compressed against this background. The commonest site for pulse rate determination is the radial artery in the lower arm. Other sites are also used (Figure 19.9) when it is difficult to use the radial artery. For example, if a patient is suffering from burns or fractures in this region.

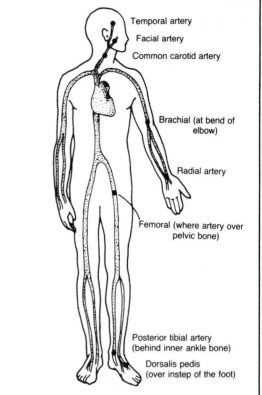

Figure 19.9 Location of alternative body sites for determining pulse rate.

19.5 Environmental health and safety

Pressure is an important factor in environmental health and safety. Its impact ranges from explosions resulting from the walls of a container not withstanding the pressure of its contents (see 6.7 APPLICATION: Explosions) to excessive pressure being applied to the body and within the body.

The close link between heat and pressure (see 19.2 Charles' law) requires personnel to be vigilant whenever sealed containers are exposed to heat. EXAMPLE: Apparently empty aerosol containers should never be heated as their thin walls are unable to withstand the pressure generated from the molecules still present in the 'empty' container.

The impact of external pressure on the body can be dramatic, such as a crush injury resulting from an accident involving a heavy object. In such an accident it is important that the correct protocol is carried out as the sudden release of large amounts of electrolytes from the crushed area can lead to further complications through the **crush injury syndrome**.

A number of factors can cause the alteration of fluid pressures within the body. Excessive loss of water in dehydration causes a change in osmotic pressure (see 21.2) while the excessive intake of a substance such as salt can lead to hypertension (see 34.4). Hypertension is also linked to sustained exposure to stress which could arise from a variety of work or environmentally related factors.

Summary

Pressure is the force applied by particles over a given area: pressure = force applied/area of application.

With solids, particles exert pressure mainly through an area in contact with another surface. The particles of gases and liquids exert a pressure by colliding with the walls of their container. Several factors may alter the rate of collision with a container's wall: temperature–Charles' law, volume–Boyle's law.

Any pressure greater than atmospheric pressure (101 kPa, 760 mm Hg) is regarded as positive pressure, and any that is less will be a negative pressure.

In a mixture of gases, each gas exerts its own pressure as if all the other gases were not present–Dalton's law. This is known as the partial pressure of a gas, e.g. PO_2.

The ability of a gas to dissolve in a liquid is proportional to the partial pressure of that gas–Henry's law.

The flow of gases and liquids through a tube is altered by the tube's diameter, length, and the difference in pressure between two regions of the tube. Fluid movement is also affected by its viscosity.

An increase in the kinetic energy of particles elevates pressure. With liquids this kinetic energy release is called hydrostatic pressure. In blood, the heart develops a hydrostatic pressure referred to as systolic blood pressure. The recoil of large elastic arteries produces a continuous diastolic blood pressure that is lower (6.6 to 12.0 kPa or 50 to 90 mm Hg) than the pulsatile systolic pressure (12.0 to 18.6 kPa or 90 to 140 mm Hg).

Chapter 20

Diffusion

Objectives

At the completion of this chapter the student should be able to:

1. describe the principle of diffusion;
2. explain how rates of diffusion may be altered within the body;
3. show how chemical gradients relate to rates of diffusion;
4. describe the effect of different substances diffusing across the same membrane;
5. describe how diffusion rates across a membrane are altered in body function.

20.1 Principle of diffusion

Diffusion is the net movement or flow of particles independent of metabolic energy from one region to another. The diffusion of non-electrolytes occurs from a region of high concentration to a region of low concentration. The process of diffusion has many applications in body function. EXAMPLES: Absorption of nutrients, exchange of oxygen and carbon dioxide, kidney function and dialysis.

Diffusion results from the energy of motion or kinetic energy of particles which are constantly colliding with each other. This constant motion of particles in random directions is called **Brownian movement**. The greater the concentration of particles in a region the greater the chance of collision. Particles in a region with a high number of collisions will be forced to a region where fewer collisions occur (Figure 20.1).

When the rate of collisions between particles in two regions is approximately equal (concentrations equal), no net movement of particles occurs. An equal movement of particles occurs between the two regions but the concentrations of particles in the two regions will remain the same.

Diffusion is rapid over short distances but slows down as distance increases. The ability of a particle to diffuse over a certain distance will be influenced by the following factors.

1. The number of particles between the given particle and its destination. The greater the number of particles, the greater will be the resistance to diffusion. Gas molecules diffuse a greater distance per unit time through a gaseous region than through a liquid. This difference between gases and liquids is due to the more dense liquid resisting movement of the gas molecules.

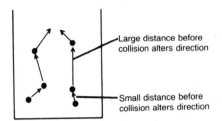

Figure 20.1   Diffusion of a substance from a
                  concentrated region to a less
                  concentrated region.

Generally, particles diffusing within gas
will move a greater distance than particles
diffusing in liquids. In the body's liquid
environment, forces such as the pressure
generated by the heart are necessary to
move the particles further than by simple
diffusion.

2. The larger the size and weight of a particle
    the greater is its inertia and the slower its
    rate of diffusion. To enable a comparison
    of the diffusion rates of different particles
    a term called the diffusion coefficient is
    used. The greater the weight of a particle
    the lower the diffusion coefficient.

3. An irregular-shape molecule may diffuse
    at a slower rate than a compact regular-
    shaped molecule that has a larger weight.
    A large globular plasma protein can dif-
    fuse faster than a long threadlike small
    molecule such as collagen.

Application: Diffusion of oxygen and
carbon dioxide

During inspiration a concentration difference develops between the lungs and
the atmosphere. This causes oxygen
and carbon dioxide to move the relatively large distance from the atmosphere to the alveoli. Differences in
concentrations of both oxygen and

---

carbon dioxide result in the diffusion of
dissolved oxygen from the alveoli to the
blood and dissolved carbon dioxide
from the blood to the alveoli (19.2). The
limited distance that substances can
diffuse in liquids is shown by the
body requiring a heart to pump blood
around the body to the tissue site. Since
diffusion in liquids occurs only through
short distances, a network of capillaries
ensures that this distance is not
too large to prevent the effective diffusion of oxygen from the lungs to the
blood and from the blood to the tissue
(Figure 20.2).

An increase in the capillary/alveoli
and capillary/tissue distance due to
oedema results in a greater resistance to
diffusion. A decreased ability of oxygen
and carbon dioxide to diffuse to the
appropriate region occurs. The greater
the degree of oedema the less oxygen
and carbon dioxide that can diffuse.

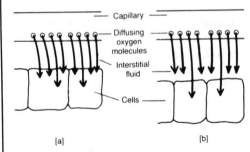

Figure 20.2   Diffusion of oxygen between a
                  capillary and cells. (a) When the
                  normal amount of interstitial fluid
                  separates the capillary and cells
                  sufficient oxygen diffuses to the
                  cells. (b) An increase in the amount
                  of interstitial fluid results in an
                  increase in resistance to the
                  diffusion of oxygen to the cells.

This lack of oxygen diffusion to the blood and tissue can be altered by increasing the difference in concentration between the alveoli/blood and blood/tissue regions. Hyperbaric chambers increase the concentration of oxygen in the lungs which results in more oxygen being able to diffuse the greater distance from the alveoli to the blood or from the blood to the cells.

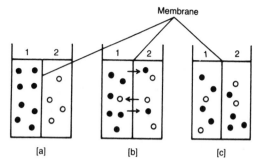

[a]   [b]   [c]

Figure 20.3 Diffusion of one substance across a membrane. (a) Solution 1 contains twice the number of oxygen molecules as solution 2, and they are separated by a membrane that allows oxygen to pass through it. (b) Twice as many oxygen molecules diffuse across the membrane from solution 1 to solution 2 than from solution 2 to solution 1; net diffusion of oxygen occurs from solution 1 to solution 2. (c) Chemical equilibrium results from the net movement of oxygen, i.e. the number of oxygen molecules in each solution becomes equal.

20.2 Diffusion across membranes

If a membrane is permeable to a solute (i.e. solute can diffuse across it) and a difference in concentration of the solute exists between the two sides of the membrane, the solute will diffuse across the membrane from the region of high concentration to the region of low concentration (Figure 20.3).

In solution 1, the greater number of oxygen molecules results in twice the chance that a given molecule will collide with the membrane than will a molecule from solution 2 (Figure 20.3a). If a particular oxygen molecule collides at the site of a hole (pore) in the membrane, it will pass through the membrane pore as long as it is smaller than the pore. This difference in the rate of collisions with the membrane results in a net movement of oxygen from solution 1 to solution 2 (Figure 20.3b). Molecules will also move from a low concentration to a high concentration but twice as many oxygen molecules move from the higher concentration. A net flow of molecules occurs until the concentration of oxygen in solutions 1 and 2 is equal (Figure 20.3c), that is, the chance of an oxygen molecule hitting a membrane pore is equal

on both sides of the membrane (chemical equilibrium). The greater the difference in concentration across a membrane, the greater is the rate of diffusion.

If the membrane separates two different solutes of neutral charge such as oxygen and carbon dioxide, these solutes will diffuse independently of each other (Figure 20.4). The oxygen molecules will diffuse down their concentration gradient by colliding with the membrane pores whilst the carbon dioxide will collide independently with the membrane pores. Diffusion of oxygen and carbon dioxide across the alveolar membrane relies on this principle.

Several factors may alter the diffusion rate of a solute across a membrane.

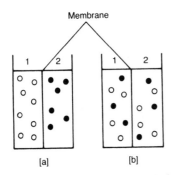

Figure 20.4 Diffusion of two substances across a membrane. (a) Solution 1 contains oxygen whereas solution 2 contains carbon dioxide. These two solutions are separated by a membrane that allows both oxygen and carbon dioxide to pass through it. (b) Both oxygen and carbon dioxide diffuse across the membrane *independently* of each other. Independent diffusion results in a chemical equilibrium between solution 1 and solution 2 for oxygen and a separate chemical equilibrium for carbon dioxide.

1. If the particles are charged, this charge will influence diffusion, as like charges repel. With charged particles the rate of diffusion depends upon the chemical and electrical gradient (difference in potential) (10.3). This balance of chemical and electrical gradients is important in the functioning of nerves and muscles (see 10.1).
2. If the surface area of a membrane separating solutions is decreased the rate of diffusion of particles across the membrane decreases. The presence of fewer membrane pores results in less particles being able to pass through the membrane at any moment.
3. An increase in membrane thickness results in a greater resistance to particles diffusing across it. The particles are also required to move a greater distance. Both of these effects can result in decreased

efficiency of respiratory gas exchange. EXAMPLE: Pulmonary fibrosis.

Application 1: Emphysema

In emphysema the total surface area of the alveolar respiratory membrane decreases due to the loss of alveolar walls. The diffusion of gases across the alveolar membrane is significantly impeded, even at rest, if the loss of total membrane surface area is greater than one-third of normal.

Application 2: Small intestine structure

The principle of an increased surface area creating an elevated rate of diffusion is shown by the extensive folding in the small intestine. This folding occurs both macroscopically and microscopically as is shown in Figure 20.5. The ultrastructure of the small intestine surface is shown in Figure 25.2. The absorptive area is increased by about 600-fold to provide a membrane surface area of 250 square metres. This large surface area enables a maximum absorption of nutrients across the small intestine and provides a large reserve for small intestine function. Removal of up to 75% of the small intestine can occur without the patient suffering serious malnutrition.

Summary

Diffusion is the net movement or flow of particles independent of metabolic energy from one region to another. Non-electrolytes diffuse from a region of high concentration to a region of low concentration. This net movement is due to the Brownian motion of particles. The ability of a particle to diffuse a certain distance will be influenced by the:

1. number of particles that it must diffuse through;
2. size and weight of the diffusing particles;
3. shape of the particle;
4. charge of the particle.

Particles will diffuse across a membrane separating two solutions of different concentrations. That is, more particles collide with the membrane on one side and then pass through it. When different non-electrolytes are in a solution, each non-electrolyte will diffuse across the membrane independent of other non-electrolytes.

The rate of diffusion across a membrane is altered by a change in the surface area of membrane and the membrane's thickness.

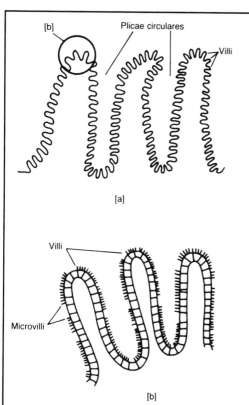

Figure 20.5 Cross-section of a small intestine wall showing folds (plicae circulares) and projections (villi and microvilli) which vastly increase the surface area. (a) Macroscopic view of the small intestine showing the deep folds of the plicae circulares which contain small projections (0.5 to 1.0 mm) called villi. (b) Microscopic view of villi shows a large number of finger-like projections from the plasma membranes of cells involved with nutrient absorption.

Chapter 21

Osmosis and body fluid balance

Objectives

At the completion of this chapter the student should be able to:

1. describe the principle of osmosis;
2. define osmotic pressure, osmol, hypotonic, isotonic and hypertonic;
3. compare and contrast the effects of isotonic, hypotonic and hypertonic solutions on cells;
4. explain how osmotic equilibrium exists between cells and the extracellular fluid;
5. describe how a balance exists between hydrostatic pressure and osmotic pressure at the capillary;
6. explain why this balance of pressure is important in the maintenance of body fluid;
7. explain how an imbalance in hydrostatic or osmotic pressure alters body fluid volume and nutrient supply.

21.1 Principle of osmosis

A large proportion of a human body consists of water. The diffusion of water is an important component of normal cell function and this diffusion is referred to as osmosis.

Osmosis is the net movement of water through a semi-permeable membrane from an area of high water concentration to an area of low water concentration. A **semi-permeable membrane** is a membrane which allows the movement of water but not other substances, through it. When a semi-

permeable membrane separates solutions of different concentrations, water will diffuse from the region of high water concentration to the region of low water concentration.

In Figure 21.1a two solutions of equal volume but different concentration are separated by a semi-permeable membrane. Solution 1 contains a larger number of water molecules than solution 2, that is, in solution 1 a greater proportion of water molecules make up the total volume. A net movement of water molecules occurs from 1 to 2 since there is a greater chance that a water molecule from solution 1 will collide with the membrane than there is from solution 2. The kinetic energy of water molecules results in a

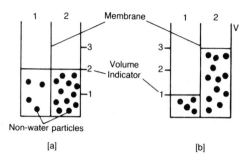

[a]   [b]

Figure 21.1 Movement of water by the process of osmosis across a semi-permeable membrane. (a) Two solutions that contain the same quantity of particles (equal volumes are separated by a semi-permeable membrane). (b) Solution 1 contains a greater proportion of water molecules than solution 2. This means that there is more chance of water molecules in solution 1 colliding with the membrane than in solution 2. A net movement of water occurs from the region of high water concentration (solution 1) to the region of low water concentration (solution 2) until the water concentrations in each are equal.

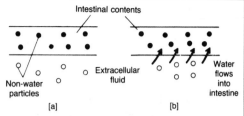

[a]   [b]

Figure 21.2 Action of purgative agents such as Epsom salts in the intestine. (a) Purgative agents are retained within the intestine since they cannot penetrate the intestinal membrane. Retention of Epsom salts results in a lower water concentration within the intestine than in the surrounding body fluid. (b) Water moves by osmosis from the high water concentration of the body fluid to the intestinal content until the water concentrations are approximately equal. This movement results in an increased fluidity of the intestinal contents which results in easier evacuation of the bowels.

movement of water molecules in both directions, but a net flow will occur until the water concentrations are equal (Figure 21.1b). In balancing the water concentrations, a change of volume has occurred. This change of volume will occur whenever a change in concentration of a solution develops.

Application: Purgative agents

Purgative (cathartic) agents such as Epsom salts (magnesium sulphate) act by increasing the water content of the faeces (Figure 21.2).

21.2   Terms relating to osmosis

Osmotic pressure

This is the pressure required to exactly oppose the net movement of water by osmosis, that is the resistance that is required to just stop the net flow of water. Osmosis results from the pressure difference developed on opposite sides of a membrane by a greater number of water particles colliding with one side of the membrane than the other side. The greater the difference in water concentration the greater is the osmotic pressure that is required to prevent water molecules moving via osmosis.

The osmotic pressure of a solution depends upon the proportion of non-electrolytes, electrolytes and colloids present compared with water molecules. Compounds that separate in solution (dissociate) into ions, create a greater osmotic pressure than compounds that remain intact in solution.

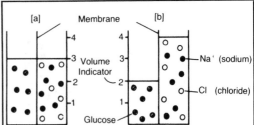

Figure 21.3 A comparison of the effect of glucose (left chamber) and sodium chloride (right chamber) on osmosis. (a) 100 mmol of glucose and a 100 mmol of sodium chloride are dissolved in water. (b) The sodium chloride solution contains twice as many particles in water as the glucose solution and the proportion of water molecules is less in the sodium chloride solution than the glucose solution. This difference in water concentration results in water diffusing from the glucose to the sodium chloride solution until both water concentrations are equal.

Application: Electrolyte and non-electrolyte influence on osmotic pressure

Glucose contains the same number of particles whether it exists as a solid or is dissolved in a liquid. Sodium chloride consists of twice as many particles in solution than when it exists as a solid. This increase in particles is a result of sodium ions and chloride ions separating (dissociating) when placed in solution. Thus 100 mmol of sodium chloride in solution contains double the number of particles and develops twice the osmotic pressure as 100 mmol of glucose (Figure 21.3).

Classically osmotic pressure was measured by the use of a hydraulic cylinder connected with a pressure gauge (Figure 21.4a). To measure the potential degree of water movement it was easier to determine the pressure that was required to prevent the flow of water. Thus, osmotic pressure was always greatest on the side with a lower water concentration. In Figure 21.4b, a net flow of water develops from the distilled water when no external forces are present. This flow is due to the greater probability of water molecules colliding with the membrane surface that adjoins the distilled water than the surface that adjoins the test solution. The pressure developed by this difference in probability can be opposed by exerting an equal but opposite pressure. This opposing pressure will increase the number of water molecules in the test solution colliding with the membrane surface. This opposing pressure is developed by compressing the piston against solution B which forces more water molecules to collide with the membrane at any given moment (Figure 21.4c). The osmotic pressure developed by solution B can be determined by measuring the pressure that is required to maintain volume of solution A at its original level (Figure 21.4c).

Osmotic pressure is always greatest on the side with the lowest water concentration and in real terms is a measure of the pressure required to oppose osmosis.

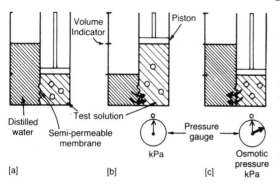

Figure 21.4 The measurement of osmotic pressure. (a) A solution of unknown osmotic pressure is placed in a cylinder containing a piston. This cylinder is separated from a measured volume of distilled water by a semi-permeable membrane. (b) Water will flow from the high water concentration to the test solution if the piston is not exerting any pressure. (c) The osmotic pressure or resistance to the flow of water is determined by applying pressure on the piston. The osmotic pressure is that pressure exerted by the piston which returns the distilled water to the original water level. That is, the required pressure that will prevent the net flow of water.

Osmol

Osmol is the measurement of a solute's ability to induce osmosis and osmotic pressure and is a measure of the total number of particles present in a solution. One osmol equals one mole (3.2) of particles present in a solution. Note that when one mole of electrolyte (e.g. sodium chloride) is placed in solution, separation into sodium and chloride ions results in a greater number of particles than occurs with a substance that remains intact in a solution. The number of osmols in an electrolyte solution is determined by multiplying the molar concentration by the number of ions present in one molecule. EXAMPLE: Calcium chloride ($CaCl_2$) contains one calcium ion and two chloride ions. A one molar concentration will therefore contain three osmols.

In physiological solutions the low concentration of particles requires the use of a term one-thousandth of an osmol, called the milliosmol (mosmol).

Osmolarity and osmolality

The osmol concentration of a solution can be described in two ways. These are osmolality when expressed per kilogram of water and osmolarity when expressed per litre of solution. These terms are interchangeable when body fluid concentrations are used. The osmolal concentration of isotonic body fluid is 280 to 290 mosmol/L. An approximate indication of correct body fluid osmolality can be found by determining if the serum sodium concentration is in the range 137 to 149 mmol/L. An elevated serum sodium would indicate a loss of water and an increased osmolality.

Isotonic or isosmotic solution

This solution will cause no shrinking or swelling of normal body cells when the latter are placed in it. The osmotic pressure in the fluid and cells is equal. No net movement of water will occur between the fluid and cell (Figure 21.5a). EXAMPLE: 50 g/L glucose solution, 9 g/L sodium chloride solution.

Hypotonic solution

This is a solution that will cause normal cells to swell. These solutions exert a lower osmotic pressure than cells. Water flows from

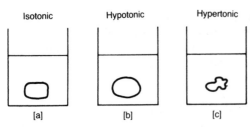

[a]   [b]   [c]

Figure 21.5 Effect of varying solution
concentrations on red blood cells.
(a) In an isotonic solution no net
movement of water occurs. Cells
retain their original size and shape.
(b) Hypotonic solution creates a net
movement of water into the cells, the
cells swell and may rupture
(haemolysis). (c) Hypertonic solution
causes cells to shrink (crenation).

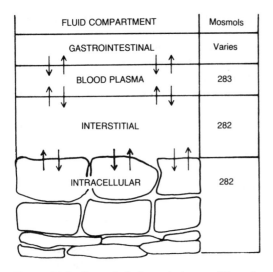

FLUID COMPARTMENT	Mosmols
GASTROINTESTINAL	Varies
BLOOD PLASMA	283
INTERSTITIAL	282
INTRACELLULAR	282

Figure 21.6 Osmotic balance between different
body fluid compartments.

the bathing solution into cells, which results
in a swelling of the cells (Figure 21.5b). When
a low osmotic pressure stretches the cell
membrane to its limit, the cell will rupture,
i.e. cells lyse. EXAMPLE: Erythrocytes (red
blood cells) will haemolyse when placed in a

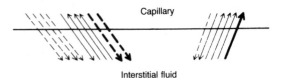

Capillary

Interstitial fluid

Figure 21.7 Exchange of fluid and nutrients at
the capillary according to Starling's
law of the capillary. The thick arrows
indicate the net movement of fluid.
The _ _ _ arrows show the relative
hydrostatic pressure and the —
arrows the osmotic pressure.

hypotonic solution such as distilled water or
4.5 g/L sodium chloride.

Hypertonic solution

This is a solution that develops a greater
osmotic pressure than cells. Hypertonic solutions have a lower water concentration
than cells, thus resulting in normal cells
losing water and shrinking (Figure 21.5c).
EXAMPLE: 18 g/L sodium chloride.

21.3 Osmotic equilibrium between cells and their surrounding fluid

The concentration of particles in the extracellular fluid compartment equals the concentration of particles in the intracellular
compartment (Figure 21.6). Throughout the
body there is an osmotic equilibrium between
these compartments. A change of concentration in one compartment also changes the
concentration in the other compartment
(Figure 21.8).

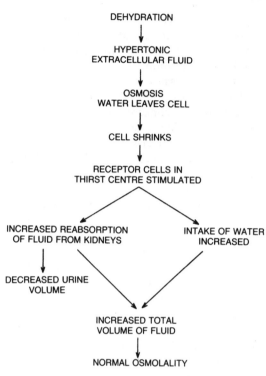

Figure 21.8 Effect of dehydration on the homeostatic mechanisms for the control of osmotic balance.

21.4 Capillary hydrostatic pressure and osmotic pressure influence on interstitial fluid concentration

In capillaries, a balance exists between differences in osmotic pressure and hydrostatic pressure. This balance enables particles to be moved to the cells and cell products to be returned to the vascular system (Figure 21.7). An imbalance in this system can result in alterations to body fluid distribution, such as oedema.

In the capillary, the hydrostatic pressure is sufficient to force solutes and water through gaps in the capillary walls. As blood flows along the capillary, an increase in resistance occurs due to both the small diameter and length of the vessel. This resistance results in a decreased hydrostatic pressure at the venule end of the capillary. The hydrostatic pressure decreases from 4.0 kPa to 1.0 kPa.

The osmotic pressure in the capillary is mainly due to plasma proteins exerting a pressure of 3.0 kPa in the opposite direction to the hydrostatic pressure. The interstitial fluid has an osmotic pressure of 1.0 kPa and no hydrostatic pressure. This results in a greater number of particles colliding with the vascular wall of the capillary than the interstitial side of the capillary. A net flow of particles into the interstitial fluid occurs. Large molecules such as the plasma proteins normally cannot pass through the capillary gaps. The retention of proteins in the blood maintains the osmotic pressure along the length of the capillary. Towards the venule end, the hydrostatic pressure decreases below the osmotic pressure. Fluid returns to the capillary by the influence of osmosis as a result of the greater number of water and solute particles colliding with the interstitial wall of the capillary.

Application: Oedema

Hypertension can result in a decreased osmotic influence. Hydrostatic pressure is greater than normal and pushes excess fluids into the interstitial space. Osmotic pressure is insufficient to overcome all of the hydrostatic influence, and thus fluid is retained in the interstitial region.

21.5 Environmental health and safety

The loss of water through the prolonged exposure to heat or through burns or fever can result in an osmotic imbalance known as dehydration.

Application: Dehydration

Diarrhoea, vomiting, fever and burns cause net water loss which results in dehydration. In dehydration, the extracellular fluid compartment loses water. This results in a hypertonic extracellular fluid when compared with the intracellular fluid compartment. Water flows via osmosis from the cell to the extracellular fluid, causing the cell to shrink. Receptor cells in the thirst centre of the brain are stimulated by shrinking. These cells initiate a homeostatic mechanism that returns the osmolality of the extracellular and intracellular fluids to normal (Figure 21.8).

Summary

Osmosis is the net diffusion of water through a semi-permeable membrane from a region of high water concentration to a region of low water concentration, that is, from a region of low solute concentration to a region of high solute concentration.

Osmotic pressure is that pressure which will oppose osmosis. The region with the lowest water concentration contains the greatest osmotic pressure.

Electrolytes can dissociate in water, creating a greater number of particles and thus a greater osmotic pressure than substances that remain intact.

The osmotic pressure of an isotonic solution is the same as intracellular fluid, whereas with hypertonic solutions the pressure is greater, and in hypotonic solutions it is less.

The ability of a substance to induce osmosis and osmotic pressure is measured in osmols. An osmol is the total number of particles present in a solution and is thus related to the molarity of a solution. In body fluids, osmolarity and osmolality are interchangeable terms describing the osmol concentration.

An osmotic equilibrium exists between the blood, interstitial and intracellular body fluid compartments. An alteration in the concentration of one compartment has corresponding affects in the other compartments.

In capillaries, a balance exists between differences in osmotic pressure and hydrostatic pressure — Starling's law of the capillary. This balance enables an exchange of respiratory gases and nutrients between the blood and interstitial fluid.

Unit Eight
Life and the Cell

This unit outlines the characteristics of life
and relates cell structure and function to life.
The role of the plasma membrane and
nucleus in cell function is treated.

Chapter 22

The cellular basis of life

Objectives

At the completion of this chapter the student should be able to:

1. describe the structure of a typical animal cell and relate this structure to cell function;
2. describe the differences between eucaryotic and procaryotic cells;
3. differentiate between cilia and flagella;
4. define cell inclusion and give examples of beneficial and harmful cell inclusions;
5. relate the use of drugs to bacterial structure;
6. relate capsules and endospores to bacterial function.

22.1 Characteristics of life

Living things consist of **protoplasm**. The protoplasm is composed mainly of water, macromolecules such as proteins, lipids, carbohydrates, nucleotide-based structures as well as inorganic substances such as electrolytes. Protoplasm is organized into cells which form the structural and functional units of life.

The main characteristics that distinguish living organisms from non-living objects are: metabolism, growth, reproduction, feeding, excretion, irritability and movement.

1. **Metabolism** reflects the overall homeostatic mechanism for regulating chemical processes within an organism. The breakdown of chemicals is called **catabolism** and provides the source of energy for organisms to sustain life through **cellular respiration**. The construction of molecules is required to form the necessary functional components required to maintain structure and allow growth to occur.

2. **Growth** refers to an increase in size or number of cells. If growth did not occur it would not be possible for an organism to reproduce and maintain the same size of organism as every cell division would result in generations of ever decreasing size.

3. **Reproduction**. As organisms die and cells die it is necessary for the cells to be copied to maintain the life of a multicellular organism and to provide a continuation of that life form following the death of an organism. Reproduction refers to the formation of new cells or the production of another generation of that organism.

4. **Feeding** is the mechanism through which the organism is able to obtain the nutrients

and energy necessary for metabolism and growth.

5. **Excretion** is the process of removing unwanted substances from the organism. These may include toxic waste products, harmful substances taken in from the environment and excessive levels of a substance.

6. **Irritability** or excitability is the ability to respond to a stimulus from the environment. This feature is necessary for organisms to make adjustments to optimize its function in a changing external environment.

7. **Movement** is more obvious in animals than plants where it is used to obtain food, defend itself and assist a wide variety of specific needs that vary between organisms. In plants movement mainly results from growth.

22.2 Classification of life

All life forms are classified according to their characteristics into a system of subdivisions commencing with **kingdoms**. A broad understanding of the overall classification process is important for Health Care Professionals as it provides a basis for the study of medical microbiology (Unit 12) and provides an insight into the relative position of humans in the living world.

Kingdoms represent major differences such as whether an organism is an animal, plant or a procaryotic organism. Each of these kingdoms have fundamental differences in their cell structure. EXAMPLE: Kingdom Animalia consist of complex cells (Figure 22.1) while Kingdom Procaryotae (Monera) consists of comparatively simple cells that lack most of the organelles (Figure 22.4). The subdivisions of the kingdoms are **division** or **phylum, class, order, family, genus** and **species**. There are over one million animal species and half a million plant species which represent only a fraction of the number that have existed. Classification systems therefore have to take into account the ancestry (evolutionary process) as well as structure, function and molecular make-up. **Taxonomy** represents the placing or **classifying** of an organism in this catalogue of past and present life. Determining the specific classification of an organism can at times, result in differences of opinion amongst scientists as new knowledge about a particular organism or group of organisms can lead to its reclassification.

Organisms within a species share the characteristic of **interbreeding** or **the capacity to interbreed**. If the organisms are asexual (35.3), they are alike in structure and function as far as can be determined. Within a species several races may occur. EXAMPLE: All humans consist of several races of the same species *sapiens*. Similar species are grouped into the next level called **genus**. EXAMPLE: Humans belong to the genus *Homo*. Each known living organism has a scientific name with the first word being the genus and the second representing the species. EXAMPLE: Humans are called *homo sapiens*.

Similar genera are grouped into **families**. EXAMPLE: Humans belong to the family *Hominidae*. Families are grouped into an order. EXAMPLE: *Hominidae* is one of eleven families in the order **Primates**. Similar orders form a class. EXAMPLE: Sixteen orders form the class *Mammalia* (Mammals). Classes form a division or phylum. EXAMPLE: Five classes form the group of animals containing a backbone or backbone-like structure and are therefore called *Chordata*. The divisions form the kingdoms which represent the umbrella of life under which all life is classified. There are five kingdoms *Procaryotae (Monera), Protista, Fungi, Planta* and *Animalia*.

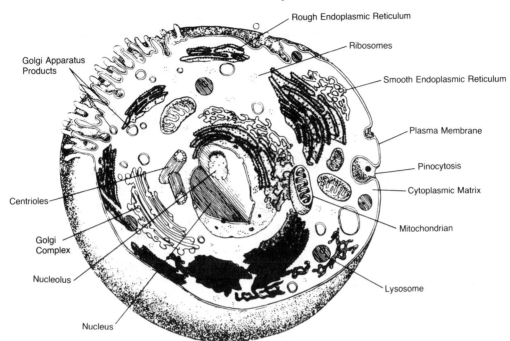

Golgi Apparatus Products

Centrioles

Golgi Complex

Nucleolus

Nucleus

Rough Endoplasmic Reticulum

Ribosomes

Smooth Endoplasmic Reticulum

Plasma Membrane

Pinocytosis

Cytoplasmic Matrix

Mitochondrian

Lysosome

Figure 22.1 The general structure of an animal cell. (After Figure 3.1 in *Principles of Anatomy and Physiology*, 3rd edition, Copyright © 1981 Gerard J. Tortora and Nicholas P. Anagnostakos, reproduced by permission of Harper and Row Publishers Inc.)

Monera are organisms with a procaryotic cell. EXAMPLE: Bacteria (Figures 22.4 and 22.5).The *Protista* kingdom consists of protozoa (35.10) while the *Fungi* kingdom represents the fungi (35.11 and Figure 35.9). *Planta* represent eucaryotic plant cells and *animalia* eucaryotic animal cells. In this chapter the structure and function of cells is discussed.The protista, procaryoticae and fungi are discussed in Chapter 35.

22.3   Cell theory

All organisms, from bacteria to humans, consist of matter that is arranged in structural and functional units called cells. A cell is generally the smallest and simplest unit of matter that has the potential to duplicate itself. The only forms of matter that do not consist of cells but which are capable of

reproducing themselves are the viruses. Viruses are termed acellular, that is, non-cellular.

All cells consist of a complex arrangement of molecules. These molecules are almost entirely composed of the elements carbon, hydrogen, oxygen and nitrogen. Cells function by altering the structure of intracellular molecules. These molecules are either broken down to provide energy or are altered into new molecules that are required by the cell or other cells in the body. Cellular homeostasis enables cells to maintain their chemical function in a changing extra-cellular environment.

The study of cells is known as cytology. Cells are divided into two types according to their internal structure. The procaryotic cells are cells that consist of a simple internal structure. Eucaryotic cells have a highly organized internal structure.

22.4   General structure of eucaryotic cells

A generalized eucaryotic cell consists of the following structures.

1. **Plasma (cell) membrane** — this separates the cell's internal contents from the extracellular environment. The term protoplasm is used to describe a cell's contents along with the plasma membrane. Protoplasm is usually divided into the nucleus and the cytoplasm.
2. **Nucleus** — a relatively large membrane-bound structure that controls and regulates cell multiplication and maintains cell function.
3. **Cytoplasm** — this is a general name for all the contents of a cell apart from the nucleus. The cytoplasm can be divided into the cytoplasmic matrix, the cytoskeleton, the internal membrane system, membrane organelles and cell inclusions.

Both animals and plants are composed of eucaryotic cells. These two forms of eucaryotic cells contain many common organelles. Each also has some unique organelles. EXAMPLE: Chloroplasts are present in plant cells but not animal cells. The general structure of an animal cell is shown in Figure 22.1.

A cell is a microcosm of life in a city. This analogy will be used to assist in understanding and remembering the function of organelles. An introductory account of the main functions of each animal cell component is described below. Note that there are many variations in the form that a cell can take. The different cell forms are described in 25.1.

22.5   Cell membranes

The plasma membrane consists of one layer of membrane. The structure of a membrane is described in 23.1. Most membranes that surround organelles also consist of one layer. Membranes play an important role in the protection and function of organelles as they control the substances that can enter an organelle thereby protecting the cell from the entry of harmful substances. The nucleus and mitochondria are surrounded by two layers of membrane and form part of the internal membrane system. ANALOGY: The membranes of a cell act as protective wrappers similar to the plastic wrappers used to seal foods.

An internal membrane system within cells provides a path for the movement of substances between the nucleus, endoplasmic reticulum, golgi complex and cell surface (22.9). The plasma membrane is described in Chapter 23.

22.6   Nucleus

The nucleus is the largest structure within a cell. It is surrounded by two membranes that contain openings or pores and form the nuclear envelope (22.7). It is possible that these pores can be closed to prevent the leakage of substances through the membrane.

Within the nuclear envelope (membrane) there exists a gel-like material called nucleoplasm, one or more spherical bodies called nucleoli (nucleolus singular) and genetic material in the shape of rods. These rods are the basis of hereditary information and are termed **chromosomes**. The chromosomes control cell reproduction whereas the nucleoli are involved in the transfer of hereditary information into a form that regulates cell chemical reactions. ANALOGY: The nucleus acts as an information resource centre from which material can be organized for use by the cytoplasmic organelles.

22.7 Cytoplasmic matrix

The cytoplasmic matrix or cytosol consists of a mixture of solutions, sols and gels. The solution component contains mainly dissolved proteins, electrolytes, fatty acids, glucose and cholesterol. The sol consists of large particles such as fat globules, glycogen granules, inclusions, secretory packages and cytoplasmic organelles dispersed in a liquid. A gel often exists near the plasma membrane.

The cytoplasmic matrix or cytosol contains all the principal structures involved in cell shape and movement, the manufacture of proteins and metabolic activity.

22.8 The cytoskeleton

Within the cytoplasmic matrix is a dynamic and spongy cytoskeleton which provides the framework necessary for maintaining cell shape as well as having a role in cell division, cell mobility and any changes in gel/sol (17.6) that may occur within the cytoplasm. ANALOGY: The cytoskeleton acts like a tent frame where the tent's shape and structural properties are determined by the frame. In a cell's movement, the cell membrane follows passively any changes in the cytoskeleton. The main cytoskeletal components are microtubules, microtubular organelles, microfilaments and intermediate filaments.

Microtubules

Microtubules are thin, rigid-like tubular structures about 25 nm in diameter consisting mainly of the protein tubulin. Microtubules can change in length rapidly by the process of polymerization or depolymerization of the tubulin building blocks which are referred to as subunits. The rapid change in cell shape allows mobile cells to move throughout the body. The unique structural shape of different cell types (25.1) is due to the microtubule arrangement within each cell form. The rapid changes that occur with cell division and the need to separate the chromosomes is achieved through microtubules which play a major role in formation of the asters and the spindle during different stages of cell division (24.2 and Figure 24.2). The spindle is responsible for the separation of chromosomes to opposite poles.

Microtubules provide a guide for the axoplasmic transport of proteins, hormones (39.3) and neurotransmitters (38.1). Microtubules may also form conducting channels through which various substances can move through the cytoplasm.

The microtubules within flagella and cilia are essential for the generation of motion by these structures (see p. 244).

Centrioles and basal bodies

Centrioles are small microtubular organelles consisting of a cylindrical structure. They exist in animal cells. They consist of nine groups of microtubule clusters arranged in a circle. Each cluster consists of microtubule triplets. Generally, a pair occurs which separate during the early stages of cell division and migrate to opposite poles of a cell where they are involved in the formation of the spindle. In plant cells the spindle is formed without them.

Basal bodies are structurally similar to centrioles but provide the anchorage base for cilia and flagella.

Cilia and flagella

These microtubular organelles are structural projections of the plasma membrane containing nine microtubule doublets arranged in a circle plus two in the centre. This microtubular shaft is referred to as the axoneme. Cilia and flagella exhibit motile properties. **Cilia** are short hair-like motile projections that occur in numerous quantities on the plasma membrane. **Flagella** (flagellum singular) are long motile projections that occur in small numbers.

Cilia usually propel material from one cell to the next by moving in coordinated waves. EXAMPLES: The respiratory tract is lined with cilia that propel mucus from the lungs. The fallopian or uterine tubes are lined with ciliated cells that move the ovum from the ovaries to the uterus. Flagella move like a whip. They are used for propelling cells. EXAMPLE: Sperm are propelled by the movement of their long tail or flagellum (Figure 25.1).

Microfilaments

The smallest cytoskeletal structures are the microfilaments. These thin structures of 4–6 nm diameter are variable in length and are mainly composed of the protein actin. The contractile properties of muscle cells is

due to actin interacting with another protein myosin (25.4 and 30.8). Cell motility in non-muscle cells appears to involve the interaction of actin and myosin. Microfilaments are also responsible for cellular cohesion.

Intermediate filaments

Intermediate filaments are so named as their size (diameter 8–12 nm) is in between the relatively large size of microtubules (25 nm) and the small microfilaments (4–6 nm). They mainly consist of a range of fibrous proteins (30.4) that provide a mechanical role in the cell such as structural reinforcement and contraction. EXAMPLE: They form the major structural proteins of skin and hair. Intermediate filaments form networks that interconnect the nucleus with the cell surface.

There are four main types: keratin filaments, neurofilaments, glial filaments and heterogenous filaments. Keratin filaments are anchored to the cell surface and are formed in the living layers of the epidermis (25.3). They form the bulk of the dead layers or stratum corneum. Neurofilaments and microtubules form the main structural framework of nerve cells (25.5). Neurofilaments form the neurofibrils that appear to be involved in transportation and support. Glial filaments are found in the cytoplasm of the astrocytes which are neuroglial cells found in the central nervous system (25.5). The heterogenous filaments are a group filaments of similar appearance but contain different proteins. One group contain the protein desmin which plays an important structural role in muscle cells where they form an interconnecting network across each muscle cell. They anchor and orient myofibrils thereby providing the basis for alignment of myofibrils into the repetitive pattens that are referred to as striations (Figure 25.4). These striations provide a basis for the unified contraction that generates the strength in a muscles action.

22.9 Internal membrane system

The internal membrane system or endo-membrane system is a system of membrane lined tubes that are interconnected through-out the cell. The system consists of the nuclear envelope, endoplasmic reticulum or ER and the golgi complex.

Nuclear envelope

The two membranes of the nuclear envelope merge at points to form pores. These pores allow the movement of large molecules carry-ing genetic instructions into the endoplasmic reticulum and cytoplasmic matrix.

Endoplasmic reticulum

The endoplasmic reticulum or ER consists of a membraneous network of canals that runs through the entire cytoplasm. The ER system of canals can be linked directly to both the nuclear envelope and the plasma membrane (Figure 22.1). The ER can be in the form of either canals or flattened canals which terminate in sac-like structures.

This canal system conveys information from the nucleus to the cytoplasm and allows intercommunication between the outside and the inside of a cell. EXAMPLE: In muscles, the ER plays an important role in the coupl-ing of muscle depolarization at the plasma membrane with the initiation of the con-tractile state deep inside a muscle cell. The presence of a canal system enables an efficient movement of substances through-out a cell which bypasses the relatively inefficient, slow movement of chemicals via diffusion through the cytoplasmic matrix.

The endoplasmic reticulum exists in two forms, either rough ER or smooth ER.

The **rough endoplasmic reticulum** bears a covering of tiny organelles called ribosomes. The ribosomes are the site of protein manu-facture. Instructions are carried from the nucleus via the ER to the areas of rough ER where the appropriate proteins are manu-factured. The proteins can then be trans-ported via the ER to storage sites or released out of the cell.

Endoplasmic reticulum that lacks a coat-ing of ribosomes is referred to as **smooth endoplasmic reticulum**. The smooth ER is involved in the production of fat and fat-soluble hormones such as steroids.

Both forms of ER in liver cells are involved in the breakdown and modification of drugs. EXAMPLE: The sedative pentobarbitone is degraded into biologically inactive com-pounds. ANALOGY: Instructions are sent from the head office or nucleus via a freeway network or ER to the manufacturing plants which are either areas of rough ER or smooth ER. This system is far more efficient than information being carried by couriers via tedious, time-consuming side streets or cytoplasmic matrix.

Ribosomes

Ribosomes are small organelles (15–20 nm) that are located on the ER. They are also spread throughout the cytoplasm, usually in the form of clusters called **polyribosomes**. As previously mentioned, ribosomes are the site of protein manufacture. ANALOGY: The sites of chemical manufacture are located on the freeway network or in industrial centres known as polyribosomes. Polyribosomes mainly produce proteins for use within

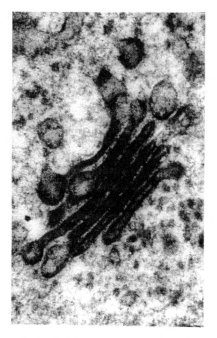

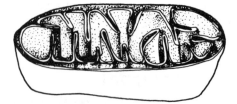

Figure 22.3 Representative mitochondrion showing the folds or cristae of the inner membrane.

Figure 22.2 Golgi complex showing a network of flattened tubes (×48 000).

the cell whereas ribosomes attached to ER are mainly concerned with manufacturing proteins for export.

Golgi complex

The golgi complex or apparatus is probably an extension of the endoplasmic reticulum. It consists of a network of flattened tubes that are stacked on top of each other in a similar manner to a group of stacked plates (Figure 22.2).

It appears that the golgi complex acts as a storage and distribution centre for the proteins and fats that were formed at the ER. These substances travel from the ER either directly or indirectly to the golgi complex. The golgi complex stores the manufactured chemicals and packages them for release. The

membrane-bound packages are released into the cytoplasmic matrix. They are then either used by the cell or are transported to the plasma membrane where they are released from the cell, that is, secreted from the cell. The golgi complex is very prominent in secretory cells. EXAMPLE: Secretory cells of the gastrointestinal tract contain a prominent golgi complex in the side of the cell that lines the tract. The packages that are utilized by the cell are usually released in the form of membrane-bound organelles called lysosomes which are described under the next heading.

The golgi complex is also involved in the manufacture of mucus which is later incorporated into the cell's membrane or secreted. Other substances that are formed and secreted, form the basis of the interstitial fluid.

In summary, the golgi complex acts as a storage and distribution centre. In addition, it is also the manufacturing site of substances such as mucus. ANALOGY: When goods are manufactured they are then stored in warehouses from which they are distributed according to demand.

22.10 Membrane organelles

Mitochondria

Mitochondria are double-membraned organelles (Figure 22.3). The inner membrane is arranged in folds or cristae which protrude into the inner mitochondrial cavity called the mitochondrial matrix. The presence of cristae result in increased surface area of the internal membrane. This relatively large surface area is important for cell function since almost all of a cell's energy is produced on the surface of the cristae (33.6). This energy is only formed in the presence of oxygen. The cristae are the end site for oxygen that has been transported through the body. Mitochondria are often referred to as the powerhouse of a cell and thus cells that require large amounts of energy contain numerous mitochondria. EXAMPLE: Cardiac muscle cells. ANALOGY: Factories can only manufacture goods when energy is present. This energy is mainly produced at powerhouses which are located in the cell at the mitochondrial cristae.

Lysosomes

Lysosomes are small organelles formed by the golgi complex. They contain powerful digestive substances that are used to break down unwanted molecules and particles such as fragments of organelles and bacteria. The lysosomes thereby remove unwanted substances and structures from the cytoplasm. These substances and structures are broken down and then are either released into the cytoplasm for recycling or are excreted from the cell. ANALOGY: Manufactured goods usually end up as waste products which have to be disposed of.

Waste disposal units break down unwanted refuse and recycle reusable goods as do lysosomes.

The rupture of lysosomal membranes releases powerful digestive substances into the cytoplasmic matrix. If sufficient lysosomes are ruptured the whole cell is broken down in the process of autolysis. EXAMPLE: Exposure to sufficient sunlight causes sunburn and the rupture of lysosomes in the skin cells. The release of the lysosomal contents kills cells near the skin's surface and leads to blistering and later to the 'peeling' of a layer of skin.

Peroxisomes

These organelles are similar in structure to lysosomes but are smaller. They occur in large numbers in liver cells. They contain enzymes related to the breakdown of amino acids and fatty acids. A by-product of these reactions is the formation of the toxic substance hydrogen peroxide which is also broken down within the organelle.

22.11 Cell inclusions

Cell inclusions are a diverse group of structures that usually contain materials retained by a cell for purposes of cellular function. Cell inclusions are used for a variety of functions. EXAMPLES: Haemoglobin for carrying oxygen in red blood cells, glycogen and fats for cell chemical reserves, melanin for cell pigmentation and mucus as a cellular secretion.

A virus is a cell inclusion that is harmful to the cell. Viruses are small acellular structures that consist of hereditary information surrounded by protein. Viruses use the cell contents for multiplication. They can remain dormant in their intracellular position until a satisfactory change affects the cell or the virus. When in the dormant or latent state they probably do not interfere with the function of their host cell.

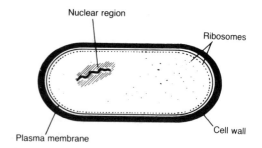

Figure 22.4   General structure of a procaryotic cell.

Application: Herpes

Herpes simplex is the virus responsible for the development of cold sores. This virus remains in a latent state in cells until some stress such as fever, emotional upset, sun exposure, being run down or ill with another disease activates it. The virus causes the formation of vesicles, especially in the skin of the lips. Rupture of these vesicles results in the release of viruses from them. Herpes can thus be transmitted by direct personal contact with the ruptured vesicles. Body defence mechanisms develop to overcome the outbreak and return the skin to normal. However, some of the virus remains in the latent state. This ensures that the virus will remain in a person for life.

---

called vacuoles. This fluid contains salts, sugars, organic acids and other soluble substances necessary for cell function.

22.13   Procaryotic cells

Procaryotic cells differ substantially from eucaryotic cells by lacking a distinct nucleus and cytoplasmic organelles (Figure 22.4). Procaryotic cells are found only in bacteria and cyanobacteria. These cells exist and function as single cells which are referred to as unicellular organisms. The important structural features of bacteria and their application to health are described below.

22.12   Important plant cell structures

Plant cells contain the above organelles plus several other structures that are necessary for plant cell function. Plants contain a cell wall which confers rigidity to the shape of a cell. Many plant cells contain chloroplast organelles. These organelles play an important role in life since they use solar energy to produce carbohydrate from carbon dioxide and water. Large cell inclusions occur in the form of membrane-bound fluid filled spaces

Cell structures

Cell membrane
The plasma membrane differs from that found in eucaryotic cells in that it probably performs the function of the mitochondria of animal and plant cells.

Ribosomes
Ribosomes are found either in the cytoplasmic matrix or are attached to the plasma mem-

brane. The ribosomes manufacture bacterial proteins.

Nuclear region

This region is not a distinct nucleus as no membrane is present. It contains one strand of hereditary information which is responsible for both reproduction and protein synthesis. Drugs such as tetracycline interfere with the growth of bacteria by interfering with the synthesis of proteins.

Flagella

These can be found on mobile bacteria, that is, rod-shaped (bacilli) and coiled (spiral forms) bacteria. Non-mobile bacteria such as spherical bacteria (cocci) lack a flagellum (Figure 35.4).

Cell wall

Most procaryotic cells contain a cell wall which has a protective function. The cell wall maintains the cell's shape during harmful environmental changes such as osmotic imbalances. Substances such as penicillin, vancomycin and bacitracin all act on cell wall manufacture, whereas enzymes such as lysozyme (found in tears, saliva) and gastric juices can rupture the cell wall.

Application: Gram positive and gram negative bacteria

Bacteria are often identified according to their reaction to the stain, crystal violet. Gram stains are widely used in medicine and are often the first step in making a bacteriologic diagnosis of an infectious disease. Bacteria that form a blue or purple colour in the presence of crystal violet are termed gram positive bacteria. This colour response results from a thick cell wall which is composed of a different chemical to the cell walls

---

of other bacteria. These latter bacteria stain red and are referred to as gram negative bacteria.

The gram positive bacteria are sensitive to penicillin and lysozyme whereas gram negative bacteria are sensitive to drugs such as ampicillin.

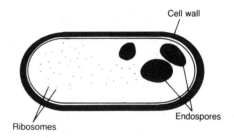

Figure 22.5   Bacterium containing endospores.

Capsules

Some bacteria have a slimy mucous-like coat surrounding the cell wall which is called a capsule. It can act as a protective structural covering, a nutrient reservoir, a site for the disposal of waste products and as a mechanism by which the bacteria can adhere to a host. EXAMPLE: The bacterium *Streptococcus mutans* causes tooth decay by being able to attach to teeth using a capsule. Capsules increase the virulence of bacteria, that is, the ability to cause disease, because they resist ingestion by the host defence cells (36.1).

Endospores

Certain bacteria produce dormant resting cells within the cytoplasm of the bacteria when the environment becomes unfavourable for normal growth and reproduction. These dormant cells are termed endospores or spores (Figure 22.5). Endospores resist harsh physical and chemical treatments and will remain in a state of suspended animation until the environment becomes favourable. When satisfactory environmental conditions exist the endospore actively grows and at this stage is referred to as a vegetative form.

Normal sterilization procedures, that is measures which destroy or remove all living organisms, can be used on the vegetative form, whereas endospores must be treated with sporicidal sterilization. EXAMPLE: Vegetative bacteria are readily killed when exposed to boiling water for a few minutes whereas spores are resistant to this measure. Spores can be killed by using an autoclave which is an apparatus that produces temperatures in the order of 121°C (see 36.5 Application: Autoclave).

The main spore-bearing bacteria include some of the most harmful bacteria. EXAMPLES: Anthrax, tetanus and gas gangrene.

Cell inclusions

Viruses are acellular structures that invade a bacterium (35.9). Viruses can live and multiply by using the cell's chemicals. A virus may lie dormant for long periods in its intracellular position interfering little, if at all, with the cell's activity. The virus remains in this latent condition until some change affects the cell or the virus, after which the virus multiplies.

Summary

Living things consist of protoplasm and exhibit the following features: metabolism, growth, reproduction, feeding, excretion, irritability and movement. Protoplasm is arranged into cells which form the structural and functional units of life.

A cell is the structural and functional unit of all organisms. Each cell has the potential to duplicate itself. Viruses are acellular structures that are capable of duplicating themselves. This duplication can only occur when they are within cells.

Animals and plants are composed of eucaryotic cells whereas bacteria and cyanobacteria consist of procaryotic cells. The contents of a cell and its surrounding membrane is often referred to as protoplasm.

The protoplasm of eucaryotic cells is subdivided into the nucleus and cytoplasm. The nucleus controls and regulates cell division and maintains cell function. The cytoplasm is the site of the manufacture, storage and breakdown of substances. It is composed of a cytoplasmic matrix, a cytoskeleton, an internal membrane system, membrane organelles and cell inclusions.

A generalized animal cell contains the following structures:

1. Membranes that act as protective barriers for cell organelles and for the entire cell; the latter is called the plasma membrane.
2. Nucleus responsible for cell reproduction and control of cell chemical reactions.
3. Cytoplasmic matrix consisting of a mixture of solutions, sols and gels.
4. Cytoskeleton which provides the framework necessary for maintaining cell shape, assisting in transport, playing a role in cell division and providing the mechanism for the action of cilia and flagella. The cytoskeleton consists of microtubules, microfilaments and intermediate microfilaments. Cellular organelles involved in this system include centrioles, basal bodies, cilia and flagella.
5. Internal membrane system consisting of a series of membrane lined tubes that are interconnected throughout the cell. The system of nuclear envelope, endoplasmic reticulum and golgi complex is involved in the production, transportation, storage and distribution of substances. Rough

endoplasmic reticulum has ribosomes embedded in it. These structures are responsible for the manufacture of proteins.

6. Membrane bound organelles are generally involved in cellular metabolic processes. Mitochondria are sites of energy production; lysosomes and peroxisomes break down substances within a cell.

An animal cell may also contain cell inclusions that can be either beneficial or harmful to the cell.

Plant cells contain the above features plus chloroplasts for converting solar energy into carbohydrates, and large fluid filled spaces called vacuoles.

Procaryotic cells differ substantially from eucaryotic cells because they lack a distinct nucleus and cytoplasmic organelles. These cells contain a nuclear region, cell membrane and ribosomes. They usually contain a cell wall which has a protective function. The composition of this wall varies between different bacteria and may be used to divide them into gram positive and gram negative bacteria. Capsules and endospores assist various bacteria in resisting harmful environments. Bacteria can also contain viruses as cell inclusions.

Chapter 23

The plasma membrane

Objectives

At the completion of this chapter the student should be able to:

1. describe the functions of the plasma membrane;
2. relate the structure of a plasma membrane to its functions;
3. list the factors that influence the diffusion of a substance through a membrane;
4. explain the difference between the diffusion of electrolytes and non-electrolytes;
5. describe the mechanisms of facilitated diffusion, active transport, pinocytosis and phagocytosis and give examples of how they are involved in body function;
6. differentiate between diffusion, facilitated diffusion, active transport, pinocytosis and phagocytosis.

The plasma membrane plays an important role in the functioning of cells. It acts as a protective barrier for the cell by restricting the entry of unwanted substances. Cells can contain slightly different membrane structures as a result of differences in cell requirements. A second function of plasma membranes is their regulation of the entry of substances required by the cell.

23.1 General structure

Fluid-mosaic model

The plasma membrane consists mainly of protein and lipid molecules. A knowledge of how these molecules constitute the plasma membrane will assist in understanding the mechanisms of how substances move through membranes. Currently, most membrane scientists believe that plasma membranes have a structure similar to the **fluid-mosaic model** (Figure 23.1). This model suggests that the membrane consists of a double layer of phospholipid that has proteins and cholesterol dispersed in it. The proteins can move within the phospholipid. Protruding like antennae from the external membrane surface of the phospholipid and protein fluid mixture are glycoproteins and glycolipids (Figure 23.1). The overall structure is asymmetrical with the external surface differing from the internal surface. This difference suggests that the ability of a sub-

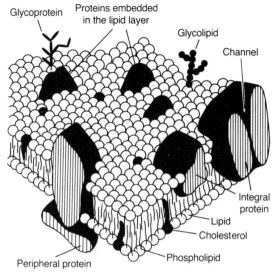

Glycoprotein — Proteins embedded in the lipid layer — Glycolipid — Channel — Integral protein — Lipid — Cholesterol — Phospholipid — Peripheral protein

Figure 23.1 The fluid-mosaic model of cell membranes proposes a double layer of lipid interspersed with mobile protein molecules.

stance to pass through a membrane may depend on the direction of the substance's movement. A substance may be able to move into, but not out of, a cell.

Phospholipids

The two layers of lipid contain phosphates attached to their outer surface. This **phospholipid** (29.2) **bilayer** has hydrophilic (5.5) outer surfaces while the opposing non-polar tails form a central hydrophobic region which repels water (5.5). This layer is self-sealing. If the layer is punctured by a needle it will seal immediately following the needles removal thus protecting the cell contents from the extracellular fluid.

Proteins

Proteins represent the main component of most biological membranes. Their main functions are:

1. transport through the formation of channels and their action as carriers;
2. providing support for the phospholipid bilayer of gel;
3. receiving signals from hormones and other chemicals in the surrounding fluid;
4. transmitting messages to the cytoplasm;
5. anchoring cytoskeletal structures;
6. providing cells with an individual identity.

Proteins are classified into two types according to their location. **Integral proteins** are proteins usually containing polar regions on both sides of the membrane. Some of these proteins span the bilayer and are called **transmembrane proteins** while others are interspersed near the inner and outer surfaces. These proteins can move within the layer. This movement is believed to be associated with the transport of substances across the membrane. The channels formed by these proteins are about 0.8 nm in diameter and provide a path for the movement of small substances such as electrolytes into and out of cells.

Peripheral proteins are loosely bound to the surface of the membrane through binding with integral proteins or the polar lipid ends. These proteins are believed to influence the shape of membranes and provide a link with the cytoskeleton.

Cholesterol

Cholesterol links with phosphate groups to make a membrane more rigid as it restricts the capacity of the phospholipid molecules to move. This increased rigidity decreases the ease with which substances can pass across the membrane.

Glycoproteins

Glycoproteins are macromolecules containing a complex of protein and carbohydrate (30.5). These structures are arranged in membranes with the carbohydrate portion protruding out of the cell. These molecules provide receptor sites that provide a cell with its identity and enable cell to cell recognition. The cell identity is an important factor in tissue rejection (37.2) and auto-immune diseases (37.3). Receptor sites also provide a mechanism for the selective action of hormones, neurotransmitters, enzymes and drugs.

Glycolipids

Glycolipids consist of branching chains of sugar attached to lipid. The carbohydrate chains form recognition sites that are important in cellular growth and development. They may also be the infection sites for several types of bacteria and viruses.

Permeability and proteins

The term **permeability** is used to describe the ease with which a substance can diffuse across a membrane. When a substance is unable to pass through a membrane, the membrane is said to be **impermeable** for that substance.

Plasma membranes are differentially or **selectively permeable**, that is, they are permeable to some substances but not to others. The selective permeability is due to specific membrane transport proteins. The channel proteins form bridges for small molecules across the entire membrane. Carrier proteins are transmembrane proteins that bind specific molecules and undergo a change in shape, enabling the molecules to move in the spaces within the protein to the opposite side.

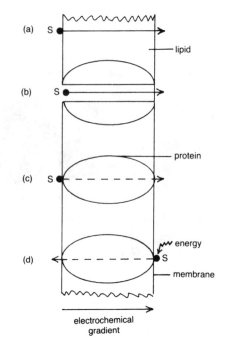

Figure 23.2 Schematic diagram of the relationship between membrane transport mechanisms and membrane transport. (a) and (b) Simple diffusion. (c) Facilitated diffusion and (d) Active transport. (S = lipid-insoluble substance.)

The functions of different membranes are therefore determined by the composition of the transport proteins they contain. The mechanisms of membrane transport can be divided into non-energy dependent (diffusion) and energy dependent (active process) (Figure 23.2).

23.2 Diffusion through plasma membranes

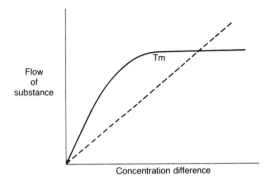

Diffusion through lipid

The plasma membrane consists mainly of lipids and this acts as a boundary between intracellular and extracellular fluid by only allowing lipid-soluble substances to pass through it. Lipids are non-polar substances and thus only non-polar substances are capable of dissolving in the lipid. EXAMPLE: Oxygen.

The rate of flow of a lipid-soluble substance across a membrane is determined by the difference in concentration that exists between the extracellular and intracellular fluids. The greater the concentration gradient, the greater is the rate of diffusion across a membrane. Remember that the net diffusion of a substance occurs from a region of high concentration to a region of low concentration (20.2).

Figure 23.3 In simple diffusion (---) the greater the concentration difference the greater is the flow of substance across the membrane. The flow of substance in facilitated diffusion (——) is controlled by protein carriers. These carriers transport substances more rapidly than simple diffusion at low concentration differences, but reach a saturation point (T_m) when all the carriers are occupied. Any further increase in concentration difference results in no change in the flow of a substance.

Facilitated diffusion

Facilitated diffusion is a process by which a lipid-insoluble substance such as glucose is rendered soluble by combining with a carrier protein within the membrane.

A carrier only facilitates the diffusion of a substance from one side of the membrane to the other. The normal requirements such as a difference in concentration are necessary for facilitated diffusion to occur (Figure 23.2).

Membranes contain many different shaped carriers. Each type of carrier is probably a protein with a unique chemical structure which enables the carrier to combine only with a complementary shaped substance. Carriers exhibit the property of specificity,

that is, they can only carry one specific substance at maximum efficiency. Other similar shaped substances may be carried less efficiently and all other substances are not able to be carried.

Facilitated diffusion differs from simple diffusion by the dependence on carriers for movement. In simple diffusion, any increase in the concentration difference results in a proportionate increase in the diffusion of a substance and there is no upper limit to the flow of a substance (Figure 23.3). With facilitated diffusion, an elevated concentration difference does not necessarily result in a proportionate increase in the flow of a substance. The rate of movement of a substance using facilitated diffusion depends upon the following factors:

1. difference in concentration between both sides of the membrane;
2. amount of carrier available;
3. time taken for the reaction with the carrier;
4. type of carrier present, as each carrier is relatively specific for similar structured substances.

There is a limit or saturation point reached in facilitated diffusion which occurs when all of the carriers are occupied. Any further increase in the concentration gradient will result in no further increase in the flow of the substance (Figure 23.3). The amount of substance that is carried when the carriers are saturated is referred to as the **threshold** or **transport maximum** (T_m) of that substance.

The transport of a substance can be altered by the presence of similar structured substances, as both substances will compete for the available carriers. When two substances with the same concentration exist in a solution, the probability of a molecule of either substance colliding with the membrane and combining with a carrier is equal.

Facilitated diffusion only transports a net flow of substance from a high concentration to a low concentration, that is, it operates on a downhill gradient. The transport of substances by combining with protein carriers does not require cell energy. Many substances that are unable to readily diffuse through the lipid barrier are carried by facilitated diffusion. EXAMPLES: Sugars, amino acids and certain ions such as sodium.

Diffusion through channels

Effect of channel size

Substances considerably smaller than a membrane pore can move at high rates through a membrane, that is, the membrane exhibits a high permeability to them. EXAMPLES: Water, chloride ions, urea, lactic acid. These substances have a small hydrated

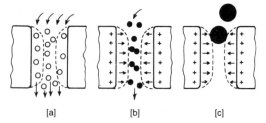

Figure 23.4 Diffusion of ions through a membrane channel: (a) Cl⁻ is able to flow through the entire diameter, (b) K⁺ can only flow through the region outside the influence of the positively-charged lining, (c) the hydrated diameter of Na⁺ is too large to allow the ion to flow through the central region of the channel.

diameter. Remember that the hydrated diameter of a substance is the combined diameter of the solute and the water molecules that are loosely attached to it (Figure 17.1). Any substance that has a hydrated diameter greater than the channel diameter of 0.8 nm is unable to move through the channel, and can therefore only penetrate a membrane if it is able to move through the lipid region. EXAMPLE: Glucose is too large to pass through the channels and so it has to move through the lipid region. The diameter of a channel therefore assists in selecting which substances can pass through a membrane.

Effect of electrical charges on the flow of ions

Small-sized positive ions such as K⁺ and Na⁺ pass with greater difficulty through a membrane channel compared with anions of a similar size. EXAMPLE: Cl⁻ passes through membrane channels approximately 500 000 times faster than K⁺. This observation suggests that the channels have positive charges surrounding them. Figure 23.4

shows how positive charges lining a channel restrict the flow of positive ions.

The field of influence of the positive charges lining a channel decreases the effective channel diameter for positive charges. Any positive charge that approaches the field of influence is repelled because like charges repel. Anions are able to move into this field of influence since opposite charges attract. This results in a channel having a greater effective diameter for anions than similar-sized cations (Figures 23.4a, 23.4b). The larger effective channel diameter for negative ions results in a faster flow of these ions through a channel.

The anions are prevented from adhering to the lining of a channel by the following factors.

1. The flow of water due to osmosis, pushes negative ions through the membrane before they can hook onto a positive charge. ANALOGY: If a person is being carried along a rapidly flowing river, the current may be too fast to enable the person to grasp objects on the river bank.
2. The hydrated diameter of anions results in the anion being separated from the channel's lining by water molecules. The presence of water molecules between the opposite charges restricts the ability of these charges to form a strong bond.

Plasma membranes have a high permeability to K^+ and a low permeability to Na^+ due to the larger hydrated diameter of Na^+ ions. This difference in permeability results in a high extracellular fluid concentration of Na^+ ions and a high intracellular concentration of K^+ ions (18.1).

23.3 Factors altering channel permeability

Effect of calcium on channel permeability

Calcium ions are thought to be present at the channel edges and involved in the positive charge of the channel's lining. An excess of extracellular Ca^{2+} results in an increased number of positive charges lining the channel, which results in a decreased channel diameter to cations. A decreased extracellular Ca^{2+} concentration results in less positive charges lining the channel and thus an increased channel diameter to cations.

Application: Hypocalcaemia

Hypocalcaemia is a deficiency of calcium which may occur as a result of dietary deficiency, decreased intestinal absorption, hypoparathyroidism or impaired kidney function. The extra demands for Ca^{2+} during pregnancy can also result in a relative deficiency of calcium, even though the calcium intake of a person may be the same as that prior to pregnancy. A deficiency of Ca^{2+} results in plasma membranes increasing their permeability to Na^+ ions (Figure 23.5). The influx of Na^+ into nerve and muscle cells can initiate nerve impulses and muscle contraction, e.g. twitching of facial muscles, 'pins and needles' and numbness in the extremities. With more severe Ca^{2+} deficiencies, spasms of skeletal muscles in the hands occur which may be followed by convulsions.

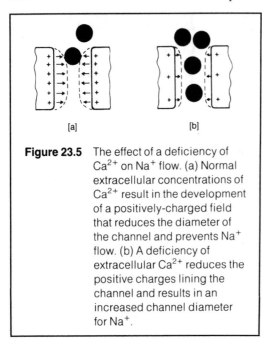

[a]   [b]

Figure 23.5 The effect of a deficiency of
Ca^{2+} on Na$^+$ flow. (a) Normal
extracellular concentrations of
Ca^{2+} result in the development
of a positively-charged field
that reduces the diameter of
the channel and prevents Na$^+$
flow. (b) A deficiency of
extracellular Ca^{2+} reduces the
positive charges lining the
channel and results in an
increased channel diameter
for Na$^+$.

23.4 Factors influencing net diffusion

Concentration difference

The rate of diffusion through a membrane is
dependent upon the difference in concentration between the two sides of the membrane.
The greater the concentration difference, the
greater is the rate of diffusion, apart from
facilitated diffusion where a maximum diffusion rate exists.

Electrical potential difference

Since opposite charges attract (4.4), an electrical force will exist across a membrane whenever a difference in charge exists between the
solutes on either side of the membrane. In
human cells the cytoplasm is negative with
respect to the extracellular fluid. This difference in charge is due to the cytoplasm
containing negatively-charged substances
that are unable to penetrate the plasma
membrane. These 'fixed' charges create an
excess of negative charges in the cytoplasm.

The negatively-charged cytoplasm attracts
positive ions across the membrane. Potassum
ions are able to move across the membrane
which results in a high intracellular K$^+$ concentration. Note that the force of attraction
is of sufficient strength so that K$^+$ ions
are pulled across the membrane from a low
concentration to a high concentration. Even
with this high intracellular concentration of
K$^+$ ions, the net intracellular charge remains
negative. The extracellular fluid is thus
positive with respect to the cytoplasm. This
positive charge repels the diffusion of K$^+$
from a high concentration in the cytoplasm to
the low extracellular concentration.

Effect of anti-diuretic hormone on channel
permeability

Anti-diuretic hormone increases the physical
diameter of membrane channels in the
kidney. The larger diameter results in an
increased reabsorption of water from the
kidney. Inhibition of anti-diuretic hormone
by substances such as alcohol and caffeine
results in less water being able to pass
through the membrane channels of the distal
parts of the kidney tubules and ducts. This
decrease in water permeability results in
excess water being retained in the tubules
and ducts. The excess water flows out of the
ducts causing diuresis, that is, an increased
excretion of urine.

The low permeability of the membrane to Na^+ ions prevents them from entering a cell. The Na^+ ions have the potential to flow but are prevented from doing so by a membrane barrier. Any increase in the membrane permeability of Na^+ will result in the flow of these positive ions into a cell.

In nerve cells an alteration in membrane permeability results in the flow of Na^+ ions into the nerve. This flow of positive ions or current results in the initiation of a nerve impulse (10.5).

Electrochemical gradient

Substances that lack a charge (non-electrolytes) diffuse down a difference in concentration or **concentration gradient**. A potential difference across a membrane has no influence on the movement of these substances.

Charged particles diffuse under the influence of two factors:

1. the chemical gradient;
2. potential difference or electrical gradient.

When the influence of the electrical gradient is greater than the chemical gradient, a net flow of ions can occur from a low to a high concentration. EXAMPLE: K^+ ions flow into cells. To determine the direction of net diffusion, the influence of the electrical gradient is compared with the chemical gradient. The combined influence of these two gradients is termed the **electrochemical gradient**. Charged substances are unable to diffuse against the direction of an electrochemical gradient, that is, against a downhill electrochemical gradient which drives ions in a specific direction.

To overcome a net force that drives substances in a specific direction requires the use of energy. Some substances have been found to move against an electrochemical gradient. EXAMPLE: Na^+ from the cytoplasm to the extracellular fluid. This suggests that an alternative mechanism to diffusion exists for the movement of substances across membranes.

23.5 Movement of substances by active processes

An active process occurs when the movement of substances across a membrane requires energy from the cell. The three main forms of active process are active transport, pinocytosis and phagocytosis.

Active transport

Active transport occurs when the movement of substances by carriers is independent of the electrochemical gradient. This independence results from the use of cell energy. The carrier mechanism is similar to that of facilitated diffusion. The difference between the two modes of transport is that active transport requires energy to enable the carrier mechanism to function. Usually the protein or glycoprotein carrier is tightly coupled to a source of metabolic energy such as ATP (31.3). An enzyme which is usually part of the carrier effects the release of energy. The energy is used to activate the carrier, to separate the substance being transported from the carrier, and to release the substance inside or outside the cell. Movement of the substance is probably brought about by the attached substance changing the three dimensional shape of the carrier.

Most plasma membranes exhibit active transport. EXAMPLES: Na^+ and K^+ in nerve transmission, absorption of nutrients from

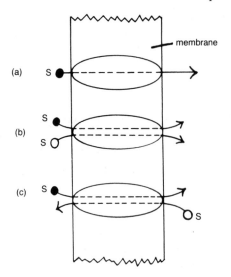

(a)

(b)

(c)

membrane

Figure 23.6 Schematic diagram of carrier proteins. (a) Unidirectional or uniport system (b) Symport system and (c) Antiport system. (S = substances being transported.)

K$^+$. Usually Na$^+$ that has 'leaked' into a cell is carried out, whereas K$^+$ is transported from the extracellular fluid into the cell by the same carrier.

Some active transport systems are driven by energy stored in ion gradients rather than directly by ATP. EXAMPLE: The active transport of glucose into the body in the intestinal and kidney cells is achieved by a coupled symport system. In this system the glucose and sodium ion bind to different locations on the glucose carrier protein. Sodium is able to bind onto the carrier and enter the cell via the altered shape of this carrier. The glucose follows into the altered shape of the carrier and subsequently into the cell. The sodium ions are pumped out on the opposite side of the cell thereby maintaining the cell's electrochemical gradient.

The movement of substances by active transport is limited by the ability of that substance to combine with, and be transported by, a carrier.

the small intestine, kidney reabsorption and electrolyte movements in muscle function.

The surface of the carrier contains a specific site for the attachment of the substance to be carried. The movement of a substance will only occur if a specific carrier for that substance is present. Similar structured substances can be used by the same carrier but these substances will be carried at different rates. EXAMPLE: There are at least five different carrier proteins for amino acids. Each carrier protein only carries a group of amino acids that have similar structure (30.9 Application: Cystinuria).

A carrier often carries a second substance in a specific direction. This is known as coupled transport (Figure 23.6) of which there are two types: symport — substances being transported in the same direction; and antiport — substances being moved in opposite directions. EXAMPLE: The most common coupled system is that of Na$^+$ and

Application: Active transport of glucose

The rate of formation and breakdown of a glucose-carrier complex restricts the quantity of glucose that can enter a cell to below the amount that is necessary for cell function. The hormone insulin increases the rate of formation and breakdown of the glucose-carrier complex. This results in an increase in glucose transport by as much as ten times the rate of transport as when no insulin is secreted.

The number of carriers available for the transport of glucose also has an influence on glucose transport. In kidney cells, the capacity of carriers to transport quantities of glucose from the tubular fluid to the blood far exceeds the normal quantities of glucose that are

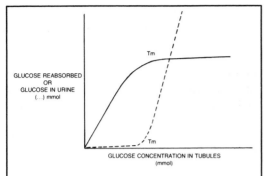

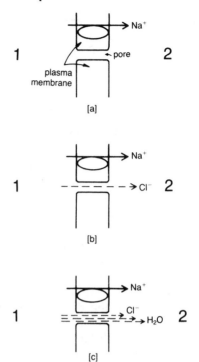

Figure 23.7 The relationship between glucose in urine and the active transport mechanism of glucose reabsorption.

filtered by the kidneys. Elevated blood sugar levels above 10 mmol/L result in a greater quantity of glucose being filtered than can be reabsorbed by the active transport carriers.

The appearance of glucose in the urine indicates the saturation of glucose carriers and is referred to as the renal threshold for glucose (Figure 23.7). The maximum amount of glucose that can be transported by carriers per minute is called the transfer maximum or transport maximum (T_m). The renal threshold varies with individuals, and in some patients the transport mechanism is defective so that glucose is found in the urine at normal blood glucose levels.

Figure 23.8 The effect of active transport on the movement of other substances. (a) Na^+ is actively transported from fluid 1 to 2, resulting in an increased positive charge in fluid 2. (b) Cl^- diffuses from 1 to 2 to neutralize the positive charges. (c) Water flows from 1 to 2 as a result of the osmotic imbalance.

Influence of active transport on moving other substances

If a charged ion is carried across a membrane, an imbalance of potential difference develops between the fluids on either side of the membrane. This alteration in potential difference changes the electrochemical gradient for other ions via diffusion down the electro- chemical gradient. EXAMPLE: If Na^+ is actively transported across a membrane as in Figure 23.8 the receiving fluid will become more positive than the donating fluid. To maintain the original balance in potential difference between the two fluids, an anion such as Cl^- is driven across the membrane. Note the movement of Cl^- is passive, that is, independent of cell energy and it can move through membrane pores instead of moving through the lipid combined with carriers (Figure 23.8b).

The movement of these ions has also resulted in an osmotic imbalance. This imbalance results in flow of water in the direction of the Na^+ and Cl^- ions (Figure 23.8c).

Application: Anion and water reabsorption in kidneys

In the kidneys, Na^+ is actively transported from the lumen of the tubules into kidney cells from which it returns to the blood. This results in the blood becoming momentarily more positive than the tubular fluid. Anions such as Cl^- are passively reabsorbed down the new electrochemical gradient. The movement of Na^+ and anions into the blood results in the development of a higher osmotic pressure in the blood. This osmotic imbalance drives water from the tubules into the blood in order to establish osmotic equilibrium. About 80% of water is reabsorbed from the kidneys by this process which is dependent on the active transport of Na^+. The inhibition of the active transport of Na^+ results in the indirect inhibition of Cl^- and water reabsorption. This is the principle behind the function of most diuretics, that is, drugs that cause increased fluid loss in urine.

Pinocytosis

Pinocytosis is a general term used to describe the active movement of substances via membrane-bound packages from the extracellular fluid to the cytoplasm or vice versa. These packages are called vesicles. The movement of substances into cells by this mechanism is used by most body cells. EXAMPLES: Absorption of macromolecules such as proteins and lipids through the wall of the small intestine. Secretion of hormones and enzymes by secretory cells.

Pinocytosis can be separated into endocytosis and exocytosis. By the process of **endocytosis** substances are taken into the cell, and by **exocytosis** they are removed from the cell.

Endocytosis is an active process where extracellular fluid containing macromolecules such as proteins is engulfed by the plasma membrane and taken into the cell. This process requires energy. The stages of endocytosis are shown in Figure 23.9. The process of pinocytosis is initiated by the plasma membrane invaginating in response to positive charges on the macromolecules. These molecules become attached to the membrane's surface by adsorption, that is, the molecules are held to the surface (17.6). The presence of these molecules causes the membrane to invaginate and eventually encircle the molecules (Figure 23.9d). The two ends of the invagination fuse forming a small sac or vesicle (Figure 23.9e). The pinocytotic vesicle then moves towards the centre of the cell (Figure 23.9f). Note that the vesicle still contains extracellular fluid with its macromolecules. Lysosomes attach to the pinocytotic vesicle (Figure 23.9g) and release their digestive agents into the vesicle causing a breakdown of the macromolecules (Figure 23.9h) after which the vesicular membrane breaks and releases its contents into the cytoplasm.

Substances can also be released or secreted by a cell using the mechanism of pinocytosis. This form of pinocytosis is called exocytosis. Vesicles that are formed by the golgi apparatus may contain macromolecules such as hormones and enzymes that need to be secreted by the cell. The size of such molecules prevents them from passing through the plasma membrane. The secretory vesicles move from the golgi complex to the plasma membrane. They then attach to the plasma

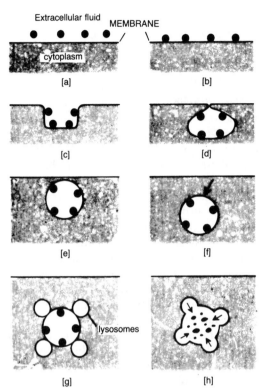

Figure 23.9 Mechanism of endocytosis.
(a) Macromolecules such as proteins approach the plasma membrane.
(b) Macromolecules are adsorbed onto the membrane.
(c) An invagination of the plasma membrane results.
(d) The invagination forms an enclosed sac or vesicle.
(e) The sac separates from the plasma membrane.
(f) The sac moves towards the centre of the cell.
(g) Lysosomes attach themselves to the sac.
(h) Lysosomes release their contents into the sac causing a breakdown of the macromolecules.

membrane. The membrane breaks releasing the contents into the extracellular fluid.

Phagocytosis

Phagocytosis is the third mechanism by which substances are moved across the membrane by active processes. It differs from pinocytosis in that only specialized cells can perform this function. **Phagocytosis** involves the ingestion of large particles such as bacteria, viruses, other cells and cell debris by white blood cells. The process is similar to pinocytosis in that the particle must be able to be adsorbed to the cell membrane. Once adsorbed, a large invagination forms around the particle which is then ingested (Figures 23.10 and 37.1). The ingested material is then digested by lysosomes.

Summary

The plasma membrane protects a cell from unwanted substances and regulates the entry of wanted substances, that is, it can maintain cellular homeostasis.

The fluid-mosaic model proposes that a plasma membrane is composed of two layers of non-polar lipid which has mobile proteins interspersed throughout it.

Membrane channels occur for small substances such as electrolytes.

The selectively permeable nature of these membranes results from:

1. the non-polar lipid region only allowing non-polar substances to diffuse through it;
2. the specific nature of membrane carriers that transport polar substances across the membrane in the processes of facilitated diffusion and active transport;
3. the small diameter of pores;

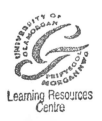

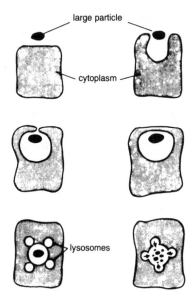

Figure 23.10   Mechanism of phagocytosis.
(a) Extracellular particle activates a
specialized cell. (b) Cell sends out
arms to engulf the particle. (c) Cell
encloses the particle by forming a
large vesicle or vacuole. (d) The
vacuole moves into the cytoplasm.
(e) Lysosomes attach to the
vacuole. (f) Lysosomes digest the
valuole's contents.

4. the positive charges lining pores result
   in cations having a relatively lower
   permeability than anions;
5. the concentration of calcium lining the

pores and thus conferring some of the
positive charge on the lining;
6. the presence of substances that can alter
   membrane structure such as anti-diuretic
   hormone.

Net diffusion of non-electrolytes is influenced by a concentration gradient whereas
electrolytes are influenced by an electrochemical gradient. Facilitated diffusion
differs from simple diffusion in that it is
also dependent upon the relative amount of
available carrier. When all the carrier is being
utilized, diffusion of a substance has reached
saturation point which is referred to as the
transport maximum (T_m) for that substance.
Active transport differs from facilitated diffusion by being independent of electrochemical gradients. Active transport also
relies on the cell's energy for the movement
of substances.

Both pinocytosis and phagocytosis differ
from diffusion, facilitated diffusion and
active transport. The latter are involved in the
movement of substances through membranes whereas the former use energy
to move substances via membrane-bound
packages. On reaching their destination
the vesicles are ruptured thereby releasing
their contents across ruptured membranes.
Pinocytosis occurs in most cells and involves
the use of vesicles whereas phagocytosis
occurs in specialized cells and involves the
use of larger membrane-bound packages.

Chapter 24

Nucleus function

Objectives

At the completion of this chapter the student should be able to:

1. describe the functions of a nucleus;
2. describe the mechanism of mitosis and meiosis in terms of chromosomes;
3. relate chromosomal abnormalities to meiotic malfunctions;
4. define a gene;
5. relate genes to patterns of inheritance;
6. list the factors that can alter gene expression;
7. explain how DNA structure is related to gene function;
8. describe the genetic code and relate errors in the genetic code to molecular-based genetic disorders;
9. explain how molecular-based mitotic malfunctions can result in cancer and how cytotoxic drugs act in the treatment of cancer;
10. explain the relationship between DNA replication and cell division.

The nucleus performs a role analogous to the head office of an organization. It controls cell multiplication and the day to day functioning of a cell. The nucleus copies its programmed, coded messages during the formation of a new cell. This information ensures that the newly-formed cell will perform its correct functions in life. This hereditary information is packaged in structures known as chromosomes.

24.1 Microscopic structure of chromosomes

Chromosome appearance

Under the microscope the nucleus is seen to contain thread-like structures which are called chromosomes. Chromosomes can only be observed with a microscope during periods of cell division. The chromosomes have been found to contain the hereditary

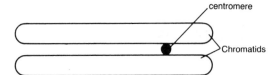

Figure 24.1   Representative diagram of a
chromosome as observed with a
microscope. The two identical
chromatids are joined by a
centromere.

information that is necessary for the growth
and maintenance of a cell. In preparation for
cell division this hereditary information is
condensed from long, very thin molecules
that are visible as a diffuse fine thread-like
network called **chromatin**, into the thick
chromosomes. Hereditary material is duplicated prior to chromosome appearance. The
result of this duplication is the formation
of chromosomes that are composed of two
identical rods called **chromatids** (Figure 24.1).
The chromatids are joined by a **centromere**.
When a chromosome consists of two chromatids it contains double the hereditary
information.

Chromosome pairs

All human cells contain twenty-three pairs of
chromosomes, except mature sex cells which
contain only twenty-three chromosomes.
Chromosomes contain the hereditary information that is necessary for the growth and
maintenance of a cell. Each pair consists of
one maternal chromosome and one paternal
chromosome, both of which contain similar
but not identical hereditary information. The
two chromosomes that belong to a pair are
termed **homologous chromosomes**. Each pair
of chromosomes has a different microscopic
size and shape to the other pairs. In twenty-
two pairs the homologous chromosomes
have the same microscopic size and shape.

These chromosomes are termed **autosomes**.
The other pair can consist of two identical
chromosomes or two different shaped structures. The twenty-third pair of chromosomes
are called the **sex chromosomes**.

Application: Karyotypes

A karyotype is a formal arrangement of
chromosomes used to identify chromosomal abnormalities and identify the
sex of an individual. This arrangement
designates a number to each homologous pair which is then used to
identify any chromosomal pair. All
human cells, apart from mature sex
cells, contain the same karyotype. A description of chromosomal abnormalities
that are detected by a karyotype is
presented in 24.4.

Sex chromosomes

The sex chromosomes of a male contain a
normal shaped chromosome in the shape of
an X and a smaller chromosome with a shape
similar to a Y. The Y chromosome contains
hereditary information that codes for the
formation of a testes. Normal males contain
an X and a Y chromosome whereas normal
females contain two X chromosomes.

Application: Barr bodies

In instances where there is a need to
determine the sex of an individual, cells
can be taken from scraping the lining of
the mouth and stained for the presence
of Barr bodies. A Barr body is a small
dark-staining area that occurs when
more than one X chromosome is present
in a cell, that is, in normal female cells.

24.2 Mitosis

Mitosis is the process of cell division where a new cell is formed that contains identical hereditary information to the parent cell. This form of cell division occurs in all body cells apart from mature sex cells. The function of mitosis is to duplicate cells for the growth and continued functioning of the body.

Mitosis consists of a series of continuous steps which are represented in Figure 24.2. The process of mitosis has been arbitarily divided into the following steps: prophase, metaphase, anaphase and telophase.

Prophase

Prophase is the earliest visible stage of mitosis. At the beginning of prophase, the chromosomes appear (Figure 24.2a) and by the end of this step they are observed as two chromatids (Figure 24.2b). In this step, the chromosomes are firstly randomly distributed throughout the nucleus and then the cell as the nuclear membrane disappears. Clearly, a splitting of the cell at this stage would result in non-identical cells (Figure 24.2c). The chromosomes need to be orientated in a single line.

Metaphase

Metaphase involves the movement of chromosomes to the centre of a cell where they are orientated in a single line (Figure 24.2d). Each double stranded chromosome attaches by its centromere to a chain called a spindle fibril. The spindle fibril is connected at each end to a centriole (22.8). The centrioles pull the chromatids apart so that identical chromatids are pulled in opposite directions. The centriole-spindle system enables a cell to divide the duplicated hereditary information

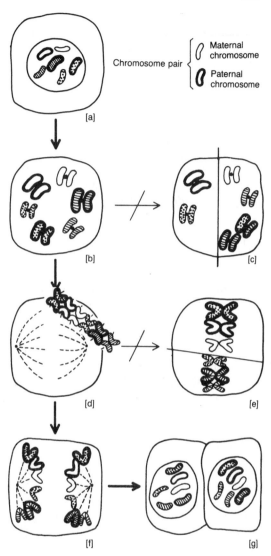

Figure 24.2 Mitosis. (a) Prophase begins with the appearance of chromosomes. (b) Prophase ends with the formation of two chromatids. (c) Dividing the cell at this stage results in non-identical cells. (d) Metaphase involves the orientation of chromosomes at the centre of the cell. (e) Lack of a spindle results in non-identical cells being formed. (f) Anaphase involves the spindle separating each pair of chromatids. (g) Telephase and formation of two identical cells.

into two distinct regions. If this spindle system fails to function or is not present the chromosomes could be split to form two non-identical regions (Figure 24.2e).

Anaphase

The separated chromatids (now called chromosomes) move along the fibrils to the appropriate centriole (Figure 24.2g). The two complete sets of chromatids are now located at opposite sides of a cell.

Telophase

This is the last step in mitosis. It involves the formation of nuclear membranes around each of the two sets of chromosomes. The chromosomes begin to become less dense and subsequently disappear from view. The cytoplasm divides, resulting in the formation of two identical cells (Figure 24.2g). These cells have the ability to undergo further mitotic divisions.

Interphase

Interphase is the period between cell divisions. It is during this step that hereditary information is transcribed into instructions for cell function. The majority of cells spend most of their existence in interphase, that is, in a state where the normal physiological and chemical activities are present. Towards the end of interphase genetic information is duplicated in preparation for cell division.

24.3 Meiosis

In the last stages of sex-cell formation, it is necessary to halve the number of chromo-

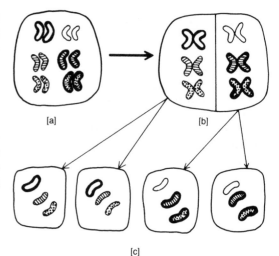

[a]   [b]

[c]

Figure 24.3 In meiosis the first division involves. (a) The alignment of chromosome pairs and (b) the subsequent separation of these pairs into two cells with half the number of chromosomes. (c) A further division occurs in which the chromatids of each chromosome separate resulting in four cells from the original single cell.

somes in a cell. If the mature sex cells contain forty-six chromosomes, the combination of male and female sex cells (sperm and ovum) would result in ninety-two chromosomes.

Meiosis is the form of cell division that results in new cells with half the original number of chromosomes. In meiotic divisions, the new generation of cells contain one of each pair of chromosomes. This confers individual differences on offspring but maintains the essential characteristics of human-cell function.

Meiosis consists of two successive division sequences. The first division involves the organization of maternal and paternal chromosomal pairs along the centre of the cell (Figure 24.3a). These pairs are arranged in a random sequence. Each chromosome wraps around its partner and attaches to a spindle fibril. The centriole–spindle complex pulls the chromosome pairs apart to opposite sides of a cell. The cell is then divided into two separate cells with half the number of chromosomes (Figure 24.3b).

The second division sequence is identical to the steps shown for mitosis apart from the fact that only half the number of chromosomes are present. Briefly, the chromosomes are orientated in a line in the centre of a cell. The centromeres of each chromosome attach to a spindle, after which the chromatids are separated to opposite sides of the cell. Splitting each cell results in the formation of two cells. Four cells result from one parent cell instead of the two cells that occur in mitosis.

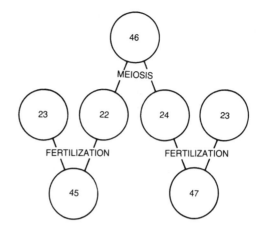

Figure 24.4 Relationship between meiotic non-disjunction and offspring chromosome number.

24.4 Chromosomal abnormalities

Meiotic malfunction

A malfunction in the meiotic process can lead to the formation of an abnormal cell which can be fertilized. Since an offspring originates from a fertilized cell, all the offspring's cells will be abnormal. The effect of a meiotic malfunction on the parent is minimal since meiosis only occurs in body cells that are involved in the formation of sex cells.

Chromosomal abnormalities can be classified according to whether a meiotic malfunction has resulted in the formation of cells with an abnormal number of chromosomes or chromosomes that have an altered structure.

Chromosomal number

Normally chromatids separate or disjoin by the influence of the centriole–spindle complex. When a pair of chromatids fails to disjoin the event is referred to as a **nondisjunction**. EXAMPLE: The non-disjunction of two chromatids in meiosis results in the formation of cells that contain either twenty-two or twenty-four chromosomes. When the twenty-four chromosome sex cell is fertilized with a twenty-three chromosome cell, the resulting offspring cells will contain forty-seven chromosomes (Figure 24.4). These cells contain one chromosome pair that has been replaced by a triplet of chromosomes. When forty-seven chromosomes are present, the syndrome is referred to as a **trisomy**.

The incidence of non-disjunction increases with the age of the mother, especially after thirty-five years of age.

Different chromosome non-disjunctions are identified by using a karyotype. The karyotype number of chromosome non-disjunctions is used to distinguish different trisomies. Autosomal trisomies usually result in abortion of the foetus in the first trimester, although trisomies of the karyotype numbers eight, thirteen, eighteen, twenty-one and twenty-two are able to live. All of these autosomal trisomies result in offspring that have multiple defects with various degrees of mental retardation. The most common autosomal non-disjunction is trisomy twenty-one or Down's syndrome.

When the non-disjunction involves a sex chromosome, the result is an alteration to the sexual development of the child. With forty-seven chromosome trisomies, three syndromes can occur as a result of sex chromosome non-disjunction. An XXX female results from a non-disjunction of one of the X chromosomes, whereas the XXY (Klinefelter syndrome) results from a non-disjunction of the mother's sex chromosome. Klinefelter syndrome is one of the common forms of hypogonadism and infertility in males as it occurs approximately once in every four hundred live male births. Fathers that have a non-disjunction of their Y chromosome propagate offspring with an XYY syndrome.

Non-disjunction results in an equal number of sex cells losing chromosomes as those gaining chromosomes (Figure 24.4). A loss of one of the autosomal chromosomes results in an embryo that is generally incompatible with life. An embyro that has one less sex chromosome can be compatible with life when one X chromosome exists. Foetuses with forty-five chromosomes including only one X chromosome are usually aborted. However some are born and this is known as Turner's syndrome. These patients exhibit a short stature and poorly developed female sex characteristics.

Chromosomal structure

Even though the total number of chromosomes is normal, the structure of one or more chromosomes could be abnormal. Structural abnormalities are mainly the result of chromosomal breakage where one part of the chromosome is lost. The loss of a section of hereditary information can result in clinical features similar to trisomies.

The term **deletion syndromes** is used to describe the group of syndromes that result from loss of a segment of a chromosome. Deletion syndromes can occur with the following chromosome numbers: four, five, thirteen, eighteen, twenty-one and twenty-two. EXAMPLE: The loss of a part of the karyotype number five chromosome results in the abnormal development of the larynx. Infants afflicted with this cry like a cat and thus this syndrome is often referred to as the Cri-du-chat syndrome (cry of the cat syndrome). These children also suffer from mental retardation and fail to thrive.

Detection of chromosome abnormalities

Patients with a suspected chromosomal abnormality may have some of their cells cultured and then karyotyped. In families where a history of chromosomal disorders is prevalent, a karyotype of a developing foetus can be performed with the view of terminating the pregnancy if necessary.

Foetal cells can be obtained from the amniotic fluid as early as the fifteenth week of pregnancy. The procedure of collecting amniotic fluid is known as **amniocentesis**. This procedure involves the insertion of a sterile needle through a locally-anaesthetized region of the mother's abdominal wall and the subsequent withdrawal of amniotic fluid.

Several tests are available to detect chromosomal abnormalities. The range of tests includes aminiocentesis and chorionic villi sampling. **Chorionic villus sampling** provides samples as early as eight weeks which are collected by a needle inserted into the vagina.

The cells from either method are then cultured until an adequate number exist for karyotyping.

24.5 Genetics

Genes

Chromosomes contain units of hereditary information called genes. A **gene** is the smallest unit which represents a single physical hereditary characteristic. EXAMPLE: Eye colour. Genes are arranged in a specific sequence along a chromosome. An understanding of meiosis assists in determining the chances of a particular gene being passed to offspring. The study of genes and their relationship to hereditary characteristics is termed **genetics**.

Alleles

When a specific gene exists in several forms the different forms are referred to as **alleles** of that gene. EXAMPLE: The absence or presence of pigment in the iris of eyes, that is, blue eyes or brown eyes. Usually only two alleles exist for a gene, with one of the alleles being dominant over the other. Each gene is represented in both chromosomes of a homologous pair. The two chromosomes can contain the same or different alleles. EXAMPLE: Two alleles for brown eyes could be present or one allele for brown eyes and one for blue eyes. When a pair of chromosomes contain the same allele a person is said to be **homozygous** for that gene. Where a gene is represented by two different alleles a person is said to be **heterozygous**.

Usually a heterozygous representation of a gene involves the occurrence of a dominant allele and a recessive allele. Whenever a dominant allele is present, it overrules the recessive allele. EXAMPLE: A person who is heterozygous for eye colour, contains one brown allele and one blue allele. The brown allele is dominant and thus suppresses the blue allele which results in brown eyes.

A heterozygous distribution of a gene results in the recessive allele being masked by the dominant allele, that is, a person is a carrier of the recessive allele. This recessive allele can be passed onto the next generation where, if the fertilized egg contains two recessive alleles, the recessive characteristic will be expressed. Most genetic abnormalities result from a homozygous recessive allele combination. EXAMPLES: Colour blindness, haemophila, muscular dystrophy and phenylketonuria. The dominant allele in these examples is normal function. Some genetic abnormalities result from the presence of a dominant allele. These abnormalities exist in people who contain either a homozygous allele combination or a heterozygous combination. EXAMPLES: The brain disorder Huntington's chorea, hypertension and diabetes insipidus.

Two terms are used to distinguish between the genetic makeup of an individual and their physical characteristics. **Genotype** describes the genetic composition of an individual. For any gene, a pair of chromosomes can contain the following combinations, that is, genotype:

$$
\left.\begin{array}{l} \text{dominant–dominant} \\ \text{recessive–recessive} \end{array}\right\} \text{ homozygous}
$$

$$
\left.\begin{array}{l} \text{dominant–recessive} \\ \text{recessive–dominant} \end{array}\right\} \text{ heterozygous}
$$

The expression of the genotype into physical characteristics is termed the **phenotype**. The following different genotypes have the same phenotype:

dominant–dominant
dominant–recessive
recessive–dominant

In these three combinations the dominant gene expresses its physical characteristics. EXAMPLE: A brown-eyed person can contain any of the following allele combinations:

brown–brown
brown–*blue*
blue–brown

The genotype is used to predict the various phenotypic possibilities of offspring.

Heredity and genes

Meiosis results in the formation of mature sex cells that contain either allele but not both. EXAMPLE: Brown or blue. Each parent produces two different sex cells that can be used in fertilization. When predicting the possible inheritance of a genetic characteristic, each possible combination of both sets of sex cells must be take into account. The relationship between hereditary and genes is illustrated by eye colour. What will the eye colour of offspring be when one parent has brown eyes while the other parent has blue eyes? The genotype of the brown-eyed parent can be either two brown alleles or one brown allele and one blue allele. Note that a general convention applies when abbreviating alleles. A dominant allele is denoted by a capital letter whereas a recessive allele is expressed by a lower case letter (brown-*B*, blue-*b*). The chances of offspring having brown or blue eyes is illustrated in Figure 24.5. If the brown-eyed person is homozygous, all offspring will have brown eyes, whereas a heterozygous brown-eyed parent would have an equal chance of producing a brown- or blue-eyed offspring.

A simpler method of determining the possible allele combinations in an offspring involves the use of special charts called punnett squares (Figure 24.6). These charts are frequently used to determine the probabilities of offspring characteristics. A chart is completed by filling in the squares which immediately indicates the different genotypes that can be formed.

A knowledge of whether the genotype of

ALLELES BROWN	BROWN	ALLELES BLUE	BLUE	OFFSPRING GENOTYPE	OFFSPRING PHENOTYPE
B	B	b	b		
B		b		Bb	BROWN
B			b	Bb	BROWN
	B	b		Bb	BROWN
	B		b	Bb	BROWN

OR

BROWN	BLUE	BLUE	BLUE		
B	b	b	b		
B		b		Bb	BROWN
B			b	Bb	BROWN
	b	b		bb	BLUE
	b		b	bb	BLUE

Figure 24.5 Relationship between eye-colour alleles and inheritance.

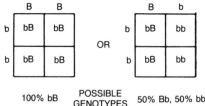

Figure 24.6 Inheritance of eye colour using punnett squares.

the brown-eyed parent is *BB* or *Bb* would enable a more precise prediction of the eye colour of the offspring.

Patterns of inheritance

Determining the phenotypes of members of a family leads to the formation of a genetic family tree. This family tree can determine the genotype of most of its members. This enables a more precise prediction of possible child phenotypes. EXAMPLE: A brown-eyed parent would be heterozygous if one of their parents was blue-eyed.

Many genetic disorders follow the simple dominant–recessive predictions, whereas some disorders such as diabetes mellitus and high blood pressure have no simple pattern of inheritance. A history of a genetic disorder in a family requires the assistance of a genetic counsellor who will inform the parents of the risks and consequences of having children. The more complex patterns of genetic inheritance probably involve genetic predispositions, that is, an individual has the genetic potential for a specific disease but this potential is only realized when certain environmental conditions exist. EXAMPLE: Obesity may act as a stress on individuals genetically predisposed to diabetes mellitus which initiates a clinical expression of the diabetes.

Sex-linked characteristics

When an allele is located on a sex chromosome, the allele will manifest itself with respect to the sex that the chromosome represents. The X chromosomes contain many genes whereas the Y chromosome has lost most of the genes. This feature of sex chromosome genes produces a pattern of inheritance that is different to that described for autosomal chromosomes. An X-linked recessive disorder will only be expressed when the normal dominant gene is absent. A female is therefore only affected if she is homozygous for that gene, since a heterozygous female contains one X chromosome with a dominant normal allele. In males, whenever a recessive allele is present on the X chromosome, the abnormal characteristic is expressed since the Y chromosome lacks

the gene. In effect, females act as carriers of sex-linked recessive characteristics.

Application: Haemophilia

Haemophilia is a sex-linked recessive disorder that results in either the failure of the blood to clot or the very slow clotting of blood following bleeding. The recessive allele is located only on an X chromosome which can be designated as X^h. The genotype for haemophilia in males is X^hY and for females X^hX^h. A female haemophiliac can only be produced from a haemophiliac male as a normal male confers a normal X^H allele to any female offspring (Figure 24.7).

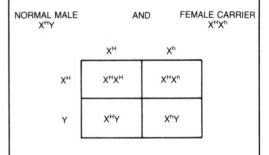

POSSIBLE GENOTYPES
25% X^HX^H, 25% X^HX^h, 25% X^HY, 25% X^hY
POSSIBLE PHENOTYPES
100% FEMALES NORMAL, 50% MALES NORMAL, 50% HAEMOPHILIACS

Figure 24.7 Inheritance of the sex-linked characteristic haemophilia. Note that a normal male is incapable of producing haemophiliac female offspring.

Multiple alleles

Some genetic characteristics contain more than two alleles. In blood groups, A and B are

Table 24.1   ABO blood group

Genotype antigen alleles	Phenotype blood group	Plasma antibodies
AA	A	bb
Ai	A	bb
BB	B	aa
Bi	B	aa
AB	AB	—
ii	O	ab

equally dominant whereas *O* is the common recessive allele. The combination of *A* and *B* results in a third equally dominant allele called AB. These capital letters refer to substances on the surface of red blood cells called antigens. An **antigen** is a substance that stimulates the production of specific immune substances called antibodies (37.2). A combination of an antigen and its specific antibody results in agglutination.

The blood of individuals is distinguished according to the type of antigen present (Table 24.1). The plasma of each blood group contains antibodies that are different to the antigen, since complementary antibodies would cause agglutination of the blood. These antibodies are represented by lower case letters.

The common recessive allele for the equally dominant *A*, *B* and *AB* is identified as *i*. The homozygous recessive blood group *ii* is called blood group *O*.

Blood transfusions require the use of blood that is compatible with the recipient's blood. If the blood is not compatible, the antigens of the donor's red blood cells will agglutinate with the antibodies of the recipient's plasma. The agglutination of blood may block blood vessels and could prove fatal if the blocked vessels supply vital areas. Whenever possible, the donor blood is the same type and has similar properties as the recipient. This compatibility is determined by cross-matching.

In emergency situations, blood group O can be used since it lacks the red blood cell antigens that combine with a recipient's plasma. Blood group O is thus referred to as the universal donor. Conversely, group AB lacks anti-A and anti-B antibodies in the plasma and thus this blood group can receive any type of red blood cells, that is, AB is a universal recipient.

24.6   Factors affecting gene expression

Effect of environment

The genotype determines the potential for growth and development of an individual. This potential is realized only when a suitable environment is present. If a person is exposed to a harmful environment the phenotype can differ from the genotype. The genotype for tallness and a large physique can be overridden by the effects of malnutrition.

Application: Environmental deafness

If a person has a gene for normal hearing, this may not be expressed if factors such as infections, exposure to excessive noise or perforation of the ear drum occur. The most common cause of deafness in new born babies is infection of the mother with Rubella (German measles) during pregnancy. In this case a person has the genotype for normal hearing but has the phenotype of the recessive allele, deafness.

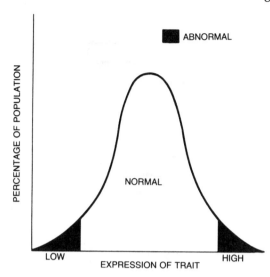

ABNORMAL

PERCENTAGE OF POPULATION

NORMAL

LOW   HIGH
EXPRESSION OF TRAIT

Figure 24.8 The distribution of a polygene characteristic in a population.

Multiple genes

Multiple genes or **polygenes** are genes that combine to produce a specific phenotypic trait. These genes determine traits that are of a quantitative nature, such as height, weight and degree of pigmentation. Many common genetic disorders such as diabetes mellitus and hypertension probably also depend on several genes. Hereditary traits that are determined by polygenes differ from those where one gene determines one characteristic, since in the former a person may have a proportion of a trait expressed, whereas in the latter an individual either has it or they do not. The distribution of a polygenic characteristic in a population is usually exhibited as a curve similar to Figure 24.8. The normal expression of the gene is usually considered to be the range of the trait that is expressed by 95% of the population. A person who is in the remaining 5% of the population is considered to be abnormal for that particular trait.

Modifier genes

Most genes in the body are probably influenced to some degree by the presence of other genes. When one principal gene is involved in determining an inherited characteristic, its expression may be influenced by other genes with effects that can be so minor that they are difficult to detect. Modifier genes differ from multiple genes in that the former modify to a varying extent a single gene's expression, whereas the latter involve several genes that act in a cumulative manner to express a hereditary characteristic.

Application: Human eye colour

Eye colour results from the presence (brown-eyed) or absence (blue-eyed) of the melanin pigment in the iris. Brown-eyed people contain the single dominant gene for the presence of melanin in the iris. The eye colour of humans can consist of various shades of blue and brown, that is, green, hazel, grey, light brown, dark brown and black. These variations in blue and brown eye colour result from the presence of modifier genes. These genes influence eye colour in the following ways:

1. amount of pigment in the iris;
2. affect the tone of the pigment;
3. distribution of the pigment throughout the iris.

It is still possible to use a punnett square when referring to a hereditary characteristic that is influenced by modifier genes. The punnett square can be used to predict the chance of brown eyes or blue eyes occurring in the offspring, but not the degree of shading of blue or brown eyes. The influence of modifier genes only alters the degree of expression of a genetic trait, they do not determine whether a genetic trait will be present.

In summary, the expressions of a gene depend on the other genes present (genetic environment) and on the physical environment.

24.7 DNA and the molecular basis of heredity

A chromosome is composed of a highly coiled molecule deoxyribonucleic acid (DNA) and proteins. Since a chromosome contains the units of hereditary information called genes, a relationship must exist between DNA structure and gene function.

DNA structure

DNA is composed of sequences of chemical structures called nucleotides (31.1). Each nucleotide contains the sugar molecule deoxyribose, a phosphate group and one of a group of nitrogen related structures known as nitrogen bases (Figure 31.1). The four types of nitrogen base are **adenine, thymine, cytosine** and **guanine**. The arrangement of these nitrogen bases are the key to hereditary information. In a DNA molecule, the nitrogen bases form the 'steps' of a spiral-shaped structure known as a double helix (Figure 24.9). The sugar molecules link with the phosphate groups to form a long DNA molecule. The double helix is a precisely-shaped molecule which requires a specific-sized nitrogen base to form the 'steps' of the helix. The only nitrogen bases that can be linked together are adenine with thymine and cyto-

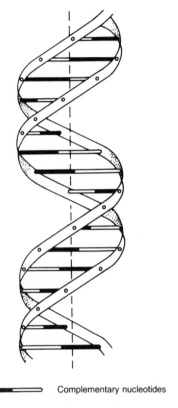

Complementary nucleotides

Figure 24.9   DNA molecule showing the double helix or spiral staircase shape of the two nucleotide strands.

sine with guanine. Any other combinations render the double-stranded helix unstable.

The only variable in a DNA molecule is the sequence of nitrogen bases. The restrictions of size result in a DNA molecule consisting of only four possible combinations (Figure 24.10a). The hereditary information is contained in the nucleotide sequences along DNA molecules.

A **gene** is a group of about 1000 pairs of nucleotides. Each gene consists of a specific sequence of nucleotides, and no two genes contain exactly the same sequence.

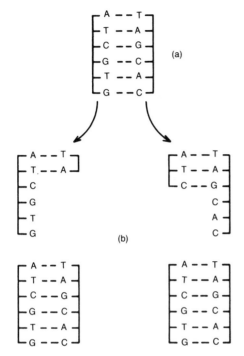

Figure 24.10 (a) The four possible combinations of the nitrogen bases adenine (A), thymine (T), cytosine (C) and guanine (G). (b) Replication of DNA.

Replication of DNA

The mechanism of DNA replication provides an understanding of the nature of life, since life depends upon the ability of chemicals to duplicate themselves.

DNA duplicates itself in the following manner:

1. hydrogen bonds that link complementary nucleotides break, resulting in the formation of two separate strands which are called the sense and antisense strands. (Figure 24.10);
2. the exposed nucleotides in each strand act as a template for free nucleotides that are present in the nucleus;

3. complementary nucleotides form hydrogen bonds with exposed nitrogen bases in each single strand;
4. the physical proximity of the recently attached nucleotides results in these nucleotides linking together;
5. the two DNA molecules are passed onto the dividing cells resulting in each cell receiving identical genetic information.

Relationship of DNA replication with cell division

The cell life cycle is useful for relating the dual roles of DNA, that is, control of cell function and mitosis (Figure 24.11). In this cycle, interphase occurs in the G, S and G_1 stages. The general control of metabolic activity occurs at the G (growth) stage. The duration of this stage varies for different cell types; nerve and muscle cells remain at this stage for years. In the S (synthesis) stage, which lasts for six to eight hours the DNA and other proteins are duplicated (Figure 24.12). The S stage is followed by the G_2 (gap) stage which does not appear to be related to DNA replication. It completes the period between mitosis called interphase.

In interphase only chromatin is present in the nucleus. Each chromatin fibre consists of a single DNA molecule. A human DNA molecule is about 5 cm long. Clearly, it needs to be compressed to fit physically within the nucleus. DNA undergoes compression by wrapping itself at regular intervals around proteins called histones. These segments are approximately 200 nucleotide pairs long and are called **nucleosomes**. A chromatin fibre can be described as a string of nucleosome beads.

For cell division to occur the strands of hereditary material must be compact. It would be physically impossible to orientate individual strands during metaphase and then successfully separate complementary

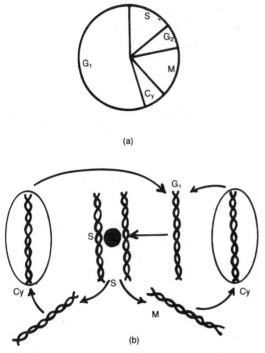

(a)

(b)

Figure 24.11 (a) Phases in a eucaryotic life cycle. (b) A DNA molecule at G_1 replicates forming two molecules at S. These molecules are compressed in the early stages of mitosis to form chromatids. Separation of the chromatids results in identical DNA molecules being passed to two new identical cells. G-growth, M-mitosis, Cy-cytokinesis.

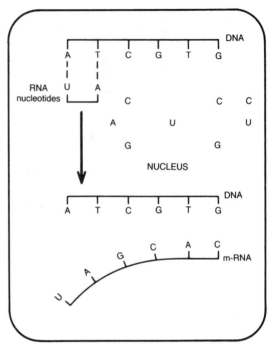

Figure 24.12 Transcription, or formation of RNA from DNA.

adjacent strands during anaphase without entanglement and breakage of the strands. In the early stages of prophase, the two identical chromatin fibres fold on themselves attached by a centromere resulting in tightly coiled condensed chromatin molecules. As chromatin molecules become shorter and thicker they become visible under a light microscope. The chromatin fibres are now referred to as chromatids which are 6000 to 10 000 times shorter than the DNA contained

within them. Two identical chromatids form double-stranded chromosomes. When two identical chromatids (chromatin fibres) separate during anaphase single-stranded chromosomes are formed. In telophase and cytokinesis (cytoplasm division) two identical single-stranded chromosomes are separated with other chromosomes and cytoplasm into new cells (Figure 24.11b).

24.8   RNA

RNA structure

RNA or ribonucleic acid is a nucleic acid which differs from DNA by containing a single helix, uracil instead of thymine and the sugar ribose (refer Table 31.1 for a comparison of the DNA and RNA features). RNA provides the means by which genetic information can be transposed into actions within the cell. Since the manufacture of chemicals and energy occurs in the cytoplasm, the RNA must be capable of transmitting the genetic information from the nucleus to the cell factories if genes are to control cell function.

The two principal forms of RNA are messenger RNA (mRNA) and transfer RNA (tRNA).

mRNA differs from tRNA in both size and function. mRNA is much larger than tRNA, and acts as a courier for genetic information from the nucleus to the cytoplasm. tRNA carries the raw materials in the cytoplasmic matrix to the factories where they are assembled according to specific genetic instructions.

RNA synthesis

For genetic information to be carried from the nucleus by RNA, a mechanism must exist where DNA is involved in the formation of RNA. DNA acts as a pattern by which RNA molecules are assembled. The formation of RNA from DNA is termed **transcription**.

In transcription, the DNA double helix splits, exposing the nucleotides. Complementary RNA nucleotides loosely attach via hydrogen bonds to their respective DNA nucleotides along the sense strand of DNA. EXAMPLE: Adenine RNA combines with thymine DNA, uracil–adenine guanine–cytosine, and cytosine–guanine. Along the sense strand are regions that are not coded for protein manufacture called intron regions. These intron regions are copied onto mRNA and have to be removed by small nuclear ribonucleoproteins (snRNPs) prior to mRNA leaving the nucleus. Since a specific RNA nucleotide can only attach to its comple-

mentary DNA molecule, a mirror image of the DNA nucleotide sequence results (Figure 24.12). The fixed position of assembling nucleotides results in adjacent nucleotides being linked by phosphate groups. As the phosphate groups form a nucleotide chain, the RNA–DNA linkages break. This break separates the DNA from the RNA chain as the latter is being assembled.

Transcription effectively produces RNA molecules that are mirror images of the gene's nucleotide sequence. This process is necessary for the maintenance and growth of a cell. Since DNA is involved in cell division, the only stage that can be used for transcription of DNA is interphase. Most cells thus exist for the majority of their lives in interphase so that the genetic information on DNA can be used for the maintenance and growth of the cell.

24.9   The genetic code

The transfer of hereditary information from one cell to another is accomplished through a series of specific nucleotide sequences called genes. These genes determine the properties of individual cells by controlling cell function, that is, the manufacture and breakdown of chemicals within cells. A knowledge of how genes control cell function is necessary for understanding such areas of cell biology as genetic disorders, virus function, and genetic engineering.

Relationship of genes and enzymes

The genetic code is the language that is used by a cell to transfer genetic information into chemical manufacture. Since genetic information is transcribed into RNA molecules, a form of communication is necessary between the RNA and the cytoplasmic substances that regulate chemical reactions. These substances are called enzymes.

Enzymes are a form of protein and, therefore, are composed of a sequence of amino acids. A specific enzyme consists of a unique sequence of amino acids which results in that enzyme only being able to regulate a specific chemical reaction (32.1).

For most cell chemical reactions to occur, a specific enzyme is required to regulate a specific reaction. Also, hereditary information from the nucleus is required to regulate specific cell chemical reactions. A mechanism must exist whereby hereditary information in the form of a gene controls the manufacture of the cytoplasmic chemical reaction regulators, that is, enzymes. By controlling the formation of enzymes, the gene is controlling the chemical reactions in the cytoplasm.

The function of a gene and an enzyme are determined by a sequence. In the case of the gene, a specific sequence of nucleotides determines its function, whereas with enzymes it is a specific sequence of amino acids. The mechanism of transferring genetic information to enzyme manufacture thus involves a relationship between nucleotide sequence and amino acid sequence. Parts of a nucleotide sequence must therefore correspond to individual amino acids if any correlation is to exist between the two sequences. The question then arises of how many nucleotides represent a particular amino acid.

Genetic alphabet

It is often convenient to represent each nucleotide by a capital letter, that is, A — adenine, T — thymine, C — cytosine and G — guanine. The **genetic code** consists of three-letter words, that is, combinations of three nucleotides. EXAMPLES: TAC, GGA and ACC. ANALOGY: The English language

is based on twenty-six letters which can be combined to form words of varying lengths. This variation in the number of letters that constitute a word and the relatively large number of letters results in virtually a limitless number of different words. In the genetic language, words are composed of only three letters. The small genetic alphabet of three letters restricts the number of genetic words to a maximum of sixty-four.

With any process where materials are to be assembled in a particular sequence, the following instructions are required:

1. words that signal the start of manufacture;
2. words that indicate the sequence in which the materials are to be assembled;
3. words that signal the completion of manufacture.

24.10   Transcription

Most of the sixty-four different nucleotide combinations represent the twenty forms of amino acid that are used as raw materials in protein manufacture. Some of the nucleotide triplets signal the start of protein manufacture whereas others stop the assembly of proteins. The genetic instructions are transcribed into complementary mRNA sequences of nucleotides. EXAMPLE: The DNA sequence TAC CGA ACC acts as a template to form the mRNA sequence AUG GCU UGG. The DNA instructions have been retained in the formation of a mirror image set of mRNA nucleotides. This process of **transcription** is necessary since the large DNA molecules are unable to move through the nuclear pores to the sites of protein manufacture. The mRNA acts as a courier of genetic information from the genetic master plan to the manufacturing plants. The nucleotide triplets in mRNA are referred to as **codons**. EXAMPLE: The mRNA sequence AUG GCU UGG consists of the three codons or words AUG, GCU and UGG.

A mRNA carries codons to initiate the formation of proteins, assemble amino acids in their correct order and stop at the end of the sequence when the protein is formed. Many of the meanings of the sixty-four codons have been resolved. EXAMPLES: The codons for the following amino acids: alanine — GCU, phenylalanine — UUU, tryptophan — UGG and tyrosine — UAU. An initiating condon is AUG whereas UAA stops protein manufacture.

A set of instructions carried by a mRNA to the protein factories could begin with the following nucleotide sequence: AUG GCU UGG UAU UAU UUU GCU.... This genetic code sentence would be interpreted at the assembly site as follows: start assembling/alanine/ tryptophan/tyrosine/tyrosine/phenylalanine/ alanine/....

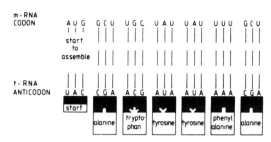

Figure 24.13 Translation of mRNA codons into an amino acid sequence.

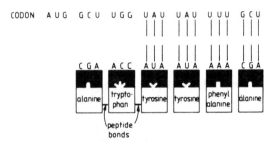

Figure 24.14 Assembling of an amino acid by linking of adjacent amino acids by peptide bonds.

24.11   Translation

The mechanism of converting genetic information into the formation of proteins is referred to as **translation**. The process of translation and thus protein manufacture occurs at the ribosomes. Ribosomes translate a sequence of codons into a sequence of amino acids with the aid of tRNA.

tRNA molecules are smaller than mRNA. They exist in approximately sixty different forms. The role of each form is that of transporting specific raw materials from the cytoplasmic matrix to the ribosomal factories. Each type of tRNA has a unique shape that is capable of carrying a specific shaped amino acid. In addition, each tRNA contains a combination of three nucleotides that are unique for that particular tRNA. These three nucleotides are termed the **anticodon** since they are able to form loose linkages with

complementary mRNA triplets. EXAMPLE: A tRNA that contains the anticodon CGA can form a loose linkage with the mRNA codon GCU.

A relationship exists between a codon and the amino acid carried by the complementary anticodon. EXAMPLE: The codon for the amino tyrosine is UAU. The tRNA that has the specific ability to carry tyrosine contains the anticodon AUA.

The mechanism by which the previously described mRNA nucleotide sequence AUG GCU UGG UAU UAU UUU GCU is translated into the amino acid sequence alanine/ tryptophan/tyrosine/tyrosine/phenylalanine/ alanine/... can now be shown (Figure 24.13). As a sequence of tRNA forms loose linkages (hydrogen bonds) with their complementary

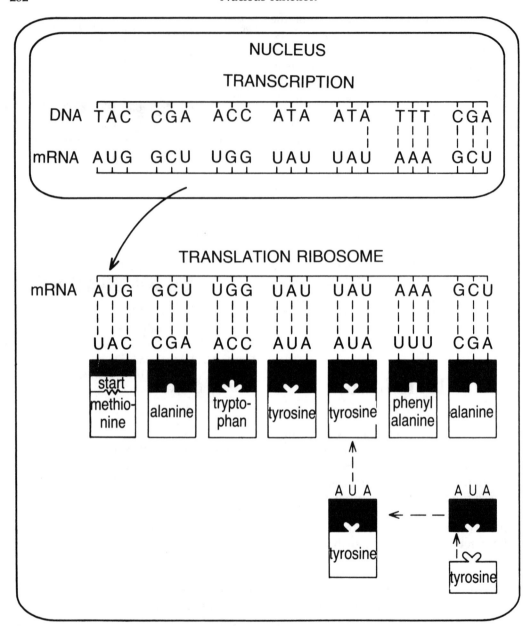

Figure 24.15 Summary of the mechanism of protein manufacture.

mRNA nucleotides, a chain of amino acids is formed.

The close proximity of oppositely charged regions of adjacent amino acids results in the formation of bonds which are known as **peptide bonds**. A peptide bond links the amine group (NH_2) of one amino acid with the carboxyl group (COOH) of an adjacent amino acid. As peptide bonds link adjacent amino acids, an amino acid chain is formed. Simultaneously, the linked amino acids separate from the tRNA carriers (Figure 24.14).

When a chain is composed of many amino acids and thus peptide bonds, the molecule is referred to as a polypeptide. Proteins are an example of polypeptides. The manufacture of proteins in a cell is schematically summarized in Figure 24.15.

24.12 Molecular-based genetic disorders

Concept of one gene – one protein

Errors in the molecular structure of a gene can result in a genetic disorder. The genetic disorder can result from an incorrect substitution of a nucleotide in the DNA molecule so that an incorrect amino acid is located within a protein molecule. Alternatively, a loss or addition of nucleotides in a gene will result in an altered instruction for the manufacture of the gene's protein. If the molecular error occurs at a functional part of the protein, a malfunction of the protein will occur. This malfunction is manifested as a genetic disorder. EXAMPLE: Sickle cell anaemia results from an alteration of only one amino acid in haemoglobin molecules.

Molecular-based genetic disorders require biochemical analysis for detection, since the chromosomes appear normal when karyo-typed. This restriction in determining a molecular defect in a chromosome resulted in a delay of half a century before a linkage could be confirmed between hereditary diseases and single proteins.

The concept that certain diseases of lifelong duration arise because an enzyme governing a single biochemical step is reduced in activity or missing altogether was first proposed in 1909 by Sir Archibald Garrod. Half a century later Garrod's hypothesis that a block in a biochemical pathway can be inherited as a single recessive trait was proven. One of the first **inborn errors of metabolism** to be recognized was phenylketonuria.

Application: Phenylketonuria

Normally the amino acid phenylalaline is converted into tyrosine which is then used for the manufacture of important body substances such as thyroid hormones and the neurotransmitters epinephrine (adrenaline), norepinephrine (noradrenaline) and dopamine. In patients suffering from phenylketonuria (PKU) a deficiency of the enzyme phenylalanine hydroxylase occurs. This enzyme is necessary for the conversion of phenylalanine into tyrosine, and thus a deficiency of this enzyme results in an accumulation of phenylalanine. The excessive accumulation of phenylalanine prevents the normal development of the brain. This abnormal development results in mental retardation of the affected infants.

The accumulation of phenylalanine can be tested in newborns by using a Guthrie test. With an appropriate low phenylalanine diet during childhood, a PKU patient can be prevented from developing the serious effects that they would have normally suffered if they had not been treated.

Consequences of gene defects

At present, over 2500 genetic disorders have been atrributed to an abnormality in the formation of proteins. The impact on the body of a particular genetic defect varies according to the functional role of the corresponding protein. The role of proteins in body function varies enormously. EXAMPLES: Membrane structure, body defence mechanisms, transporting oxygen, hormones and the control of biochemical pathways by enzymes. It is currently estimated that every individual is a carrier of between five and eight recessive deleterious genes that would have serious phenotypic effects if present in the homozygous state. As knowledge of disease mechanisms increases, the number of genetic disorders known to be present or carried by a person could be expected to be even higher than at present.

Many genetic defects may only be detected when a patient is exposed to an environmental agent that requires the normal functioning of that gene. In such cases the patient has a genetic predisposition, for example, an abnormal response to a drug.

Application: Pseudocholinesterase deficiency

Patients with pseudocholinesterase or serum cholinesterase deficiency only manifest this deficiency in the presence of the muscle relaxant succinylcholine (scoline). In the presence of this drug a patient will remain in transient paralysis for several hours instead of minutes. This response is due to the deficiency of the enzyme that normally breaks down this drug.

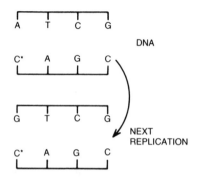

Figure 24.16 Genetic defect formed at one site in a DNA molecule where T has been replaced by a C*.

Molecular sites of genetic disorders

The replication of DNA is the probable site of most genetic disorders. For instance, the pairing of two nucleotides that are not complementary results in the erroneous nucleotide directing the combination of nucleotides complementary to itself in subsequent generations (Figure 24.16). Another failure of the genetic mechanism is the incorporation of similar structured substances into a DNA strand. These substances can cause erroneous replication of a nucleotide sequence. EXAMPLE: A substance that is structurally similar to thymine but pairs with guanine rather than adenine. Subsequent generations would have cytosine incorporated in the DNA sequence instead of thymine.

24.13 Molecular-based mitotic malfunction

Difficulty arises in determining whether a malfunction in DNA replication in somatic cells is due to the direct effects of a harmful environmental agent or is a consequence of a genetic predisposition. Mitotic molecular malfunctions result in the formation of abnormal proteins in a certain type of body tissue. The genetic defects may result in the failure of the normal processes that control cell division. In such cases a cancer may occur. Various agents known as carcinogens can initiate this uncontrolled multiplication of cells. EXAMPLE: Pollution, ultraviolet radiation, cigarette tar and viruses. A current approach to the elimination of cancer is the use of drugs that hinder cell division, and thus the growth, of the rapidly dividing cancer cells.

Application: Cytotoxic drugs

An understanding of the mechanisms of cell division has enabled the development of a range of drugs that interfere with cell division mechanisms. Drugs that have a toxic action upon cells are known as cytotoxic drugs. Many of these drugs act by interfering with the mechanism of DNA replication. These drugs usually have a similar structure to one of the nucleotides. This similarity enables the drug to combine with a replicating DNA molecule and cause mutations that are incompatible with cell life. Since most cells divide at a relatively slow rate when compared with cancer cells, the cytotoxic drugs mainly influence the rapidly-dividing cancer cells. These drugs will also cause abnormalities in the frequently-dividing sex cells and foetal cells.

Summary

The nucleus controls cell multiplication and the day-to-day functioning of a cell. The hereditary material is packaged in chromosomes.

Human cells contains twenty-three pairs of chromosomes, apart from the mature sex cells which contain only twenty-three chromosomes. Each of the twenty-three homologous pairs of chromosomes contains one chromosome from the maternal parent and one from the paternal parent. One pair are involved in the expression of sexual characteristics and are thus called sex chromosomes whereas the other twenty-two pairs are termed autosomes.

Mitosis is the process whereby hereditary information (DNA) is separated to form two identical cells. The duplication of cells is necessary for the growth and continued functioning of the body. Meiosis is a form of cell division that results in new cells with half the original number of chromosomes. This process is used in the last stages of sex cell formation for the separation of the homologous pairs of chromosomes.

Malfunction of the meiotic apparatus results in cells being formed with either abnormal quantities of chromosomes or chromosomes that have an altered structure. These abnormalities can be detected in the foetus by the combined processes of amniocentesis or chorionic villus sampling, cell culture and karyotyping.

Individual units of hereditary information are represented as genes. Each gene represents a single physical hereditary characteristic which is usually expressed in two forms, although on some occasions more than two forms exists. These forms or alleles are usually either dominant or recessive. An allele of a particular gene is found in both chromosomes that constitute a homologous pair. When the two chromosomes contain an identical allele a person is said to be homozygous for that particular gene. When the two alleles are different the person is heterozygous and is often referred to as a carrier of the recessive allele.

The genotype refers to the genetic composition of an individual whereas the phenotype expresses the physical characteristics of that person.

Genetics is the study of genes and their relationship to hereditary characteristics. The patterns of inheritance for a particular gene can be determined by taking into account the possible combinations of the parents' genotypes.

The potential genotypic combination's expression can be altered by the environment and the presence of other genes. The expression of a gene depends on the other genes present (genetic environment) and on the physical environment.

Each chromosome is composed of a long strand of DNA. The DNA is in the form of a double helix, with the two strands being linked by complementary nucleotides; adenine links with thymine and cytosine links with guanine. The sequence of these nucleotides determines the coding of hereditary information. A gene is represented by a specific sequence of approximately 1000 pairs of nucleotides.

When the two strands of DNA are split, the exposed nucleotides link with complementary free DNA nucleotides which results in the formation of two identical strands of DNA. This doubling of genetic information is necessary for cell division.

During periods between cell division or interphase the DNA splits and the exposed nucleotides or the sense strand act as a template for the formation of mRNA in the process of transcription. This mRNA is single-stranded and contains uracil in place of thymine. The mRNA carries the genetic information in the form of nucleotide triplets or codons to the ribosome. These codons form loose linkages with complementary triplets or anticodons of tRNA. Each tRNA has a specific amino acid attached to it, and thus the aligning tRNA molecules line up their corresponding amino acids into a specific sequence. This process of translating mRNA genetic information into proteins is called translation.

Alterations to the nucleotide sequence result in malformation of proteins, such as in the genetic disorder phenylketonuria. Many of these molecular-based genetic defects can only be detected when a patient is exposed to an environmental agent that requires the normal functioning of the gene. Various agents can cause a malfunction in mitotic DNA duplication which can lead to cancer. Rapidly dividing cancer cells can be acted upon by cytotoxic drugs whose site of action is usually the interference of the molecular cell division mechanism.

Unit Nine
Extracellular Structure and Function

This unit relates the different specialized functions of cells to body homeostasis. The relationship between cellular organization and function is discussed, with particular reference to the impact of abnormal cell function to body homeostasis.

Unit Nine
Extracellular Structure and Function

Chapter 25

Cellular organization

Objectives

At the completion of this chapter the student should be able to:

1. describe the similarities and differences between tissues, organs and systems;
2. list the types of tissue;
3. relate the structure of each tissue type to its function;
4. explain how the function of tissues maintains homeostasis;
5. compare the different functions of each type of tissue;
6. describe how cellular specialization and organization differ within each tissue type.

25.1 Cell forms

Human cells arise from a single cell. During the process of human development many cells are formed, and groups of these cells undergo cell differentiation. This process results in cells being altered into specialized types such as blood, nerve and muscle cells. These cells have each acquired specific functions from the same genetic makeup.

Following differentiation, specialized cells can be identified by their particular structure and function. The structure of different cells varies from the relatively simple red blood cell to the complex nerve cell (Figure 25.1). Some cells, such as the phagocytic white blood cells have a variable shape. This variable shape enables these cells to engulf nearby microbes and cell debris.

The size of cells varies from the relatively small red blood cell or erythrocyte with a diameter of 7.5 µm to the large fat cells with a diameter of 120 µm. A large variation of size can occur with the same cell type. EXAMPLE: The length of nerve cells varies from a few millimetres in the brain to over a metre in some spinal cord nerves.

Certain cells exhibit a specialized surface that consists of cytoplasmic extensions called microvilli (Figure 25.2). These extensions or folds increase the surface area of cells thus enabling a greater efficiency in the absorption of materials. EXAMPLE: Cells lining the surface of the small intestine.

The variety of cell types in the body indicates the high degree of specialization that exists in body structure and function (Table 25.1).

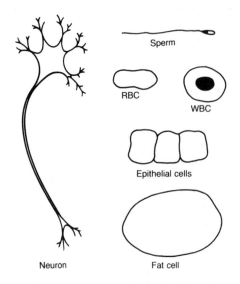

Sperm

RBC

WBC

Epithelial cells

Neuron   Fat cell

Figure 25.1   Diversity of size and shape of cells.

Table 25.1   Examples of the specialized function of cells

Cell	Function
Epithelial	Absorption and secretion of chemicals; protective barrier to the external environment
Fat	Storage of energy
Goblet	Secretion of mucus
Muscle	Moving parts of the body
Nerve	Conduction of information
Red blood cell	Transporting oxygen and carbon dioxide
White blood cell	Helps protect the body against foreign material

25.2   Levels of cellular organization

Cells are organized into tissues, organs and systems. Tissues contain cells with similar structure and function whereas organs consist of several different tissues grouped together to form a structural and functional unit. EXAMPLES: Kidneys or liver. A system consists of a group of interacting organs that cooperate as a functional unit in the life of an organism. EXAMPLES: Endocrine and nervous systems.

Tissues

A **tissue** is a combination of many cells that have a similar structure and function, that is, a tissue has a characteristic structure and function. EXAMPLE: Muscle tissue is composed of muscle cells that combine together to act as a structural and functional unit. Traditionally all animal tissues are divided into the four basic categories of epithelial tissue, muscular tissue, nervous tissue and connective tissue. Blood or vascular tissue is discussed in Chapter 26.

Organs

An **organ** consists of several tissues that act in a unique, coordinated functional manner. EXAMPLE: The kidney consists of dense and loose connective tissue, epithelial tissue, vascular tissue, nervous tissue and muscle tissue. Each of these tissues individually contributes to the total function of the kidney. Muscle tissue in the arterioles regulates the arteriole diameter and thus the flow of blood into and out of the kidney.

The unique specialized properties of different organs enables organs to play an important role in body homeostasis. EXAMPLE: The kidney has the ability to act as a filter for the body. It is thus able to regulate the removal and retention of important body substances such as water and electrolytes. It also acts as a site for the removal of toxic cellular waste materials.

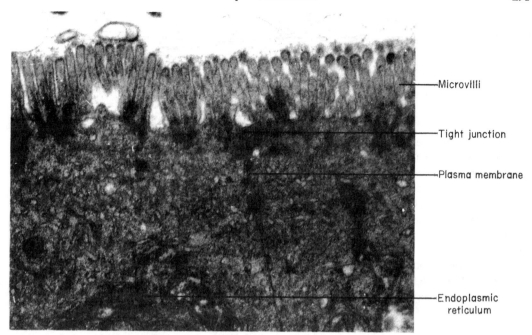

— Microvilli

— Tight junction

— Plasma membrane

— Endoplasmic reticulum

Figure 25.2 Surface of the small intestine showing microvilli, tight packing of cells and cell connections via plasma desmosomes. (×5000).

Systems

The combined action of several organs is required for the effective function of many organs. EXAMPLE: The ability of the kidneys to function relies upon a mechanism for the physical excretion of kidney filtrate from the body. The kidney along with the ureters, urinary bladder and urethra form the urinary system. This system has the ability to remove water, electrolytes, waste products and other substances from the body.

A **system** relies upon the efficient functioning of all its constituent structures. EXAMPLE: Any factor that blocks the urinary tract will result in a diminished effectiveness of the entire urinary system.

25.3 Epithelial tissue

Epithelial tissue covers the surface of the body and organs. It also lines body cavities and organs and is found in secretory structures or glands.

The general functions of epithelial tissue are to act as a protective barrier for underlying tissue, secretion and absorption of substances. The function of this tissue is closely related to structure.

Epithelial cells provide the body with a protective barrier from the external environment. EXAMPLE: Surface of skin. Within the body these cells restrict the movement of foreign substances across the walls of the gastrointestinal tract, urinary tract and respiratory tract. In order that they can function as a protective barrier, it is necessary for these cells to be packed so as to form an effective seal (Figures 25.2 and 25.3). The tight packing of cells results in only small

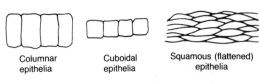

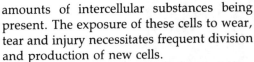

| Columnar epithelia | Cuboidal epithelia | Squamous (flattened) epithelia |

Figure 25.3 General structure of epithelial tissue.

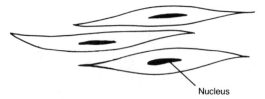

Nucleus

Figure 25.4 The structure of smooth muscle fibres.

amounts of intercellular substances being present. The exposure of these cells to wear, tear and injury necessitates frequent division and production of new cells.

Epithelial cells also perform the important functions of absorption and secretion, that is, the intake or removal of substances from the body. EXAMPLE: All digested nutrients are absorbed into the body across a layer of epithelial cells that line the gastrointestinal tract.

The structure of epithelial tissue is arranged in such a way so as to maximize the movement of substances across it. This tissue is usually arranged in thin sheets of cells in structures that are involved in absorption or secretion. EXAMPLES: Cells lining the gastro-intestinal tract, respiratory system, urinary and reproductive tracts.

The structure of epithelial cells varies from flat or squamous cells to cubes and column-shaped cells. The squamous cells are the most efficient cells for allowing substances to diffuse across them. Their thin shape offers minimal resistance to diffusing particles. These cells are therefore used to line capillaries where a minimum barrier to diffusion of oxygen and carbon dioxide is required.

All glands are composed of epithelial cells. A gland may consist of one cell or a group of highly specialized epithelial cells that secrete substances into ducts or into the blood. All glands are classified as either **exocrine** which secrete their products into ducts or **endocrine** which secrete their products directly into the blood. Goblet cells (secrete mucus) and parietal cells (secrete hydrochloric acid) are examples of secretory cells that are often interspersed throughout epithelial layers.

These single-cell exocrine glands enable epithelial layers to perform a variety of secretory roles.

Epithelial tissue has nerves penetrating it but not blood vessels. The lack of blood vessels requires epithelial cells to obtain their nutrients either from the region that they are lining or from blood capillaries in underlying connective tissue. Connective tissue also acts as a support for the epithelial tissue since the thin cell layers of epithelial tissue can be easily torn when not attached to a rigid structure.

25.4   Muscular tissue

Muscular tissue has the ability to shorten or contract. It is responsible for locomotion and for movement of various parts of the body with respect to one another. Muscle cells are elongated, relatively large cells that can be up to 40 cm in length. The size and length of these cells has resulted in their being referred to as fibres. Muscle tissue is divided into three categories: smooth, skeletal and cardiac.

Smooth muscle

Smooth muscle is the contractile tissue of all internal structures except for the heart. EXAMPLES: Walls of blood vessels, gastro-intestinal tract, respiratory tract and uterus.

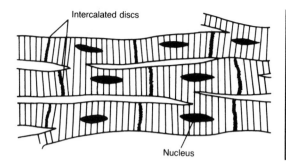

Intercalated discs

Nucleus

Figure 25.5 Cardiac muscle fibres showing the intercalated discs and the repetitive striations.

Smooth muscle fibres may occur singly or in small groups. Each fibre is characterized by its long spindle shape (Figure 25.4). These fibres are able to contract spontaneously or they can be controlled by the internal nervous system which is known as the autonomic nervous system. This nervous system is an important component of the body's internal communication network as it links the brain to tissues (38.4). The contraction of smooth muscle in response to autonomic stimulation is usually not under voluntary control. For this reason, smooth muscle is often called **involuntary muscle**. The slow sequential contraction of smooth muscle along a tube such as the gastrointestinal tract results in the mixing and continual movement of materials.

Application: Peristalsis

Peristalsis is the rhythmic movement of smooth muscle contractions that mix and propel the contents of various tubular smooth muscle structures. EXAMPLES: Gastrointestinal tract, ureters and most glandular ducts. The usual stimulus for peristalsis is disten-

---

tion, that is the stretching of a tube wall due to the accumulation of fluid.

Various factors such as emotional stress can cause an elevated peristaltic rate in the small intestine. This increased frequency of waves propels the intestinal contents to the bowel and results in diarrhoea.

Cardiac muscle

Cardiac muscle is the tissue that gives the heart its electrical and contractile properties. It is similar to smooth muscle in that it is automatic and can also be controlled by the autonomic nervous system.

Cardiac muscle is similar to skeletal muscle in that both exhibit cross bands or transverse striations along the length of their fibres (Figure 25.5). Cardiac muscle has a unique thickened region that connects the ends of adjacent muscle fibres. These thickened regions are called **intercalated discs**. They are responsible for the conduction of impulses to adjoining muscle fibres. The individual fibres contract in response to the spread of an electrical impulse along the surface of muscle cells. These impulses are similar to nerve impulses.

Under normal conditions the heart contracts in a rhythmic movement of about seventy-two times a minute. This rate can be altered by the autonomic nervous system in order to maintain homeostasis. The rhythmic contraction of muscle throughout the heart results in blood being forced from the heart and into the large arteries that emanate from it.

Cardiac muscle can exhibit three different physiological properties:

1. The automatic property of the heart spontaneously contracting at regular intervals

is often referred to as **autorhythmia**. Cells that have highly developed autorhythmic properties are located at the pacemaker, the region that determines the rate of muscle contraction. Pacemaker muscle cells have little contractile ability, their main function being to initiate impulses that are conducted to the rest of the heart.

2. Coordinated contraction of the heart requires the rapid conduction of impulses throughout the heart. Since ordinary cardiac muscle cells can only conduct impulses at a slow rate, a network of specialized rapidly conducting cardiac cells exists. This is called the **Purkinje network**.

3. The vast majority of cardiac muscle cells exhibit the ability to contract. Both the pacemaker and Purkinje fibres have little contractile ability even though they are cardiac muscle fibres.

The efficiency of the heart to pump blood depends on a coordinated contraction that is initiated at the pacemaker at the top of the heart in a region called the sino-atrial (SA) node. The SA node sets the basic pace for the heart rate. Following the initiation of an electrical impulse, it spreads over the filling chambers of the heart or atria from top to bottom leading to a contraction of the atrium. This action forces blood into the two large chambers which are known as the ventricles. The spread of the impulse by the Purkinje fibres enables the ventricles to contract in a coordinated manner, thus forcing blood into the vessels that emanate from the ventricles.

Application: Cardiac arrythmias

Efficient heart function relies on the development of electrical impulses and their subsequent conduction through the heart. Disturbances of impulse

---

formation, conduction or a combination of both can result in a lack of rhythm in the heart's action. Abnormal rhythmic contractions are termed cardiac arrhythmias.

Asynchronous contraction and quivering of the atria or ventricles are referred to as atrial fibrillation and ventricular fibrillation respectively. Fibrillation results in regions of muscle contracting at different rates forming a quivering effect or rippling of the surface. This uncoordinated contraction reduces the effectiveness of the heart. In ventricular fibrillation failure to reverse the arrhythmia quickly will result in circulatory failure and death.

The process of defibrillation is achieved by applying strong electric shocks to the heart by defibrillators. If the normal pacemaker is still functioning and viable, it may take over the rhythm, and then normal coordinated cardiac contractions resume.

Skeletal muscle

The muscles of the body that are attached to the skeleton are composed of **skeletal muscle**. It is similar to cardiac muscle in that it contains transverse striations. Large numbers of these long parallel fibres group together to form bundles (Figure 25.6). Many of these bundles are bound together by connective tissue to form large and small muscles.

Skeletal muscle differs from cardiac and smooth muscle by its inability to spontaneously contract, that is, it only contracts when it is stimulated by the nervous system. Skeletal muscle is controlled by the somatic nervous system. This nervous system involves the nerves that connect the spinal cord to the external regions of the body (38.4).

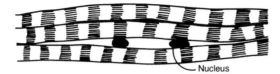

Figure 25.6 A bundle of skeletal muscle fibres showing repetitive striations.

This nervous system is under the influence of conscious control and thus skeletal muscle can be contracted at will.

Skeletal muscle fibres in a muscle will contract as one unit. They act in coordination with bones (levers) to move parts of the body. The rate of contraction can be rapid in the case of muscles used in locomotion, or slow in the case of muscles that are used for the maintenance of posture in which case they maintain long periods of sustained contraction.

Application: Disorders of skeletal muscle

Disorders of skeletal muscle are known as myopathies. The dependence of skeletal muscle on nerve stimulation is shown when this stimulation is lost. The resulting disuse of the muscle results in some degree of muscle wasting which is referred to as muscular atrophy. EXAMPLE: Long-term immobilization of a limb will result in some muscle atrophy.

The most advanced cases of muscular atrophy are characterized by a substantial reduction in affected muscle size, along with a loss of tone of the muscle. This severe form of muscle atrophy occurs when the nerve supply to the muscle is disconnected. EXAMPLES: Poliomyelitis, peripheral neuritis and

---

peripheral nerve injury cause the removal of nerve connections to regions of skeletal muscle.

Various forms of myopathies have a genetic origin and usually result in muscle weakness. EXAMPLE: The muscular dystrophies are a group of genetic abnormalities characterized by a progressive weakness and atrophy of muscles.

25.5 Nervous tissue

Nervous tissue is composed of cells capable of rapidly conveying information to different regions of the body. These nerve cells or neurons are an essential component of body homeostasis. The **neuroglia** (glial cells) comprise another group of cells which support, protect and assist the function of neurons.

Neuroglia

The neuroglia can be separated into three functional cell types. The first group forms part of the blood–brain barrier, that is, the barrier which restricts the movement of certain substances into the brain. Another group helps hold the neurons together. This group contains cells that produce a substance called myelin which forms a sheath around most neurons. Myelin serves the important function of increasing the velocity of nerve impulses. A third group of neuroglial cells is involved in the removal of microbes and cell debris from nervous tissue by the process of phagocytosis (23.5).

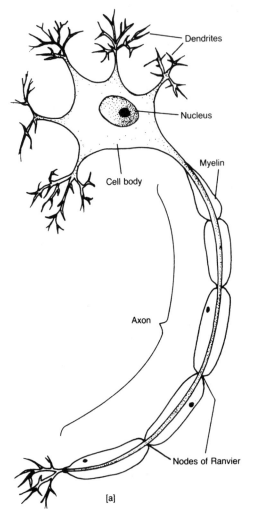

General structure of neurons

Neurons are cells that exhibit:

1. **irritability** — ability to respond to alterations in the environment;
2. **conduction** — ability to conduct impulses along their length;
3. **neurotransmission** — ability to transmit impulses to adjacent nerve, muscle or endocrine gland cells.

The structure of neurons is markedly different from all other cell types. A neuron consists of a cell body with projections extending from it. These projections are either numerous and relatively short or singular and up to 1 m in length (Figure 25.7a). The former are referred to as dendrites while the latter is known as an axon.

The cell body

The **cell body** contains a nucleus and cytoplasmic organelles. It is the site of most of the cell's chemical reactions and thus damage to it results in the death of the neuron. The cell body is located in either the grey matter of the spinal cord and brain or in the ganglia of neurons associated with the autonomic and somatic nervous systems. The dendrites receive signals and transmit them to the cell body.

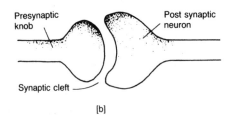

Figure 25.7 (a) Structure of a neuron.
(b) A synapse.

The axon

The **axon** carries impulses away from the cell body and to other cells. These long structures are able to conduct nerve impulses to relatively distant cells. The conduction of these impulses can be assisted by covering the axon with a myelin sheath. The term **nerve fibre** is used to describe an axon and its sheaths. Axons containing these sheaths are myelinated whereas those lacking a covering are unmyelinated. Myelinated axons have an appearance similar to a string of sausages (Figure 25.7a). The myelin prevents sodium ions and potassium ions from entering and leaving the axon. This restriction results in impulses only being formed at points where the myelin sheath is absent, that is, at the nodes of Ranvier. A nerve impulse is thus required to jump from one node to the next node in a process called saltatory conduction (10.5). The importance of myelin to nerve function is highlighted in multiple sclerosis. This debilitating disease is characterized by a breakdown of the myelin sheath.

The axon terminates as a branched region with individual branches containing knobs at their ends (Figure 25.7b). These knobs form close associations with adjacent nerve, muscle or endocrine cells.

The synapse

A **synapse** is the region where two neurons make close contact with each other. The axon located before the synapse forms the presynaptic region with the neuron being called a presynaptic neuron. The dendrites of another nerve form the postsynaptic region and the neuron is thus referred to as the postsynaptic neuron. The presynaptic knobs are separated from the postsynaptic dendrites by a minute gap of about 20 nm. This gap is called the synaptic cleft.

The region where a nerve and muscle make functional contact is known as a **neuro-muscular junction**. The distance separating the two cells is also approximately 20 nm.

Neurotransmission

The electrical nerve impulse is unable to directly cross the 20 nm gap of synapses and neuromuscular junctions. A mechanism known as **neurotransmission** is used in both situations to indirectly transfer the nerve impulse across the cleft. This mechanism is initiated by the release of chemicals called **neurotransmitters** in response to a nerve impulse arriving at the presynaptic terminals. The released neurotransmitter diffuses from the presynaptic knob across the cleft to the adjacent cell's membrane. The neurotransmitter alters the nature of this membrane so that a nerve impulse is either generated or is prevented from being formed. The effect of a neurotransmitter is either the stimulation or inhibition of the postsynaptic membrane or muscle terminal. The main neurotransmitters are acetylcholine, norepinephrine, dopamine and serotonin. Each of these neurotransmitters can only exert their influence on specific membranes. Following their brief effect on the postsynaptic membrane, the neurotransmitters are removed or broken down by enzymes. Failure to remove or break down a neurotransmitter will result in it exerting a continued effect on the postsynaptic neuron. Any alteration of the neurotransmission mechanism by drugs can either enhance or inhibit the actions of nerves.

Forms of neurons

Neurons vary in size and shape according to their function. One of the main functions of nerves is their ability to form nerve impulses from alterations in their extracellular environment. Some neurons contain highly specialized dendrites that are receptive to specific changes in the extracellular environment. These neurons are referred to as sensory neurons and the specialized dendrite region is called a **sense organ or receptor**. Except for pain receptors, each receptor responds to a specific stimulus, such as light. Receptors play a vital role in body homeostasis as they detect variations in such things as chemical concentration, pressure changes and tissue stretching.

Neurons that are required to conduct impulses over relatively large distances contain axons of up to 1 m in length. Some neurons contain very short axons. These neurons usually link nerves in the grey matter of the spinal cord and brain. Neurons that contain specialized axon terminals for functional connection with muscles or glands are referred to as motor neurons.

White and grey matter

A nerve is a combination of many bundles of nerve fibres. The axons of a myelinated nerve appear white, and hence the term **white matter** is given to the regions of the brain and spinal cord that contain a predominance of axons. A cluster of cell bodies results in a slightly grey colour. The large regions of the brain and spinal cord that consist mainly of cell bodies are known as **grey matter** (Figure 38.3).

25.6   Connective tissue

This is the most abundant tissue in the body. It binds, supports and protects other body tissue. The common features of **connective tissue** are the rich blood supply and the extensive intercellular material between the widely scattered cells. The intercellular substances form a matrix that may be a liquid, a solid, or a semi-rigid gel. The composition of the matrix determines the characteristics of that particular connective tissue. EXAMPLE: Blood is a connective tissue composed of a liquid matrix, whereas bone contains a solid matrix. The wide diversity in structure and function of connective tissue has resulted in the need to classify connective tissue into four categories which are known as connective tissue proper, cartilage, bone and vascular tissue.

Connective tissue proper

Connective tissue proper consists of cells and extracellular fibres embedded in a semi-fluid matrix called tissue fluid.

Several types of cells are found in this tissue. Some remain in a relatively fixed position. EXAMPLE: Fibroblasts which are responsible for production of collagen and the maintenance of extracellular components. Other cells have the ability to move. EXAMPLES: Plasma cells for antibody production, mast cells for heparin and histamine production, and macrophages for engulfing cell debris and bacteria.

The three forms of fibres embedded in the matrix are:

1. **Collagenous** fibres — composed of the protein collagen. These fibres are flexible but offer great resistance to a pulling force, that is, they are difficult to stretch. They have a wavy appearance and are composed of intertwined units of collagen. When collagen is broken down by boiling, gelatin results.
2. **Elastic** fibres — composed of the protein elastin. These fibres are easily stretched and they will return to their original shape when the force is removed. They are thus similar to a rubber band.
3. **Reticular** fibres — composed of collagen. These fibres are very thin and form the framework of many soft organs such as the spleen and pancreas.

The relative quantity of various kinds of cells, fibres and matrix is found to differ greatly from one body region to another. The classification of connective tissue proper is thus difficult and inexact. The connective tissue proper is separated into two forms according to the relative density of fibres. These forms are termed loose connective tissue and dense connective tissue. In many regions of the body these two forms may overlap.

Loose connective tissue is continuous throughout the body and consists of a loose network of collagen and elastic fibres. It is located beneath the skin, around blood vessels, organs and nerves. The intercellular matrix is mainly composed of a gel, which forms a predominant proportion of the interstitial fluid. The loose spongy arrangement of collagen and elastic fibres is used to support body structures. This spongy nature enables this tissue to hold water. Most of the cells of loose connective tissue are involved in the repair and defence of body tissue. Examples of these cells are:

1. fibroblasts — formation of collagen following injury;
2. macrophages (histocytes) — phagocytic cells (Figure 37.1);
3. plasma cells — produce antibodies;
4. mast cells — produce histamine and heparin;
5. white blood cells — various functions (26.1);
6. adipose cells — fat storage.

Adipose tissue is a specialized form of loose connective tissue which is involved in the production and storage of fat and thus energy (see 33.11). As fat is a poor conductor of heat, the layers of fat under the skin prevent excessive heat loss. Adipose tissue also supports and physically protects various organs by being arranged as protective pads around these organs. About 10% of the body weight of an average person is fat which represents approximately forty days of reserve energy.

Dense connective tissue can be subdivided according to the arrangement of the fibres:

1. Dense irregular connective tissue is composed of the same cell types as loose connective tissue. However, these fibres are interwoven in an irregular dense framework between small amounts of intercellular matrix. This tissue forms the

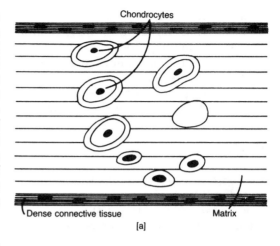

[a]

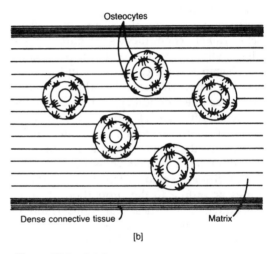

[b]

Figure 25.8 (a) Cartilage (hyaline) tissue.
(b) Bone tissue.

capsule that protects and supports organs. It is also located in the dermis and constitutes the sheaths of nerves and tendons.

2. Dense regular connective tissue consists of fibres arranged in a regular dense framework with little intercellular matrix. The orderly arrangement of the fibres is indicative of the mechanical requirements of the tissue. Several forms of arrangement

and therefore function exist in the body. EXAMPLES: Ligaments — flexible, strong cords connecting bones at joints which consist of parallel bundles of elastic and collagen fibres. Tendons — strong cords connecting bones to muscles which consist of parallel bundles of collagen fibres.

Cartilage

Cartilage consists of a gel-like matrix enclosed in a layer of dense connective tissue. The considerable degree of stiffness of this matrix enables cartilage to be used as a specialized supportive tissue. Embedded within the matrix are large quantities of fine collagen and elastic fibres and specialized cells called **chondrocytes** (Figure 25.8a). These cells are responsible for the production of collagen and the constituents of the intercellular matrix. This tissue lacks blood vessels, and thus the chondrocytes rely upon the efficient diffusion of nutrients and toxic waste products through the intercellular matrix to the blood vessels in the surrounding dense connective tissue.

The firmness and flexibility of cartilage varies according to the proportion of fibres embedded in it. These variations result in cartilage being found in a wide range of locations in the body. EXAMPLES: Large tubes of the respiratory tract, discs between vertebrae, menisci in the knee joint, articulating surfaces of bones, foetal skeleton.

Bone tissue

Bone tissue differs from other forms of connective tissue since it contains calcified extracellular components. The calcified matrix confers the hard and unyielding nature to bone that makes it an ideal tissue to act as a skeleton. The rigid property of bony tissue enables bone to be used as a lever for mechanical movement.

Embedded within the calcified matrix are bone cells or osteocytes (Figure 25.8b). These cells perform the specialized function of producing the intercellular material. When diminished levels of calcium and magnesium occur in the blood, some of the matrix is broken down to release the required quantities of calcium and magnesium.

Bone is subdivided into one of two forms according to the nature of the matrix. **Spongy bone** contains relatively large spaces within the matrix. These spaces are occupied by bone marrow, the site of blood cell production (26.1). **Compact bone** appears as a solid mass with microscopic sized spaces. The proportion of spongy and compact bony tissue in a bone depends upon its function. A bone such as the femur requires great strength to support the body weight and is thus composed of a higher proportion of compact bone than the skull bones.

Bone has the ability to replace itself throughout the life of a person. This ability is shown in the healing of fractures.

Application: Fractures of the bone

A fracture is a break in a bone. It results from a bone being unable to resist an excessive force being applied to it. It is important for the fragments of bone to be returned and then maintained in their pre-injury position. Failure to do this can lead to the healing of the fracture in an abnormal position and/or delayed healing. The process of fracture repair can take several months. Various immobilization methods such as traction and plaster are used to maintain the fragments in a relatively fixed position.

Fracture repair involves the following steps:
1. broken blood vessels at the fracture site form a clot;

2. dense connective tissue forms a collar around the gap between the bones;
3. the collar helps to stabilize the fragments as its surrounding bony regions are gradually replaced with new bone; at this stage the healing bone is not strong enough to bear weight;
4. the region inside the collar is joined and then the thickened collar region is remodelled; the complete healing process has resulted in the fractured bone being similar to its pre-fracture structure.

25.7 Tissues and homeostasis

Tissues are combinations of many cells with a similar structure and function. These similarities enable tissues to serve a variety of roles in maintaining body homeostasis such as:

1. **Movement** — muscles produce actions that assist the movement of substances throughout the body. EXAMPLE: Cardiac muscle.
2. **Transportation** — blood acts as a medium for the transportation of substances to different regions of the body.
3. **Filtration** — epithelial tissue acts as a filter for the movement of substances from the blood to cells.
4. **Absorption** — epithelial tissue acts as a selective barrier for the movement of substances into the body. EXAMPLE: Walls of the small intestine.

5. **Secretion** — glandular tissue secretes specific substances for the regulation of other cells. EXAMPLE: Endocrine glands secrete hormones.
6. **Protection** — loose connective tissue protects organs from both physical damage and infection.

Summary

The body consists of three levels of cellular organization:

1. Tissues are combinations of many cells that have a similar structure and function. The four main tissue forms are epithelial tissue, muscular tissue, nervous tissue and connective tissue.
2. Organs consist of several tissues that act in a unique coordinated functional manner. EXAMPLES: Kidney, heart, liver.
3. Systems are composed of a group of interacting organs that operate as a functional unit. EXAMPLES: Endocrine and nervous systems.

Cells are categorized into a particular type of tissue according to their structure and function. The four types of tissue exhibit specific characteristics.

Epithelial tissue consists of cells that form protective layers. Being packed closely together, these cells act as a barrier between the body and the external environment. These cells also line vessels, tubes and ducts within the body in order to prevent leakage. EXAMPLES: Cells lining the respiratory tract, blood vessels. Epithelial cells that can secrete substances are known as gland cells and exist as single secretory structures such as mucous membrane cells. Gland cells can also exist as multicellular structures that either secrete substances into ducts (exocrine glands) or blood vessels (endocrine glands).

Muscular tissue consists of cells that can contract. These cells are responsible for locomotion and for the movements of various body structures. This tissue can be divided into smooth muscle, skeletal muscle and cardiac muscle. Smooth muscle is the contractile tissue of all internal structures, apart from the heart which consists of cardiac muscle. Both smooth and cardiac muscle can contract automatically or be controlled by the autonomic nervous system. Skeletal muscle is controlled by the somatic nervous system. Skeletal muscle is attached to the skeleton and is used in locomotion, posture, facial expression and any other similar coordinated action.

Nervous tissue is composed of neurons and neuroglia. The neurons rapidly conduct information in the form of nerve impulses whereas the neuroglia support, protect and assist the function of neurons. A neuron consists of a cell body and projections from the cell body. The short projections receive information and are called dendrites, whereas a long projection or axon carries information away from the cell body. Axons form synapses with other nerves and neuromuscular junctions with muscles. These functional connections conduct information via a mechanism referred to as neurotransmission.

Connective tissue consists of cells, fibres and extensive amounts of intercellular material or matrix. This tissue binds, supports and protects other body tissue. The four main forms of connective tissue are connective tissue proper, cartilage, bone and vascular tissue. Each of these forms differs according to the intercellular matrix.

Chapter 26

Blood

Objectives

At the completion of this chapter the student should be able to:

1. list the constituents of blood;
2. describe the functions of the various blood constituents;
3. explain the effects of abnormal concentrations of these constituents;
4. explain the mechanisms of oxygen and carbon dioxide uptake, transport and release;
5. relate blood gas measurements to abnormal body function.

Blood is a body fluid that comprises about 8% of the total body weight. Blood is composed of a solution and a colloid of various substances which is called plasma, and a suspension of cells, among which the red blood cells (erythrocytes) predominate.

Blood plays a vital role in the function of complex multicellular organisms such as humans. It is the medium of transportation of nutrients and chemical regulators to the cell, and of removal of cellular excretions. Blood also plays an important role in the defence of the body against foreign microorganisms (37.2). (The normal values of blood constituents are listed in Appendix I.)

26.1 Constituents of plasma

Plasma is the fluid component of blood. It comprises about 55% of total blood volume.

Plasma consists of approximately 91.5% water, 7% protein and the remaining 1.5% a mixture of a variety of substances such as electrolytes, lipids, hormones, carbohydrates and vitamins.

Plasma proteins

The three major groups of protein present in plasma are **albumin**, **globulin** and **fibrinogen**. Their combined concentration is normally in the SI unit range of 66 to 82 g/L (6.6 to 8.2 g per cent). All plasma proteins perform the following functions in blood:

1. Exert osmotic pressure and so play an important role in the prevention of fluid loss from the capillaries (21.4).
2. Act as a mobile storage medium for amino acids. Whenever a particular tissue is depleted of protein the required amino acids can be readily supplied by the rapid breakdown of plasma protein.

3. Buffer increased concentrations of acid and base. Plasma proteins constitute the greatest quantity of plasma buffers and thus play an important role in the homeostasis of blood acid–base balance (16.5).

Albumin is the most abundant plasma protein, with the normal range of plasma concentration being 42 to 58 g/L (4.2 to 5.8 g per cent). It accounts for over 90% of the colloid osmotic pressure and thus plays the principal role in blood capillary fluid regulation.

Plasma globulin is a collective term for three types of proteins known as globular proteins. These globulins constitute about 44% of the total protein concentration of plasma. They exist in a concentration of approximately 25 g/L (2.5 g per cent). The three forms of globulin are alpha (α), beta (β) and gamma (γ). The γ globulins are produced by cells in the reticuloendothelial system and form the antibody component of the body defence system (37.2). The α and β globulins are produced by the liver and bind with various substances for the purpose of transportation in plasma. These substances include electrolytes (EXAMPLES: Iron and copper) hormones (EXAMPLES: Thyroid hormone thyroxin) lipids and fat-soluble vitamins.

Fibrinogen exists in small quantities in the order of 3.0 g/L (0.3 g per cent). This protein is essential for the formation of clots.

Non-protein nitrogens

Non-protein nitrogens (NPN) are substances that contain nitrogen but are not proteins. Some of the important NPNs are urea, creatinine and uric acid. All of these substances are waste products of nitrogen metabolism.

Urea is the main end product of protein breakdown and it occurs in normal concen-

trations of between 3.2 to 7.5 mmol/L (19 to 45 mg/100 mL). Urea is normally removed from the body by the kidneys. An elevated plasma urea concentration can indicate a decreased efficiency in kidney function. The urea concentration will also be raised as a result of any factor that elevates the rate of protein breakdown. EXAMPLES: Low protein intake, injury and infection.

Creatinine is a waste product formed as a result of muscle activity. Its normal concentration range is 0.06 to 0.12 mmol/L (0.68 to 1.40 mg/100 mL) in males and 0.04 to 0.10 mmol/L (0.45 to 1.10 mg/100 mL) in females. Creatinine concentration is increased by muscle disuse, trauma and steroid therapy. The plasma level of creatinine depends directly on the efficiency of the kidneys. As the ability of the kidneys to filter creatinine falls, due to impaired renal function, the plasma concentration of creatinine rises.

Uric acid is a nitrogen-containing compound that results from nucleic acid breakdown. The normal plasma uric acid range is 0.18 to 0.47 mmol/L (3 to 8 mg/100 mL). Uric acid has a low solubility in water and thus any elevation in the concentration of uric acid can result in precipitation. The formation of crystals in the kidney can lead to renal failure. Crystal formation of uric acid in joints results in gout, in which case foods such as meat that are rich in nucleic acids should be avoided.

Electrolytes

Plasma contains a variety of electrolytes. The predominant cations are sodium, potassium, calcium and magnesium. The principal anions are chloride, bicarbonate and phosphate.

Sodium (Na^+) is the most abundant plasma electrolyte, with normal plasma concentration ranging from 137 to 149 mmol/L (137–149 meq/L). Sodium plays an important role in nerve and muscle function, the homeostasis of fluid and electrolyte balance. Abnormally low sodium concentrations are referred to as hyponatraemia and may be caused by burns, certain diuretics and excessive perspiration. The effect of hyponatraemia is muscular weakness, decreased blood pressure, tachycardia and circulatory shock. Hypernatraemia causes cellular dehydration which causes thirst. The dehydration of the brain cells results in mental confusion and coma if not treated. The net effect of hypernatraemia is water depletion, and thus reversal is achieved by giving water orally and placing the patient on a low sodium diet. Another method is the intravenous administration of 5% glucose in water.

Potassium (K^+) occurs in concentrations of 3.8 to 5.0 mmol/L (3.8 to 5.0 meq/L) in the plasma. It is essential for the normal function of nerve and muscle, especially cardiac muscle. Potassium depletion or hypokalaemia results in arrhythmias which may progress to cardiac arrest. Care must be taken when alleviating hypokalaemia by injecting intravenous potassium since hyperkalaemia may occur. Hyperkalaemia causes disordered cardiac function that may progress to ventricular fibrillation and cardiac arrest.

Calcium (Ca^{2+}) concentrations in plasma range from 2.25 to 2.60 mmol/L (4.5 to 5.2 meq, 9.0 to 10.4 mg/100 mL). About half this calcium exists as free dissolved ions while the remainder is bound to substances such as plasma proteins. Calcium plays an important role in blood clotting. It also influences nerve and muscle function and the permeability of plasma membranes. A calcium deficiency or hypocalcaemia results in an increase in the permeability of nerves and muscle cells to sodium (23.2). The result is an increased activity of nerves and muscles which is manifested as increased nervous activity and twitching. In severe deficiency, spasms of skeletal muscles and convulsions can occur. Hypocalcaemia may also inhibit the clotting process thus protracting any

bleeding. Hypercalcaemia can cause vomiting, nausea, loss of muscle tone and confusion, and if untreated it may lead to coma.

Magnesium (Mg^{2+}) exists in normal plasma concentrations of 0.80 to 1.05 mmol/L (1.6 to 2.1 meq/L, 19.5 to 25.5 mg/L). Magnesium is essential for the functioning of many enzymes, particularly those relating to carbohydrate metabolism. Magnesium also plays an important role in neuromuscular function. Hypomagnesaemia or magnesium deficiency in the blood causes symptoms similar to those of hypocalcaemia, that is, twitching and tremors which may lead to convulsions. Cardiac arrhythmias may also develop. Hypermagnesaemia depresses nerve and skeletal muscle activity.

Chloride ions (Cl^-) are the most predominant anions found in plasma. Their relatively large plasma concentration of 95 to 105 mmol/L (95 to 105 meq/L) indicates that they play an important role in the maintenance of extracellular osmotic pressure and body water homeostasis. Chloride ions are also used in acid–base regulation. A close association exists between chloride and sodium ions. Often, changes in chloride concentration are closely linked to changes in sodium concentration. A loss of sodium ions is usually accompanied by chloride depletion. Disturbances of the gastrointestinal tract can result in hypochloraemia or a chloride deficit which is independent of sodium concentration. In such cases, an elevated bicarbonate ion concentration develops along with alkalosis.

Hydrogen carbonate (bicarbonate) ions (HCO_3^-) occur in normal plasma concentrations of 21 to 32 mmol/L (21 to 32 meq/L). Their principal role in blood is that of acid–base regulation and the indirect transport of carbon dioxide. Their function in acid–base balance is discussed in 16.5. The effect of altered hydrogen carbonate ion concentration is described in 16.6.

Phosphate ions (PO_4^{2-}) exist in normal plasma concentrations of 0.80 to 1.5 mmol/L (2.5 to 4.6 mg/100 mL). They play an important role in energy production, and thus depleted plasma phosphate concentration or hypophosphataemia results in lethargy and muscle weakness. A close association exists between phosphate and calcium. This association is shown in cases of hyperphosphataemia where plasma calcium concentrations usually fall and the resulting hypocalcaemia manifestations occur. The role of phosphate as a buffer is described in 16.5.

Non-electrolytes

The main non-electrolyte present in plasma is **glucose**. Its normal plasma concentration following fasting is 5.0 to 6.6 mmol/L (80 to 120 mg/mL). Glucose plays a vital role in the supply of energy to cells (33.2). Hypoglycaemia or depleted glucose results in a diminished supply of energy to the brain. This is manifested as dizziness, faintness or lethargy which can rapidly lead to coma and if untreated, death. Hyperglycaemia or elevated blood glucose results in loss of appetite, nausea, vomiting, thirst and drowsiness which can lead to acidosis and coma if not treated. A more detailed discussion of blood glucose concentrations occurs in 28.4.

Lipids

Lipids are a group of organic compounds that have the general property of insolubility in water (29.1). The four main forms of lipid that are present in plasma are fatty acids, triglycerides (fats), phospholipids and cholesterol. Most lipid is transported in blood by combining with protein to form a water-soluble lipoprotein.

Fatty acids are straight-chained organic acids that are either saturated or unsaturated (carbons linked by double or triple bonds — 7.2). Fatty acids are mainly transported in combination with albumin. They are the main building block of many lipids. Their normal fasting concentrations are very low, but an increased breakdown of fat will result in elevated plasma levels.

Triglycerides or fats consist of fatty acids and the alcohol glycerol (Figure 29.1). Fat that is absorbed across the small intestine is transported as an emulsion. The emulsion consists of droplets of fat surrounded by proteins. These droplets are known as chylomicrons (17.6). Triglyceride can also be formed in the liver. This triglyceride is transported by lipoproteins to the adipose tissue. The normal range of plasma triglyceride concentration is 0.05 to 2.30 mmol/L (4.4 to 203 mg/100 mL). Elevated triglycerides would be expected to occur following ingestion of a meal and in situations where excessive amounts of fats are being formed by the liver.

Phospholipids are lipids that contain phosphate. They are the main constituent of cell membranes. They are transported throughout the body by lipoproteins.

Cholesterol is used by body to form steroids. It is transported mainly by lipoproteins. The accepted cholesterol concentration ranges from 2.6 to 6.5 mmol/L (100 to 250 mg/100 mL). A diet containing saturated fatty acids will elevate plasma cholesterol, whereas polyunsaturated diets tend to lower cholesterol levels.

Lipoproteins play an important role in the transport of lipids. They are mainly involved in the transport of lipids from the liver to other tissues. Various types of lipoproteins occur, and each type carries specific lipids. EXAMPLE: β lipoproteins (low density lipoprotein — LDL) carry cholesterol.

Application: Atherosclerosis

Atherosclerosis is a disease of large and medium-sized arteries where a lipid–protein deposit decreases the diameter of the artery. The deposit is called a plaque or atheroma and is mainly composed of cholesterol combined with proteins. Raised plasma cholesterol levels and thus elevated low density lipoprotein levels have been strongly correlated with atherosclerosis.

26.2 Formed elements of blood

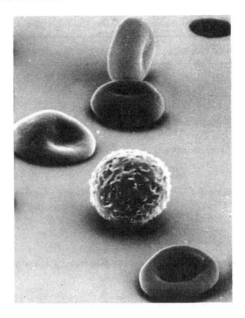

Figure 26.1 Biconcave erythrocytes with a lymphocyte (× 4000).

Formed elements constitute the other major constituent of blood. They consist of blood cells and cell-like bodies suspended in the plasma. The formed elements can be placed into the following categories: erythrocytes (red blood cells), leucocytes (white blood cells), platelets (thrombocytes).

The formed elements enable the blood to perform important homeostatic functions such as transporting oxygen, combating inflammation, halting haemorrhages and fighting infection.

Erythrocytes

Erythrocytes are commonly called red blood cells (RBCs). These cells lack a nucleus and have a biconcave shape (Figure 26.1). The average life span of a red blood cell is 120 days and the production of erythrocytes in the bone marrow is approximately equal to the rate of destruction. The normal concentration of erythrocytes differs in women and men, with the normal female range being 3.9 to 5.6×10^{12}/L (3.9 to 5.6×10^{6} μL/mm^3) and the male range being 4.5 to 6.5×10^{12}/L (4.5 to 6.5×10^{6} μL/mm^3). These cells represent the greatest concentration of any formed element in plasma. They influence the viscosity of blood and thus the relative ease with which blood flows through the vascular system.

Red blood cells contain large quantities of haemoglobin which carries most of the oxygen in the blood. Haemoglobin therefore plays a vital role in body homeostasis, since normal cell function relies upon oxygen. Haemoglobin is also involved in the transport of carbon dioxide away from the tissues. Related to this transport is the role of haemoglobin as a buffer in blood pH homeostasis (16.5). The relationship, between haemoglobin and the transport of oxygen is discussed later in this chapter.

The production of erythrocytes is termed erythropoiesis. Red blood cell production

Table 26.1 Classification of the main forms of anaemia

Form of anaemia	Mechanism affected	Cause
Aplastic	Sites of production	Destruction or inhibition of red bone marrow caused by toxins and medications
Blood loss (haemorrhagic)	Demand exceeds production capability	Acute or chronic haemorrhage
Folic acid deficiency	Maturation of red blood cell altered	Dietary insufficiency, malabsorption and increased requirements during pregnancy
Haemolytic	Faulty red blood cell production and excessive breakdown	Faulty red blood cell membranes or enzymes result in a marked decrease in red blood cell life, agents such as parasites and toxins
Iron deficiency	Relative deficiency of raw material	Inadequate diet, malabsorption, increased body utilization such as occurs with pregnancy
Pernicious (vitamin B_{12} deficiency)	Maturation of red blood cell altered	Lack of gastric intrinsic factor (assists absorption), dietary insufficiency and disease in the intestine
Sickle cell	Faulty haemoglobin production leads to short life span, demand exceeds supply	Heredity
Thalassaemia	Faulty haemoglobin production	Heredity

depends upon the supply of raw materials such as iron, sufficient manufacturing sites (bone marrow) and correct production and release of red blood cells. Alterations to any of these factors can result in a relative deficiency of haemoglobin in the blood. Such a deficiency is called anaemia.

Application: Anaemia

Anaemia is a relative deficiency of haemoglobin that may result from alteration in the production of red blood cells, excessive destruction in the blood or losses as a result of haemorrhage.

The net effect of any of these alterations is an imbalance between the rate of formation and destruction of red blood cells. Anaemia results in a lack of oxygen being supplied to the tissues. This leads to fatigue, weakness and pallor. Anaemia can be classified according to the location of the abnormality (Table 26.1).

Leucocytes

Leucocytes or white blood cells (WBCs) occur in a variety of forms and perform functions

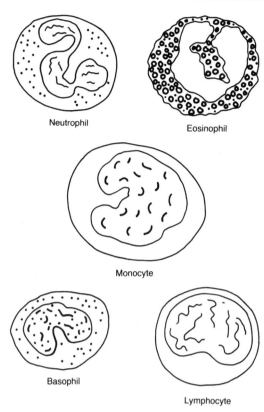

Neutrophil

Eosinophil

Monocyte

Basophil

Lymphocyte

Figure 26.2   Different types of leucocytes.

associated with the body defence system. The total leucocyte concentration is less than that of the red blood cells, with the normal range being 4.0 to 11.0 × 10^9/L (4000 to 11 000/mm^3). Leucocytes originate from either lymphatic tissue or red bone marrow. The lymphatic tissue produces while blood cells that contain a non-granular cytoplasm and a regular-shaped nucleus. Red bone marrow produces some of these cells, but is mainly involved in the production of cells that have a granular cytoplasm and irregular-shaped nucleus. The latter cells exist in three forms: neutrophils (polymorphs), eosinophils and basophils. The non-granular white blood cells are classified as either lymphocytes or monocytes (Figure 26.2).

Neutrophils are phagocytic cells that respond to inflammation and tissue destruction. They account for 60 to 70% of the total white blood cell count. They increase in number in response to infection and inflammation.

Eosinophils account for about 2 to 4% of the leucocyte count (Figure 26.3). They appear to be involved in combating substances responsible for causing allergies. A high eosinophil count usually indicates an allergic condition, although some parasites such as hookworms can cause an elevated count.

Basophils account for only 0.5 to 1% of the leucocyte count. Little is understood about the function of basophils although it is believed that they are involved in allergic reactions.

Lymphocytes comprise a group of different cell types, all of which appear similar when observed under a microscope. Most lymphocytes appear to play specialized roles in the immunity of the body to foreign agents. Lymphocytes represent 20–25% of a normal total white cell count. A comprehensive discussion of their functions in immunity is given in Chapter 37.

Monocytes represent 3–8% of the total white cell count. Monocytes are able to move into tissues and phagocytose foreign material and are thus referred to as the scavenger cells of the body. They appear to clean up the remains left by the phagocytic neutrophils.

Generally, white blood cells remove debris and foreign material from the extracellular fluid. It would be reasonable to think that the more leucocytes present, the greater is our body's ability to fight infection and inflammation. However, in cases where an uncontrolled production of white blood cells occurs, the result is often infection!

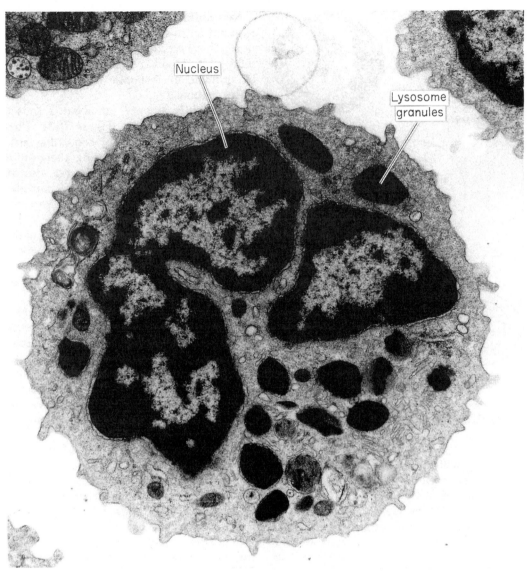

Figure 26.3 Eosinophil containing numerous lysosome granules (×16 000).

Application: Leukaemia

Leukaemia is a blood disease in which an uncontrolled production of white blood cells occurs. A marked increase of a specific white cell type occurs in the blood. EXAMPLE: Lymphocytes. Many of these white blood cells are abnormal, immature and lack the ability to perform their normal functions. Even though the number of white blood cells is elevated, the presence of large quantities of abnormal and immature cells restricts the body defence mechanisms, thus resulting in an increased susceptibility to infection. The relative proportion of other white blood cell forms decreases due to the cancerous spread of the abnormal leucocyte into their regions of formation.

The leukaemia tissues form new cells at a rate that places a drain on the nutrients circulating in the body. In particular, amino acids and vitamins are depleted, thus leading to a rapid deterioration of body proteins. This eventually results in death of the patient.

Platelets

Platelets (thrombocytes) are tiny disc-shaped cells that lack a nucleus. Platelets have a life span of about one week and thus a continual turnover of platelets is necessary for the maintenance of normal concentrations of 150 to 400×10^9/L (150 000 to 400 000/mm^3).

Platelets initiate the clotting mechanism by their ability to:

1. release vasoconstrictor substances;
2. provide a temporary plug capable of controlling flow in small vessels;
3. contribute to the coagulation mechanism which eventuates in a blood clot.

Application: Haemostasis

Haemostasis refers to the arrest of bleeding. Platelets are the key factor in the haemostatic mechanism (Figure 26.4(a)). Following vascular injury, platelets near the damaged region adhere to the exposed collagen fibres of the vascular well. The platelets immediately release substances that cause the aggregation of new platelets and constriction of the vessel. The constriction limits the flow of blood through the damaged region. The aggregation of more platelets at the traumatized site results in the formation of a platelet plug which covers the vascular break. These platelets assist the formation of the enzyme thrombin from its inactive form prothrombin. Thrombin formation also requires the presence of various plasma coagulation factors and calcium.

Thrombin converts the plasma protein fibrinogen into long fibrous threads called fibrin. This is achieved by the process of coagulation, that is, the formation of suspended particles by combining colloid particles. These suspended particles coat the plug, giving it strength to resist being dislodged by the moving blood. The platelet plug–fibrin complex is referred to as a blood clot (Figure 26.4(b)).

26.3 Haemoglobin and oxygen transport

A knowledge of how oxygen enters the blood, is transported through the vessels

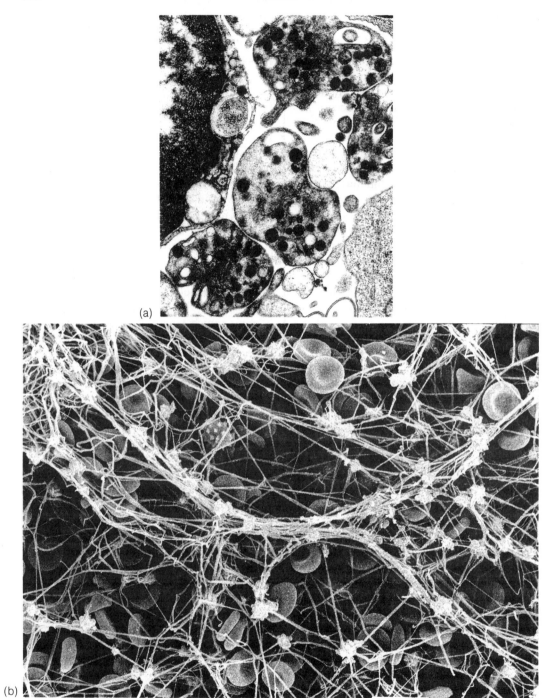

Figure 26.4   (a) Platelet cell structure (×14 700) (b) blood clot showing fibrin thread network trapping
blood cells.

and then released in the region of tissue, is important in gaining an understanding of the homeostasis of tissue oxygen supply. The homeostasis of oxygen is an essential component of body homeostasis since nearly all of the energy produced in the body requires the presence of oxygen.

Haemoglobin

The non-polar nature of oxygen results in oxygen having a low solubility in water and thus plasma (17.2). The amount of dissolved oxygen normally transported in blood is about $0.5\,mL$ $O_2/100\,mL$ blood or $15\,mL/min$. The body tissues usually require $20\,mL$ $O_2/$ $100\,mL$. Clearly an alternative method of transport is required for oxygen to travel from the lungs to the tissues. Nearly 97% of oxygen transported in the blood is carried by the substance haemoglobin which is the main constituent of red blood cells.

Haemoglobin is a pigment that consists of the protein globin wrapped around four haem groups. A **haem** group is a chemical structure that has iron located in its centre. An oxygen molecule is carried in the crevice between each haem group and the globin molecule. Since four haem groups exist, one haemoglobin molecule can therefore carry four oxygen molecules.

An important feature of haemoglobin is its ability to combine with oxygen in a loose, weak association. This enables haemoglobin to readily pick up oxygen and easily release oxygen without requiring the use of large amounts of energy. This ability is essential if a carrier is to pick up oxygen from the lungs and then readily release it in the tissue capillaries.

Each haem group does not become oxygenated simultaneously. The binding of an oxygen molecule to one haem group enhances further binding of oxygen with the remaining haem groups. The effect of this binding mechanism is the sequential uptake and release of oxygen. This sequential binding plays an important role in the mechanism of oxygen release at the tissue capillaries.

The ability of oxygen to be sequentially combined with haemoglobin and sequentially released is determined by the difference in the partial pressure of oxygen (PO_2) in the blood. The high PO_2 in the pulmonary capillaries results in large quantities of oxygen binding with haemoglobin, whereas the low PO_2 in the tissue capillaries causes oxygen to be released from the haemoglobin.

Uptake of oxygen

Oxygen uptake is dependent upon a high PO_2 in the blood. The site of oxygen intake is the lungs, therefore a high PO_2 is required in the pulmonary capillaries if oxygen is to be transported to the tissues. Diffusion of the oxygen from the lungs to the blood is dependent upon the relative difference in the concentration of oxygen between the lungs and the blood.

In 19.2 a relationship was described between PO_2 in the alveoli of the lungs and the pulmonary capillaries. The normal diffusion of oxygen from an alveolar PO_2 of $13.3\,kPa$ ($100\,mm\,Hg$) to the blood results in blood leaving the lungs with a PO_2 of $12.6\,kPa$ ($95\,mm\,Hg$). At this blood PO_2 all the haemoglobin is carrying its maximum amount of oxygen. The haemoglobin is said to be saturated.

Any condition which causes less oxygen to enter the pulmonary capillaries, thus a lower PO_2, can result in haemoglobin not being saturated. The relative uptake of oxygen is reflected in the degree of saturation of arterial blood, that is its PO_2. The measurement of blood arterial PO_2 is thus an important diagnostic aid in detecting conditions that result in the low uptake of oxygen in the blood.

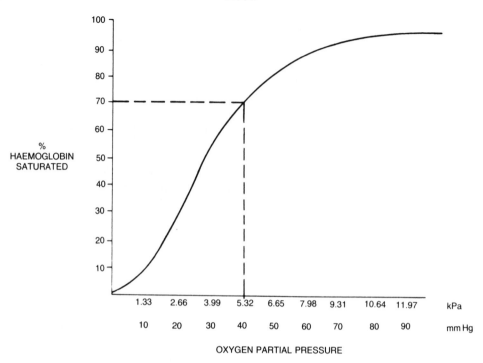

Figure 26.5 The oxygen–haemoglobin
dissociation curve.

Release of oxygen

Haemoglobin releases oxygen in accordance
with tissue needs. Consumption of oxygen
by tissue is reflected by a lower tissue capillary PO_2. A decrease in this capillary PO_2
results in the release of oxygen from the
haemoglobin molecule. The normal relationship between oxygen release and capillary
PO_2 is shown in Figure 26.5. The response of
haemoglobin to PO_2 is often referred to as the
oxygen–haemoglobin dissociation curve.
The percentage of haemoglobin saturated is
the proportion of oxygen bound to haemoglobin compared with the total amount of
haemoglobin present. The PO_2 of tissue capillaries under normal conditions is 5.32 kPa
(40 mm Hg). Under these conditions, 25%
of the total amount of haemoglobin-bound
oxygen is released and 75% is therefore
retained. This retention acts as a readily
accessible reserve of oxygen.

When oxygen utilization of tissues increases rapidly such as during strenuous
exercise, the PO_2 in the interstitial fluid can
decrease to levels of 2.0 kPa (15 mm Hg).
These low PO_2 levels cause the release of
most of the oxygen reserve. In the curve, a
level of 2.0 kPa results in haemoglobin only
being able to retain approximately 20%
oxygen saturation.

The result of normal levels of oxygen dissociation from haemoglobin is a venous
PO_2 of 5.32 kPa (40 mm Hg). On arrival at
the lungs, the difference in partial pressure
results in a diffusion of oxygen from the
alveoli to the blood and subsequently combination with haemoglobin.

26.4 Carbon dioxide transport

Uptake of carbon dioxide

The PCO_2 of arterial blood is 5.3 kPa (40 mm Hg). The production of carbon dioxide by cells results in a tissue PCO_2 of 6.0 kPa (45 mm Hg). This relative difference in carbon dioxide concentration causes carbon dioxide to diffuse from the tissues into the blood in the capillaries until the concentrations are equal. The venous blood thus has a PCO_2 of 6.0 kPa (45 mm Hg).

Carbon dioxide is carried in the blood by three mechanisms: dissolved in plasma (7%), combined with haemoglobin (23%), converted into the hydrogen carbonate ion (70%).

The non-polar nature of carbon dioxide results in a low solubility in plasma and therefore only about 7% of carbon dioxide is transported by this mechanism.

Approximately 23% of carbon dioxide combines with haemoglobin. The weak bonding of carbon dioxide to haemoglobin is reversible, that is, the carbon dioxide can readily be released when a decrease in dissolved carbon dioxide concentration occurs.

$$CO_2 + \text{haemoglobin} \rightleftharpoons \text{haemoglobin } CO_2$$
$$\text{Eqn 26.1}$$

Seventy per cent of carbon dioxide combines with water to form hydrogen carbonate ions (Eqn 26.2).

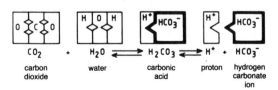

$$CO_2 + H_2O \rightleftharpoons H_2CO_3 \rightleftharpoons H^+ + HCO_3^-$$

carbon dioxide + water ⇌ carbonic acid ⇌ proton + hydrogen carbonate ion

$$\text{Eqn 26.2}$$

The reaction occurs in the plasma and in the cytoplasm of the red blood cells. Only about 10% of hydrogen carbonate is formed in the plasma. In the red blood cells an enzyme called carbonic anhydrase effects the rapid formation of carbonic acid from carbon dioxide and water. About 90% of the carbonic acid dissociates into hydrogen and hydrogen carbonate ions. The high concentration of hydrogen carbonate ions in the cell results in large quantities diffusing from the cell into the plasma. This diffusion results in a loss of negative ions by the red blood cells. To maintain the negative charge, chloride ions move from the plasma into the cytoplasm in a process known as the chloride shift.

The hydrogen ions or acid formed as a result of carbonic acid dissociation are buffered by haemoglobin (16.5). Some hydrogen ions, however, remain in their free state, thus conferring greater acidity. For this reason the pH of venous blood (7.36) is lower than arterial blood pH (7.40).

Release of carbon dioxide

When blood arrives at the lungs, a difference in concentration exists between the venous carbon dioxide concentration and the alveolar carbon dioxide concentration. The alveoli have a PCO_2 of 5.3 kPa (40 mm Hg) compared with the returning blood carbon dioxide of 6.0 kPa (45 mm Hg). This difference results in carbon dioxide diffusing from the blood into the lungs. As carbon dioxide is removed from the plasma, an imbalance develops between the proportion of carbon dioxide, carbonic acid and hydrogen carbonate ions. The lowered carbon dioxide levels result in a proportionate change of hydrogen carbonate and hydrogen ions to carbonic acid resulting in decreased hydrogen carbonate ions, and a proportionate conversion of carbonic acid to carbon dioxide and water.

The continued removal of carbon dioxide by diffusion thus results in a sustained conversion of hydrogen carbonate ion to carbonic acid and thence carbon dioxide, that is, a reversal of Eqn 26.2.

The carbon dioxide combined with haemoglobin is removed as a result of the higher affinity of haemoglobin for oxygen and the relatively larger concentration of oxygen.

26.5   Use of blood gases

The determination of blood PO_2 and PCO_2 can be a useful aid in detecting abnormal respiratory function, blood function and metabolic function. Blood gas studies are also useful as an assessment of the therapy.

Blood gases are usually obtained from arterial blood. It is essential that the sample of blood is free of air bubbles since this results in false readings.

Hypoxia

Hypoxia is a diminished amount of oxygen in the tissues. The general cause of this is **hypoxaemia**, that is, an insufficient concentration of oxygen in the blood. The effect of hypoxaemia ranges from decreased mental, emotional and muscular stability at 6.65 kPa (50 mm Hg) to unconsciousness at 4.3 kPa (32 mm Hg) and circulatory failure at 3.7 kPa (28 mm Hg). Hypoxaemia can occur with either a normal PCO_2 or an elevated PCO_2.

Some of the common causes of hypoxia are:

1. Decreased alveolar PO_2 due to either inhalation of low oxygen gases or inadequate respiratory function. EXAMPLES: Impaired lung movement and chronic obstructive airways disease (COAD).

2. Altered diffusion rates between the alveoli and pulmonary capillaries. EXAMPLES: Emphysema, pulmonary oedema, pneumonia and pulmonary fibrosis.
3. Decreased transport capacity of blood EXAMPLES: Anaemia, inadequate circulation.
4. Abnormal tissue metabolism. EXAMPLES: Severe oedema, and toxicity due to substances such as cyanide.

Arterial PCO_2 levels

The normal arterial PCO_2 ranges from 4.8 to 5.8 kPa (36 to 44 mm Hg). Alterations in the PCO_2 can assist in the identification of the cause of hypoxia. An elevated PCO_2 suggests that either the lungs have difficulty in eliminating carbon dioxide or that abnormal metabolism results in the excessive production of carbon dioxide.

PCO_2 can be normal even when the ability of oxygen to diffuse from the alveoli to the pulmonary capillaries has been altered. This is because carbon dioxide has a better ability to diffuse from the blood to the alveoli than oxygen has to diffuse from the alveoli to the pulmonary capillaries.

Measurements of arterial PCO_2 can also be used in conjunction with acid–base measurements to determine acid–base status. A description of the various forms of acid–base imbalance is given in 16.6.

Compensated metabolic acidosis has low PCO_2 levels, whereas uncompensated metabolic acidosis has normal PCO_2. In compensated and uncompensated respiratory acidosis an elevated PCO_2 occurs. Both uncompensated and compensated respiratory alkalosis cause a decreased PCO_2, whereas metabolic alkalosis usually has a normal PCO_2.

Summary

Blood consists of a fluid called plasma which contains a variety of suspended particles referred to as formed elements. Plasma consists of:

1. colloids in the form of proteins and lipoproteins;
2. an aqueous solution of electrolytes and non-electrolytes.

The three major plasma protein groups are albumin, globulin and fibrinogen. They influence blood osmotic pressure and are important blood buffers. These proteins also act as a mobile storage medium for amino acids. Globulin proteins play important roles in body defence mechanisms (immunoglobulins) and in the transportation of substances in plasma. Fibrinogen is an essential component of the blood-clotting mechanism.

Non-protein nitrogens refer to substances in the plasma that contain nitrogen but are not proteins such as urea, creatinine and uric acid.

Electrolytes play important roles in body homeostasis. EXAMPLE: Sodium in fluid and electrolyte balance. Abnormal concentrations of electrolytes can greatly influence the health of a patient. EXAMPLE: Low levels of potassium cause cardiac arrhythmias which may progress to a cardiac arrest.

The main non-electrolyte present in blood is glucose which is vital for brain function.

Most lipids are transported in the blood as either lipid–protein complexes (lipoproteins) or as droplets known as chylomicrons.

Suspended particles in blood are referred to as formed elements. These formed elements are:

1. Erythrocytes or red blood cells are small haemoglobin-containing cells that constitute the greater proportion of formed elements. The haemoglobin carries 97% of oxygen transported in the blood, and thus a lack of haemoglobin or anaemia results in a lack of oxygen being supplied to tissues.
2. Leucocytes or white blood cells occur in a variety of forms and perform functions associated with the body defence system. Leucocytes that contain granules in their cytoplasm are called granular leucocytes. They exist as either neutrophils, eosinophils or basophils. Non-granular leucocytes exist as either lymphocytes or monocytes. Leucocytes either phagocytose unwanted material or they produce substances that are involved in body defence mechanisms. Leukaemia is the uncontrolled production of white blood cells.
3. Platelets or thrombocytes are tiny cells that lack a nucleus. They form an important part of the clotting mechanism.

The transport of oxygen in the blood is dependent upon the ability of haemoglobin to pick it up in the pulmonary capillaries and release it according to tissue demand in the tissue capillaries. Haemoglobin requires a lower PO_2 than the alveoli to pick-up oxygen and a greater PO_2 than the tissues to release oxygen. Any factor that alters the difference in PO_2 can alter the amount of oxygen transported in the blood.

Carbon dioxide is transported in the blood dissolved in plasma (7%), or combined with haemoglobin (23%), or converted into the hydrogen carbonate ion (70%).

The greater the concentration of carbon dioxide in the blood, the greater is the quantity of carbonic acid, hydrogen carbonate ion and hydrogen ion. Release of carbon dioxide to a lower PCO_2 in the alveoli results in lowered carbonic acid, hydrogen carbonate ion and hydrogen ion.

The determination of blood PO_2 and PCO_2 can indicate respiratory and cardiovascular function. Hypoxia or decreased amounts of oxygen in the tissues can result from inadequate respiratory function, restricted diffusion between alveoli and pulmonary capillaries, inadequate transport capacity in blood or abnormal tissue metabolism. Elevated PCO_2 suggests that lungs have difficulty in removing carbon dioxide or that abnormal metabolism results in excessive carbon dioxide production. Altered blood PCO_2 also influences the acid–base balance of blood.

Unit Ten
Human Nutrition I: Nutritional Principles and Biomolecule Groups

In this unit, the general principles of nutrition and the properties of the major biochemical groups are related to health care and body function.

Chapter 27

General concepts of nutrition

Objectives

At the completion of this chapter the student should be able to:

1. relate nutrition to health;
2. define the terms nutrition, digestion, absorption, metabolism, anabolism, catabolism, and diet;
3. describe the food groups and relate the effects of food storage, food preservation and food preparation to the nutritional value of these food groups;
4. describe the specific methods used to supply patients with nutrients.

27.1 Introduction to nutrition

Nutrition encompasses the relationship between the provision, assimilation and utilization of substances and the maintenance of health. These substances or nutrients include carbohydrates, lipids, proteins, vitamins, minerals and water. They contribute to health by supplying the necessary proportions of raw materials required for maintaining the structure and function of the body. Most molecules in food are used for growth, to provide energy (Table 27.1), maintain and repair the body's structure and maintain the body's homeostatic mechanisms.

A person's daily intake of food and drink is referred to as a **diet**. The nutritional requirements of individuals vary according to factors such as age, sex, size and current health status. To meet these requirements a person eats a selection of foods, as no single food contains the necessary levels of raw materials to meet all the needs of the body. A balanced diet is therefore necessary to give the required daily allowance of nutrients.

A diet can be planned, usually by a dietician, to meet the specific requirements of an individual. The use of a diet to manage and treat a specific medical condition is called diet therapy. EXAMPLE: A high protein diet is used for individuals with a large amount of tissue damage. Diet therapy can be used to overcome the condition called malnutrition where the body fails to receive all of the essential nutrients.

Assimilation and utilization of nutrients depend upon their absorption across the wall of the intestine. The selective permeability of plasma membranes limits the number of substances that can be absorbed in this way (23.2 and 23.3). Generally only small molecules can pass freely across the intestinal wall, although a limited quantity of large molecules can be absorbed by pinocytosis. As foods are generally composed of combina-

Table 27.1 Energy per gram of nutrient (values represent averages because chemical composition of nutrients varies)

Nutrient	kJ/g	Calories/g
Protein	17	4.1
Fat	37	8.8
Carbohydrate (expressed as monosaccharide)	16	3.8
Alcohol	29	6.9

Table 27.2 The food groups

Food group	Examples of foods
Milk	Milk, buttermilk, cream, cheeses
Meat and meat substitutes	Beef, fish, poultry, eggs, beans, peas, lentils and nuts
Vegetables/fruit	Carrots, potatoes, spinach, pumpkin, oranges, apples, pears, bananas and apricots
Bread/cereals	Breads, rice, macaroni, spaghetti, breakfast cereals and cakes
Butter/margarine (fifth group)	Butter, margarine

tions of large molecules, the body needs to process most foods so that they are able to be absorbed across the intestinal wall. The breakdown of food into an acceptable form for absorption is called **digestion**. The importance of effective digestion and absorption to health is shown in Malabsorption syndrome. Individuals with this syndrome suffer disturbances in the normal mechanism of either digestion or absorption, and although they eat the correct quantities of food for a well balanced diet can yet suffer from deficiencies of certain nutrients.

After absorption into the lymph or blood, the nutrients are transported to various tissues to be processed into other molecules, stored or immediately utilized. The first organ to receive recently absorbed food is the liver, the main biochemical processing organ for the body. The liver is involved in metabolism, that is, the manufacture and breakdown of many of the body's biochemicals, and it influences the biochemical processes of other tissues by acting as a storage and distribution centre.

Metabolism is the mechanism which produces homeostasis of body chemical processes. Normal body metabolism involves a balance between the manufacture or synthesis of chemicals and their breakdown. The synthesis of any biochemical is referred to as **anabolism**; their breakdown into simpler structures is called **catabolism**. The balance between anabolism and catabolism varies according to the demands of individual tissues.

Body homeostasis is dependent upon metabolism since the rate of chemical synthesis and breakdown controls body function. Normal metabolism requires an adequate supply of nutrients and the biochemical regulators known as enzymes and hormones.

27.2 Composition of foods

Food groups

Food is usually subdivided into four or five groups. A summary of the main foods in each group is listed in Table 27.2.

Factors affecting food composition

The nutritive values of food can be altered by factors such as storage conditions, processing and the way in which a meal is prepared (Table 27.3). It is important for individuals to be aware of the potential nutritive difference between natural, unpreserved foods and the food which is served following food preparation.

Food storage

The loss of nutritive value during storage is attributed to factors such as temperature, humidity, length of time and exposure to light. As a general principle, food should be eaten as soon after purchase as possible in order to minimize a loss of nutritive value. Many vegetables and fruit need to be stored in a humid atmosphere. The best substitute for this is a refrigerator. Light can change the nutritive value of some foods and it can also increase chemical changes resulting in the accumulation of harmful substances. EXAMPLE: Potatoes must be stored in the dark.

Food preservation

The spoilage and deterioration of food is caused by microorganisms, enzymes and oxidation (see 6.6). Most food is preserved by one of the following methods.

1. The presence of an unfavourable environment for the growth and multiplication of bacteria. EXAMPLES: Salting, drying, smoking and freeze drying all remove water. Fermentation produces acidic conditions that are inhospitable to most microorganisms. Freezing and refrigeration employ cold temperatures to slow down or stop bacterial reproduction.
2. Destruction of microorganisms. EXAMPLES: The use of high temperatures in canning and the use of ionizing radiation (11.8) in sealed containers.
3. The inactivation of enzymes by methods such as freezing and high temperatures.
4. Prevention of oxidation. EXAMPLE: The addition of antioxidants prevents oxygen

from reacting with fats and oils and thus prevents food from turning rancid.

Food preparation

The loss of nutrient value can be minimized by proper food preparation. Nutrients can be lost in cooking if excessive amounts of water and prolonged high temperatures are used. EXAMPLE: Vitamins such as thiamine, which are water-soluble and susceptible to high temperatures, (34.1) are destroyed in cooking. Food should be cooked in only small quantities of liquids or in their own juices to minimize the loss of water-soluble nutrients when the liquid is discarded. EXAMPLE: Only 50% of ascorbic acid is retained when cabbage is cooked in large quantities of water, whereas up to 90% is retained when small quantities of water are used. Other methods of reducing losses of soluble nutrients are: minimizing surface area by using pieces as large as possible; cooking foods with skins on wherever possible; and avoiding long periods of soaking in water which is to be discarded. EXAMPLE: Cooking potatoes in their skin results in only a small loss of ascorbic acid whereas cooking potatoes in water means a loss of about 40% of the vitamin. Care should be taken to prevent overcooking. Correct planning is important when preparing a meal so that foods do not cool and have to be reheated. Vegetables should be served immediately after cooking.

27.3 Nutrition and health

Daily dietary allowances

It is important for both health team workers and patients to understand the close relationship between nutrition and health. A well-

Table 27.3 Effect of food preservation and food preparation on energy content and nutrient content of selected foods

Food (100 g quantity)	Edible portion of purchased mass (% or g)	Energy (kJ) (C)	Water (g)	Protein (g)	Fat (g)	Carbohydrate (g)	Calcium (mg)	Iron (mg)	Sodium (mg)	Thiamine (mg)	Ascorbic acid (mg)
Chicken											
boiled	—	829 (198)	63.6	26.3	8.4	0	14	1.9	98	52	0
fried	—	1059 (253)	53.9	28.6	13.1	2.9	15	2.1	94	69	0
roasted	—	833 (199)	60.4	29.1	9.4	0	16	2.1	79	78	0
Eggs											
raw whole	88	670 (160)	73.8	12.5	11.6	0.7	54	2.4	122	102	0
boiled	88	670 (160)	73.8	12.5	11.6	0.7	54	2.4	122	87	0
fried	—	942 (224)	67.2	11.7	19.4	0.6	52	2.2	200	83	0
omelette	—	1038 (248)	64.8	11.4	22.6	0.8	52	2.2	1036	86	0
poached	88	670 (160)	73.8	12.5	11.6	0.7	54	2.4	722	89	0
scrambled	—	883 (211)	70.0	9.4	17.7	2.6	90	1.6	763	79	0
Honey	100	1348 (322)	19.3	0.5	—	80.0	6	0.8	10	31	1
Wholemeal bread	100	963 (230)	40.0	8.1	2.4	46.7	35	3.0	529	274	—
Table margarine	100	3044 (727)	15.5	0.4	81.2	0.6	20	0	1250	—	0
Peas											
green, raw	43	335 (80)	78.0	6.3	0.4	15.5	24	1.9	2	321	26
boiled	43	293 (70)	81.0	5.4	0.4	13.5	20	1.8	1	250	20
canned (minus liquid)	100	339 (81)	77.0	3.8	0.3	16.8	23	1.8	236	112	9
dried, raw	100	1403 (335)	9.5	22.8	1.3	60.2	63	4.9	37	670	Trace
dried, boiled	100	431 (103)	71.6	7.4	0.3	19.6	20	1.6	12	166	0
frozen, raw	100	310 (74)	80.7	5.4	0.3	12.8	20	1.9	129	320	19
frozen, boiled	100	293 (70)	81.9	5.2	0.3	11.9	19	1.9	120	286	14
Potato											
baked	—	762 (182)	64.8	2.3	10.1	21.9	11	0.8	7	95	13
boiled	—	335 (80)	77.8	2.0	0.1	19.1	9	0.7	6	103	11
fried	—	1122 (268)	47.4	3.8	14.2	32.6	15	1.1	223	100	11
mashed (milk added)	—	268 (64)	82.6	2.0	0.7	13.2	24	0.4	300	85	8
dehydrated	100	1499 (358)	6.1	7.5	0.6	82.8	28	3.2	89	276	31
frozen, raw	100	327 (78)	78.0	1.8	0.1	19.0	10	0.7	6	80	9
frozen, fried	100	1005 (240)	52.8	3.0	12.2	30.0	18	1.2	299	75	8
Tuna											
canned in water	100	699 (167)	70.0	28.0	5.8	—	10	1.6	875	50	—
canned in oil	100	1206 (288)	52.6	25.6	19.5	—	7	1.2	800	45	—

Based on *Metric Tables of Composition of Australian Foods* by the Commonwealth Department of Health, Australia (1982).

balanced diet is essential for maintaining health. The World Health Organization and the Food and Agriculture Organization of the United Nations have adopted recommendations for the daily allowance for many nutrients. These allowances should provide a level of nutrition that maintains good health for substantially all the world's population. Allowances differ from country to country because of differences in climate and occupation. The allowances may not meet the specific needs of those persons who have had various nutrients depleted through illness or who require additional nutrients for the repair of tissues (Table 27.4).

Physical health

Some general signs of good nutrition are average weight for body size, good muscles, smooth and clear skin, glossy hair, clear and bright eyes, good posture, alert facial expression, good appetite, good digestion and good elimination.

Improper dietary intake can initiate diseases or predispose a person to them, e.g. heart disease, atherosclerosis, diabetes mellitus, and hypertension. EXAMPLES: The prolonged excessive intake of kilojoules (29.1 — Application: Obesity) and the excessive intake of sodium (34.2 — Application: Salt intake). The ability of the body to overcome or minimize the effects of improper diet is determined by genetic factors and the individual's relative state of health.

Personal needs

Humans often eat to satisfy personal or social needs. Emotional disturbances can lead to the eating of excessive amounts of food which, if the emotional upset is prolonged, will lead to obesity. Some individuals suffer from a condition called anorexia nervosa, which is believed to involve psychological factors and which is characterized by the persistent desire to lose weight. The condition can be fatal unless normal eating habits are restored.

Another psychologically related nutritional disorder is alcoholism in which the individual is unable to control the urge to drink alcohol. The long-term effect of alcoholism is liver damage and the diminished ability of the liver to act as a metabolic organ. Other effects are malnutrition due to a combination of inadequate diet and the interference of nutrient absorption by alcohol. Alcohol also damages brain tissue and may cause foetal abnormalities.

Physical and psychosocial needs determine nutritional requirements, which vary between age groups and sexes. EXAMPLE: The requirements for minerals are increased during infancy, childhood and pregnancy.

Needs of hospitalized patients

Specific attention to nutritional intake is required for hospitalized patients. Failure to provide adequate nutrition may prolong convalescence, predispose to infection, and interfere with wound healing. In the management of patients it is important to maintain normal body function during reduced nutrient intake, increased metabolic needs or altered metabolic mechanisms. EXAMPLES: An accelerated rate of protein catabolism occurs with burns, injuries and infection; the normal intake of nutrients can be altered by disturbances of the gastro-intestinal tract and in the post-operative state.

When a patient is unable to take food orally one of the following feeding methods is used.

1. *Gastric gavage or tube feeding*. A nasogastric tube can be used to pass a specially prepared solution of essential nutrients

Table 27.4 Recommended dietary allowances (RDA) of certain food constituents for selected age groups in Australia and USA

Age (years)	Protein (g)	Vitamin B$_{12}$ (μg)	Ascorbic acid (mg)	Riboflavin (mg)	Thiamine (mg)	Calcium (mg)	Iron (mg)
Infants							
0.5–1.0	2.5 ± 0.5 per kg	0.3	30	0.5	0.4	500–700	4–8
	(2.0 per kg)	(1.5)	(35)	(0.6)	(0.5)	(540)	(15)
Children							
1–3	20–39	0.9	30	0.7	0.5	400–800	5
	(23)	(2.0)	(45)	(0.8)	(0.7)	(800)	(15)
Boys							
7–10	37–66	1.5	30	1.1	0.9	600–1100	10
	(34)	(3.0)	(45)	(1.4)	(1.2)	(800)	(10)
Girls							
7–10	36–63	1.5	30	1.1	0.8	600–1100	10
	(34)	(3.0)	(45)	(1.4)	(1.2)	(800)	(10)
Males							
15–18	67–90	2.0	50	1.5	1.2	500–1400	12
	(56)	(3.0)	(60)	(1.7)	(1.4)	(1200)	(18)
18–35	70	2.0	30	1.4	1.1	400–800	10
	(56)	(3.0)	(60)	(1.7)	(1.5)	(800)	(10)
35–55	70	2.0	30	1.2	1.0	400–800	10
	(56)	(3.0)	(60)	(1.6)	(1.4)	(800)	(10)
55–75	70	2.0	30	1.0	0.8	400–800	10
	(56)	(3.0)	(60)	(1.4)	(1.2)	(800)	(10)
Females							
15–18	60–66	2.0	50	1.1	0.9	500–1300	12
	(46)	(3.0)	(60)	(1.3)	(1.1)	(1200)	(18)
18–35	58	2.0	30	1.0	0.8	400–800	12
	(44)	(3.0)	(60)	(1.3)	(1.1)	(800)	(18)
35–55	58	2.0	30	0.9	0.7	400–800	12
	(44)	(3.0)	(60)	(1.2)	(1.0)	(800)	(18)
55–75	58	2.0	30	0.8	0.6	400–800	12
	(44)	(3.0)	(60)	(1.2)	(1.0)	(800)	(10)
Pregnant	66	3.0	60	1.1	0.9	900–1300	15
	(74)	(4.0)	(80)	(1.5)	(1.4)	(1200)	(40–70)

Figures in brackets are US values.
Values from *Dietary Allowances for Use in Australia* by the Commonwealth Department of Health 1982, and *Recommended Dietary Allowances (USA)* 1980, National Academy of Sciences, Washington.

directly into the stomach. This temporary form of feeding is used for patients who have difficulty chewing or swallowing food. The patient is elevated sufficiently to allow gravity to move the fluid slowly to the stomach. The food must be liquefied and is prescribed according to the individual needs and tolerance of the patient.

2. *Gastrostomy*. This is the surgical insertion of a tube into the stomach through the abdominal wall and is necessary for patients with an oesophageal obstruction. Patients can be fed temporarily through the tube during a period of corrective surgery or this can be the permanent method when an inoperable oesophageal obstruction occurs or when an oesophagotomy has been performed. The patients require special care as they are denied the pleasures of taste and the sociability of eating. The opening or **stoma** and the channel through the layers of tissue are well established after one to two weeks. Long-term feeding by gastrostomy requires that the patients learn how to feed themselves, or that a member of the family or another acceptable person is instructed in the preparation of the food and the care of the stoma. Liquefied food is used as in **gastric gavage or** else normal foods, put **through a blender.**

3. *Parenteral nutrition*. Parenteral refers to the introduction of substances into the body by a route other than the gastrointestinal tract. Parenteral nutrition involves the delivery of nutrients directly into the bloodstream via a catheter into a large vein. It is used for patients who are: unable or unwilling to take food orally or by gastric gavage; unconscious for an extended period; lacking sufficient absorptive area in the intestine or who are in a state of high catabolic activity such as burns. Short-term intravenous feeding, carried out for a period of several days to a week, supplies sufficient glucose to meet the needs of the nervous system (28.4) and the maintenance of fluid and electrolyte balance (18.1).

Long-term intravenous nutrition is referred to as total parenteral nutrition or parenteral hyperalimentation. The solutions of food are individually prescribed and contain preparations of a commercial protein hydrolysate or synthetic amino acid mixture which is combined with a concentrated dextrose solution. The need to supply large quantities of nutrients in a small volume results in the use of hypertonic solutions (21.2). This in turn means the preparation must be fed into a large vein as hypertonic solutions are likely to cause thrombosis in smaller peripheral veins.

Summary

Nutrition encompasses the relationship between the provision, assimilation and utilization of nutrients and the maintenance of health. The six main categories of nutrients are carbohydrates, lipids, proteins, vitamins, minerals and water. Nutritional requirements vary between individuals but a minimum daily allowance for each nutrient is recommended by authorities for maintaining good health. These minimum allowances differ in different countries due to climate and occupation. A balanced diet is required, as no single food contains the necessary levels of raw materials. A variety of factors such as a change in health status may necessitate the use of specific diets requiring particular proportions and quantities of nutrients. Improper dietary intake can predispose a person to or initiate diseases.

Food is usually subdivided into either four or five groups. The four food groups are: milk; meat, eggs and fish; vegetables; fruit and bread–cereals. The five group subdivision includes an additional category, butter–margarine. The nutritive value of each food can be decreased by storage conditions, processing and method of meal preparation, which can substantially alter the actual quantities of nutrients ingested by a person.

Following ingestion of food, the nutrients

are digested and absorbed; then assimilated and utilized by the body in the processes of anabolism and catabolism. Metabolism is a general term covering the processes of anabolism and catabolism. Body homeostasis is dependent upon metabolism since the rate of chemical synthesis and breakdown controls body function.

Hospitalized patients require special diets, as inadequate nutrition may prolong convalescence, predispose to infection and interfere with wound healing. When food is unable to be taken orally the individual can be supplied with the required nutrients by one of the following means: gastric gavage or tube feeding, gastrostomy, parenteral nutrition and total parenteral nutrition.

Chapter 28

Carbohydrates

Objectives

At the completion of this chapter the student should be able to:

1. explain the relationship between photosynthesis and the utilization of energy;
2. describe the general structure of carbohydrates;
3. describe the digestion and absorption of carbohydrates;
4. list the main sites of glucose utilization.

28.1 Biochemicals and photosynthesis

The ability of the body to assimilate nutrients and utilize them is an essential component of nutrition. The main substances involved are carbohydrates, proteins, lipids, vitamins, minerals and water. It is important for health team members to understand the general features and differences of these substances, their role in body function, their involvement in major metabolic pathways and their participation in the production of energy. The carbohydrates, lipids and proteins are organic compounds. The removal of hydrogen atoms from these biochemicals can release chemical energy. Before this energy can be utilized it has to be transferred to specific biochemicals called nucleotides. EXAMPLE: ATP or adenosine triphosphate. The nucleotides have the capacity to release energy in a form acceptable for general body function (31.3). The energy stored in the hydrogen bonds of carbohydrates, some lipids and proteins has originated from photosynthesis (Figure 11.1). The eating of plants or animals transfers the energy, originally from the sun, to the human body via a food chain (Figure 28.1).

The recycling of carbon via the **carbon cycle** reflects the transfer of energy through the living world. **Photosynthesis** occurs in two general stages. In the first stage (**light reaction**) oxygen, energy and hydrogen ions are released in a light-dependent reaction occurring in photosynthetic pigments such as chlorophyll (Eqn 28.1). The second stage, called the dark reaction or **Calvin cycle**, involves the incorporation of the released energy and hydrogen ions into molecules of carbon dioxide. The reaction results in the formation of glucose (Eqn 28.2). The overall balanced equation for plant photosynthesis is shown in Equation 28.3. The glucose can subsequently be converted into proteins and lipids by plants or animals.

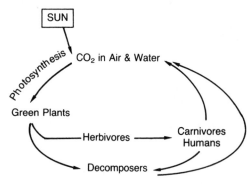

Figure 28.1   General cycle for carbon. Herbivores eat plants to obtain energy from C — H bonds whereas carnivores obtain energy from the C — H bonds of animal biochemicals.

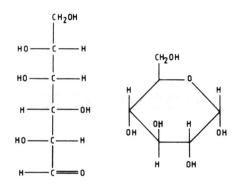

Figure 28.2   The structure of glucose can be represented as either a straight-chain molecule or as a cyclic molecule.

$$\text{Water} + \text{ADP} + \text{Phosphate} \xrightarrow[\text{chlorophyll}]{\text{light}}$$

$$\text{Hydrogen ions} + \text{electrons} + \text{oxygen} + \text{ATP}$$

$$\text{Eqn 28.1}$$

$$\text{Carbon dioxide} + \text{hydrogen ions} + \text{electrons} + \text{ATP} \rightarrow \text{glucose} + \text{ADP} + \text{phosphate}$$

$$\text{Eqn 28.2}$$

$$6CO_2 + 6H_2O \rightarrow C_6H_{12}O_6 + 6O_2 \quad \text{Eqn 28.3}$$

28.2   Carbohydrate structure and function

Structure

Carbohydrates contain carbon, hydrogen and oxygen. The basic structural unit of a carbohydrate is the sugar molecule. Most sugar molecules important to humans contain six carbon atoms and are commonly referred to as **hexoses**. There are sixteen different hexose isomers with the molecular formula $C_6H_{12}O_6$ (7.4 and Figure 5.10). Body function relies almost entirely on the glucose isomer of $C_6H_{12}O_6$ (Figure 28.2).

A large variety of carbohydrates occur in nature. A classification system has been devised to identify individual carbohydrates. Firstly, only carbohydrates contain the suffix **-ose**.

The following method is used to determine the quantity of sugar units in a particular carbohydrate: **mono** — one sugar unit, **di** — two sugar units, **poly** — many sugar units.

The suffix **saccharide**, which simply means sugar base, is added to the above prefixes: monosaccharide, EXAMPLES: Glucose, galactose; disaccharide, EXAMPLES: Maltose, lactose; polysaccharide, EXAMPLES: Starch, glycogen.

Function

The principal function of carbohydrates is to supply energy in the form of glucose to tissues such as nerve tissue. A temporary

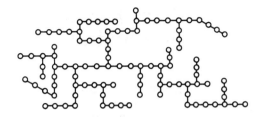

Figure 28.3 The structure of glycogen showing the chains and branches of glucose molecules.

store of body carbohydrate exists in the form of the polysaccharide, glycogen (Figure 28.3). **Glycogen** is composed of large chains of glucose molecules. When blood glucose decreases, sufficient glucose is released from the glycogen to return the blood levels to normal.

28.3 Digestion and absorption of carbohydrate

Carbohydrate digestion and absorption involves the breakdown of polysaccharides to monosaccharides, since only monosaccharides are able to pass through the plasma membrane at the site of absorption.

Digestion

Mouth and oesophagus

Saliva contains an enzyme (salivary amylase) that acts on polysaccharides to produce small quantities of the disaccharide maltose. The enzyme simply acts by slicing two glucose units at a time off the polysaccharide chain. The action of the enzyme continues in each bolus (ball) of food as it passes down the oesophagus.

Stomach

The highly acidic gastric contents (pH 1.2 to 3.0) inactivate the enzyme. The stomach acts as a temporary reservoir for the carbohydrates and controls their rate of entry into the small intestine. This action of the stomach assists in maximum digestion of carbohydrate in the small intestine.

Small intestine

The small intestine is the site of most carbohydrate digestion. The pancreas secretes an enzyme (pancreatic amylase) into the first part of the small intestine or duodenum via the pancreatic duct. This enzyme has a similar action to the salivary enzyme, that is, it forms maltose from polysaccharides.

The small intestine is permeable to monosaccharides and impermeable to disaccharides. This membrane property thus necessitates the breakdown of maltose to monosaccharides for the absorption of carbohydrates into the body.

Two other disaccharides occur in the small intestine: sucrose which is common table sugar, and lactose which is derived from milk. Both these disaccharides are digested only in the small intestine.

The final step in carbohydrate digestion involves the breakdown of maltose, sucrose and lactose to their constituent monosaccharides. The specific enzymes involved in their digestion are released from the surface of the intestinal cells (maltase for maltose, sucrase for sucrose and lactase for lactose).

Absorption

Absorption of monosaccharides across the small intestine is enhanced by its folded structure. The villi and microvilli markedly increase the surface area of available intestinal membrane (20.2). The enzymes responsible for breaking down disaccharides are located in the microvilli. The primary monosaccharides absorbed across the membrane are glucose, fructose and galactose. These are derived from maltose — two glucose molecules, sucrose — one glucose and one fructose, lactose — one glucose and one galactose.

There appear to be two processes by which monosaccharides are absorbed across the intestinal wall: facilitated diffusion which requires a concentration gradient, and active transport (23.5) which is independent of concentration gradients but requires energy.

Both these transport mechanisms involve the use of carriers since monosaccharides are too large for diffusion through membrane pores and they are relatively insoluble in the lipid component of the plasma membrane (23.2 and 23.3). All carriers have a specific preference for a particular substance, other similarly structured substances being transported at slower rates. The carriers involved in the transport of monosaccharides appear to be glucose carriers since glucose is transported at a faster rate than galactose or fructose.

Application: Lactose intolerance

A deficiency in the enzyme lactase results in an inability to digest and absorb milk. The undigested lactose causes:

1. an osmotic imbalance between the intestinal contents and the body which results in additional water entering the intestinal contents;
2. bacteria break down the lactose to lactic acid which causes an increase in intestinal mobility.

Both these factors cause pain and diarrhoea. Elimination of milk from the diet usually overcomes the pain and diarrhoea.

28.4 Sites of absorbed carbohydrate

Following ingestion of a carbohydrate, the glucose concentration in blood rises for about thirty minutes, but after three hours has usually returned to the original pre-meal level. Monosaccharides absorbed into the body are mainly used for energy supply. The intermittent dietary supply of sugar necessitates a reserve of body sugar. Without this reserve, an insufficient supply of glucose would occur between meals. The carbohydrate reservoir in humans is in the form of glycogen which is stored in the liver and skeletal muscle. Once this reservoir is full, any excess sugar absorbed into the body is converted into fat. The carbohydrate is thus indirectly stored in another form of energy.

When entering the body, monosaccharides are either utilized by tissue immediately or stored as glycogen or fat. The liver, brain, blood cells, skeletal muscle and adipose tissues are the most important utilizers of glucose. The uptake and use of glucose is controlled by hormones (4.2).

Liver

When glucose, fructose and galactose enter the blood stream after absorption, they are transported via the portal vein to the liver. The liver is the major metabolic organ and its blood supply is closely linked to that of the small intestine.

The liver is a major site of monosaccharide uptake. Most of the monosaccharides that have been taken up by the liver are converted into glycogen. Since glycogen is composed of chains of glucose molecules, fructose and galactose must be converted into glucose before being stored as glycogen.

Brain

The brain requires a continual supply of glucose. It uses about 120 g of glucose per day which is approximately 25% of the energy requirement of a normal resting adult. An interruption to the supply of glucose will result in brain damage. Following a meal, a proportion of the glucose will be immediately utilized by the brain. During periods between meals, the brain receives glucose by the breakdown of glycogen and the subsequent release of glucose into the blood. The brain relies upon liver glycogen since no glycogen is formed in the brain.

Application: Glycogen storage disease

The reliance of the brain on liver glycogen is shown in glycogen storage disease. Children with glycogen storage disease are able to form glycogen but are unable to reconvert glycogen into glucose. Without constant feeding, brain damage will occur as a result of decreased blood glucose levels (hypoglycaemia) during intervals between meals.

Blood cells

Blood cells have a small but constant demand for glucose. The total demand on the body is approximately a quarter that of the brain.

Skeletal muscle

Skeletal muscle can either use glucose immediately for energy or it can store it as muscle glycogen. The amount of glucose used by skeletal muscles varies according to the work they perform. At rest or with mild exertion this muscle only utilizes about a quarter of the quantity used by the brain. During times of vigorous exercise the demand for glucose is elevated. The increased glucose is supplied by the increased blood supply to the muscle, and the conversion of glycogen to glucose increases. Muscle glycogen represents the major reserve of body carbohydrate.

Adipose tissue

Adipose tissue converts excess sugar into fat. There is only an excess of sugar when both the immediate tissue demands are satisfied and the glycogen reserves are restored to their normal levels.

Kidneys

The kidneys actively reabsorb glucose from the kidney filtrate back into the blood. When the blood sugar level exceeds this capacity, glucose appears in the urine and its presence is referred to as **glycosuria**.

The digestion and absorption of large quantities of carbohydrate can result in blood sugar concentrations that exceed the ability of adipose tissue to convert into fat. The inability of adipose tissue to utilize all the excess glucose results in greater concentrations of sugar being filtered by the kidneys. If the blood sugar level exceeds 10 mmol/L, the threshold or T_m is exceeded and glycosuria results (23.5). This form of glycosuria is referred to as temporary or alimentary glycosuria. It is not considered to be pathological in the short term.

In diabetes mellitus the ability of tissues to remove sugar from the blood is decreased. This can result in blood sugar levels far in excess of what would be expected for a particular carbohydrate intake. The elevated blood sugar level will often exceed the T_m

following meals, and thus glycosuria occurs more frequently. The measurement of glyco-suria and a knowledge of the carbohydrate intake can be used to diagnose diabetes mellitus.

Application: Testing for glycosuria

Simple, quick methods of testing urine for sugar exist. Tablets, powder and strips of paper can all have a specific colour changing reagent impregnated into them. EXAMPLES: Clinitest tablets and clinistix paper strips. The presence of glucose causes the reagent to change colour. The intensity of colour is indica-tive of the amount of glucose present. A semi-qualitative measurement can be performed by comparing the colour intensity with that in the chart ac-companying the product. If glucose is found, a blood sugar test may be ordered to confirm the observation.

Summary

The ability of the body to assimilate nutrients and utilize them is an essential part of nutri-tion. The main nutrients are carbohydrates, proteins, lipids, vitamins, minerals and water. Photosynthesis incorporates light and hydrogen into molecules of carbon dioxide. The resulting nutrients release energy for body use following the removal of hydrogen.

Carbohydrates are compounds that contain carbon, hydrogen and oxygen arranged into structural units known as sugars.

The principal function of carbohydrates is the supply of stored energy in the form of glucose to cells. Glucose can be stored in the liver and muscles in the form of the polysaccharide glycogen.

Carbohydrates are partially digested in the mouth due to a salivary enzyme, and completely digested in the small intestine by the action of pancreatic and intestinal enzymes. The primary monosaccharides absorbed across the small intestine are glucose, fructose and galactose. They are absorbed by facilitated diffusion and active transport.

Following absorption, monosaccharides are transported to the liver where any depleted glycogen reserves are replaced. Since glycogen consists of only glucose molecules, fructose and galactose are con-verted into glucose. When the requirements of liver and other tissues are met, the remain-ing glucose is converted into fat and stored in adipose tissue.

Carbohydrates are an important source of energy for the body, and in particular the brain. The energy released from breaking hydrogen bonds is used in a series of reac-tions to form ATP from ADP and phosphate. Energy in the form of ATP is used by cells for membrane transport, synthesis of chemical compounds and mechanical work.

Chapter 29

Lipids

Objectives

At the completion of this chapter the student should be able to:

1. list and briefly describe the features of the different forms of lipid;
2. describe the process of fat digestion and absorption;
3. list the major sites of fat utilization.

Lipids are a diverse group of organic substances which share the property of being relatively insoluble in water and readily soluble in organic solvents such as ethanol, ether and chloroform. The diverse nature of lipids in both structure and function has necessitated the classification of lipids into several groups. The important lipid groups found in the body are fats (triglycerides), phospholipids, prostaglandins, steroids and waxes. These lipid groups have a range of functions such as the storage of energy, membrane structure and chemical stimulants and inhibitors. Fats constitute the major form of dietary lipid and body lipid. This chapter will therefore place an emphasis on their metabolism.

29.1 Fats

Structure

Fats or triglycerides consist of three fatty acids bonded to a molecule of alcohol called glycerol (Figure 29.1). These substances vary in size according to the length of the hydro- carbon chains of the fatty acids. Animal fats contain saturated fatty acids whereas plant fats are polyunsaturated (7.2).

Digestion

Large quantities of triglyceride are unable to move across the wall of the gastrointestinal tract. It is therefore necessary for fat to be digested.

Digestion begins in the stomach where a small quantity of fatty acids are liberated from the glycerol. This breakdown of triglyceride is due to the action of an enzyme (gastric lipase). The greater the acidity of the gastric contents, the lower is the ability of this enzyme to release fatty acids.

The small intestine is the major site of lipid digestion. The undigested triglycerides are exposed to bile and pancreatic juice when they enter the first section of the small intestine or duodenum.

Bile is a secretion of the gall bladder which enters the duodenum via the bile duct. Bile emulsifies fat, that is, forms an emulsion by breaking down the ingested fat into droplets (17.6). This formation of the emulsion is assisted by the churning effect of peristalsis.

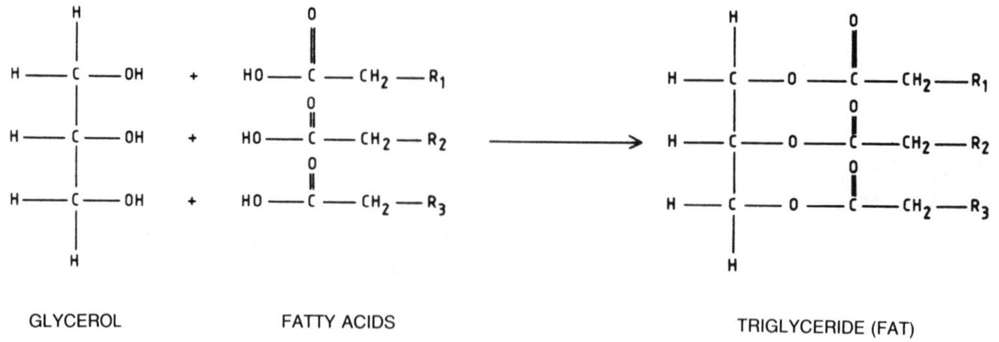

GLYCEROL   FATTY ACIDS   TRIGLYCERIDE (FAT)

Figure 29.1 The structure of fats showing glycerol and three fatty acid molecules.

Both obstruction of the bile duct and the removal of the gall bladder result in incomplete lipid digestion.

The formation of an emulsion of tiny fat droplets assists the action of a pancreatic enzyme (lipase) in breaking down triglyceride into fatty acids and glycerol. The enzyme acts on the surface of a fat droplet. The greater the number of small droplets, the greater is the surface area, and thus the available lipid, for enzymatic digestion.

Absorption

The products of fat digestion, that is, glycerol and fatty acids are absorbed across the walls of the small intestine. Fatty acids appear to be absorbed by active transport (23.5). In addition some undigested droplets are absorbed as a temporary emulsion (17.6). These large molecules are absorbed across the membrane by pinocytosis (23.5). The rate of digestion and absorption of fat is slower than that of carbohydrates and proteins. However, most ingested fat is absorbed in normal circumstances. Only a small amount of undigested fat should be present in the faeces.

Application: Steatorrhoea

The occurrence of large amounts of fat in the faeces is known as steatorrhoea. This can indicate maldigestion due to either deficient secretion of pancreatic lipase or bile salts. If digestion is normal, the steatorrhoea may be due to malabsorption of fat as a result of disease of the small intestine wall. EXAMPLE: Coeliac disease.

Sites of absorbed fat

Following absorption, most fat is transported in the plasma as droplets of fat known as **chylomicrons** or as fatty acids attached to albumin.

Muscles

Muscles usually use fat as their source of energy. During periods of vigorous activity they stop fat use and switch over to glucose utilization. Some of the absorbed fat is immediately utilized by muscle.

Liver and body tissue

The liver can immediately utilize fat to produce energy or form other substances according to the metabolic needs of the body.

Fat is found in most cells in the body. In

adipose tissue the stored fat occupies most of the cell. In other cell types fat is normally dispersed throughout the cytoplasm in combination with phospholipid and proteins.

Adipose tissue

Most absorbed fat is stored in adipose tissue in various regions of the body (25.6). Most fat is stored in fat depots in subcutaneous tissue, around the kidneys and in the abdomen. The fat depots are the major sites for the storage of energy, that is, they act as a reservoir of potential chemical energy. This depot fat does not remain stationary for long periods. It is continually being mobilized and shifted from one depot to another. During periods of either fasting or poor nutrition, sufficient quantities of mobilized fat are released and sent to the liver. In the liver the fat can be converted into other substances such as glucose. In addition, sufficient quantities of fat are sent to tissues such as muscle so as to maintain their production of energy. When excessive amounts of nutrients are taken into the body, the nutrients are stored as fat in adipose tissue.

Application: Obesity

Obesity can be defined as a condition where more kilojoules (calories) are taken in than the body requires over a period of time. The excess energy is stored as fat. As the obese person more frequently develops metabolic disease than a person who is the same age and has a normal body weight, obesity is now considered to be a disease. This disease is likely to start in middle age. Some of the diseases that an obese person has a greater chance of developing are mature onset diabetes mellitus, atherosclerosis, hypertension, heart disease and phlebitis. The enlarged de-

---

posits of fat can also impair organ function by crowding the organ, restricting circulation or placing the organ in an abnormal position.

Other functions of fat

Fat acts as an insulator and thus conserves the body's normal temperature. Adipose tissue also protects organs from mechanical injury and determines the figures of women and men. It also serves the function of an 'overflow reservoir' since excess dietary intake of carbohydrates is converted to fat for storage.

A special form of adipose tissue is used to produce energy in the form of heat in newborn babies.

29.2 Other forms of lipid

Phospholipids

Phospholipids consist of glycerol combined with two fatty acids and one phosphate group. All living cells contain a plasma membrane composed of phospholipid. The phosphate region is polar whereas the remainder of the molecule is non-polar. The non-polar nature of plasma membranes acts as a barrier for many ions and polar substances (23.2).

All tissues apart from blood and skin are capable of synthesizing their own phospholipids. The liver acts as a major source of phospholipid for the body. Unlike fats, phospholipids appear not to be involved in the storage and release of energy.

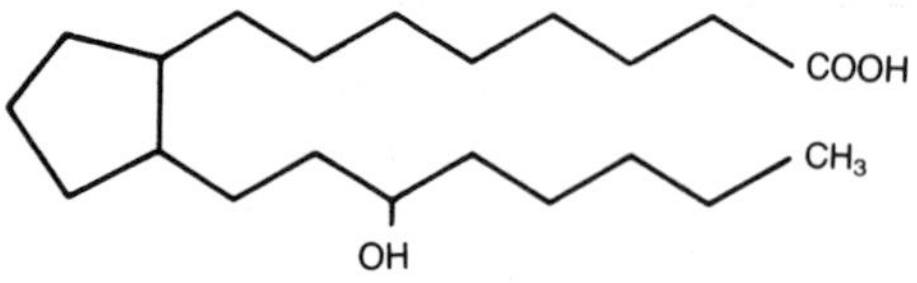

Lipids

Figure 29.2 The general structure of many prostaglandins.

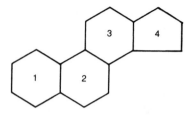

Figure 29.3 The general structure of steroids.

Prostaglandins

Prostaglandins are twenty carbon fatty acids containing a five carbon ring (Figure 29.2). They appear to be present in virtually all tissue and are released from membrane phospholipid. Their actions are diverse and only just beginning to be discovered. EXAMPLES: Induction of labour, decreasing gastric secretion of hydrochloric acid, altering blood vessel diameter opening respiratory passages, regulating body temperature. Prostaglandins act as messengers for many hormones (see 31.3). Prostaglandins are presently categorized into the following groups: PGA, PGB, PGC, PGD, PGE, PGF, PGG and PGH. In the future this list is likely to expand even further. Most of these groups appear to be derived from a substance known as arachidonic acid. The effect of prostaglandins on the body is shown by their inhibition. The marvels of aspirin and indomethacin are attributed to their ability to block the formation of prostaglandins from **arachidionic acid**.

Prostaglandin groups often act in opposition to each other. EXAMPLES: PGF inhibits platelet aggregation whereas PGB accelerates aggregation, PGF causes vasoconstriction whereas PGE causes vasodilation. The role of prostaglandins in body function is only just beginning to be understood. In future years, an understanding of their complex variety of actions is likely to lead to these substances playing an important role in arresting disease.

Steroids

Steroids are a group of substances that include cholesterol, bile salts, sex hormones and hormones secreted from the adrenal cortex. They contain four carbon rings as illustrated in Figure 29.3.

Cholesterol

Cholesterol plays an important role in body metabolism. It is an essential component of membranes and is also used to form bile salts, steroid hormones and vitamin D. It is normally abundant in nervous tissue, the adrenal glands and the skin. About 90% of cholesterol is made by the liver and regions of the intestine. The liver also serves as the chief agent for removing cholesterol by converting it into bile salts.

Bile salts

Bile salts are formed from cholesterol in the liver and secreted via the gall bladder and bile ducts into the duodenum. Bile salts act as the emulsifying agent for facilitating lipid digestion.

Steroid hormones

Steroid hormones have a variety of actions in the body. They are secreted from the adrenal cortex and gonads. EXAMPLES: Cortisol and aldosterone from the adrenal cortex and oestrogens and androgens from gonads. The actions of some steroid hormones are described in Chapter 40.

Waxes

Waxes are hydrophobic substances that are less greasy than fats. They are secreted by the skin to reduce water loss. They are used in ointments, cosmetics and a variety of pharmaceutical preparations.

Summary

Lipids are a diverse group of organic substances which share the property of being relatively insoluble in water. There are several categories of lipids:

1. Fat or triglycerides consist of three fatty acids and glycerol. They are the major reserves of energy and are stored in adipose tissue.
2. Phospholipids contain two fatty acids, a phosphate group and glycerol. They are the main constituents of plasma membranes.
3. Prostaglandins are twenty carbon fatty acids containing a five carbon ring. They appear to have a wide variety of actions on the body and are sometimes referred to as tissue hormones. Their actions on the body are blocked by aspirin.
4. Steroids contain four carbon rings. They are groups of substances that include cholesterol, bile salts and steroid hormones.
5. Waxes are hydrophobic substances secreted by the skin to reduce water loss.

Fat digestion begins in the stomach where a small quantity of fatty acids are released from glycerol. The major site of fat digestion occurs in the small intestine where the actions of bile and pancreatic juice complete the digestive process. The products of fat digestion, that is fatty acids and glycerol, are then absorbed across the wall of the intestine. Some fat is absorbed as a temporary emulsion by the process of pinocytosis.

Absorbed fat is transported as chylomicrons and fatty acids are transported by attaching to albumin. The sites of absorbed fat are muscles, liver, adipose tissue and most other cells. The principal site of stored fat is adipose tissue.

Objectives

At the completion of this chapter the student should be able to:

1. describe the structure of amino acids;
2. relate the structure of proteins to their function;
3. list the groups of proteins based on function;
4. describe the process of protein digestion and absorption;
5. explain the difference between essential and non-essential amino acids.

Proteins are one of the most important groups of body chemicals. They have many functions within the human body, notably as enzymes responsible for regulating biochemical processes, as structural proteins (such as in cell membranes and collagen), as hormones (such as insulin) and as antibodies for body defence. Even though proteins perform a wide variety of body functions, they all are composed of the same fundamental chemical units which are known as amino acids.

30.1 Amino acids

Amino acid structure

There are twenty different amino acids that commonly make up proteins. All of these amino acids contain an amine group $(-NH_2)$ and an acid group $(-COOH)$ (Figure 30.1). These amino acids differ only by the atoms

that are present in the R group, that is, side chain. The names of these amino acids are listed in Table 30.1. Note that the amino acids have been grouped according to their acid/base properties and hydrophilic/hydrophobic properties. Remember that **hydrophilia** means water attracting whereas **hydrophobia** means water repelling.

Properties of amino acids

The properties of amino acids play an important role in determining the structure and function of a protein.

Ionization

Amino acids ionize in aqueous solutions by the weak acid (COOH) donating its proton (H^+) to the weak base, amine (NH_2). The result is the formation of an amino acid that contains a negatively charged region (COO^-) and a positively charged region (NH_3^+) (Figure 30.2). This negatively and posi-

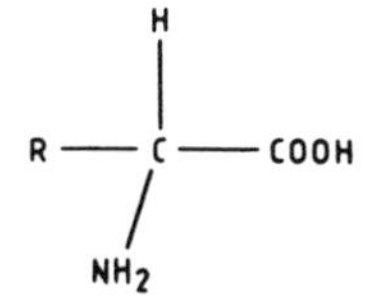

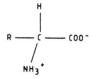

Figure 30.1 General formula of amino acids where NH$_2$ represents an amine group, COOH an acid group and R varies according to the amino acid.

Figure 30.2 The ionized form of an amino acid.

Table 30.1 The twenty common amino acids that are present in proteins

Group	Name
Basic	Lysine
	Argine
	Histidine
Acidic	Aspartic acid (aspartate)
	Glutamic acid (glutamate)
Hydrophilic	Glycine
	Serine
	Threonine
	Asparagine
	Glutamine
	Cysteine
	Methionine
Hydrophobic	Alanine
	Valine
	Leucine
	Isoleucine
	Proline
	Phenylalanine
	Tyrosine
	Tryptophan

amino acids. Some amino acids contain an amine as the R group. EXAMPLES: Lysine and histidine. The ability of these amino acids to accept protons from the solution and combine them with the extra amine group renders these amino acids bases. Since proteins are composed of amino acids, some of which are weak acids or bases, proteins are able to perform an important role as buffers.

Affinity for water

The nature of the R group or side chain can influence the affinity of an amino acid for water. Side chains with a high affinity for water are polar and are described as hydrophilic. EXAMPLES: Glycine and cysteine. In contrast, hydrophobic side chains are non-polar and repel water. The relative affinity of these side chains for water plays an important role in determining the physical shape of proteins.

30.2 Protein structure and function

tively charged compound is referred to as a zwitterion. When amino acids exist as zwitterions they can function as buffers (16.5).

Amino acids such as aspartic acid and glutamic acid contain as the R group an additional carboxyl (COOH) group. These acids can donate the additional proton into the solution, thus conferring the title of acidic

Proteins consist of large chains of amino acids that are joined together by bonds that are referred to as **peptide bonds** (Figure 8.12c). Hence proteins are called polypeptides. The arrangement and number of amino acids determine a protein's structure. The shape of proteins is fundamental to the processes of life. The three-dimensional structure of proteins can be described in terms of a struc-

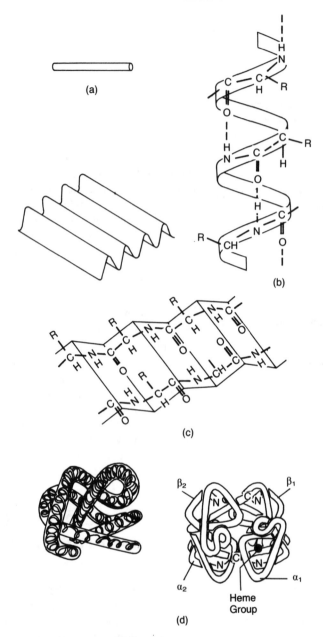

Figure 30.3 Levels of protein structure (a) primary, (b) helix, (c) pleated sheet, (d) tertiary and (e) quaternary structure of haemoglobin showing the four subunits: two α and two β, terminal carboxyl (c) and amino (N) functional groups.

tural hierarchy going from simple to complex that is, **primary**, **secondary**, **tertiary** and **quaternary**.

30.3 Levels of protein structure

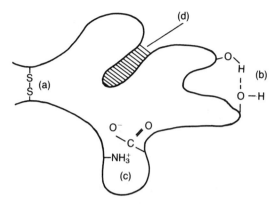

Figure 30.4 The native conformation of a globular protein showing cross linkages (a) disulphide bridge, (b) hydrogen bonds, (c) salt bridges and (d) hydrophobic interaction.

Primary structure

The primary structure represents the simplest protein structure. Primary structures refer to the amino acid sequence held together by peptide bonds (Figure 8.12c). It is the sequence of amino acids that determines the shape or **native conformation** (5.11) and hence the function of a protein.

Secondary structure

The secondary structure represents individual polypeptides forming repeating patterns such as the α-helix shape (Figure 30.3b) as seen in DNA (Figure 24.9) and the pleated sheet (Figure 30.3b). The shape of the helix is due to hydrogen bonds (5.2) linking amino acids from different locations along the chain. Each turn of the helix consists of an average of 3.6 amino acids. The spring-like structure of helixes provides a high degree of flexibility and elasticity. EXAMPLE: Hair. Pleated structures are flexible but not elastic. EXAMPLE: Silk. Where a repeating pattern is not present a random coiling of the chain occurs (Figure 30.3c). Proteins usually contain regions of repeating patterns with the remainder of the chain forming a random coil.

Tertiary structure

The tertiary structure of a protein represents the folding of polypeptide chains into specific fibres or layers (Figure 30.3d). The ability for many proteins to act in a selective manner is due to their unique shape or **native conformation**. EXAMPLES: Enzymes (32.1), antibodies (37.2) and cell surface proteins (23.1). The unique shape of each protein is determined and maintained by linkages between different parts of polypeptide chains (Figure 30.4). These **cross-linkages** result from interactions between different side groups of amino acids along a polypeptide. The different forms of bonding are:

1. **Covalent bonds** (5.2) such as the covalent bond linking two sulfur atoms. These bonds are known as **disulfide bridges**.
2. **Hydrogen bonds** (5.2) are formed between polar groups on side chains.
3. **Ionic bonds** are formed between acidic and basic side groups. These bonds are called **salt-bridges**.
4. **Hydrophobic interactions** result from the repelling of water over an area by regions of non-polar groups. These regions form pockets or caves as non-polar groups are turned inwards away from water.

Application: Collagen structure and function

Collagen is the most abundant protein in the body being the major protein of connective tissue (25.6). It provides strength to body structures through its triple helix structure (Figure 30.5). These helixes are linked together by bonds at various points along the chains. These **cross-linkages** determine the relative flexibility and strength of collagen fibres. The greater the number of cross-linkages, the greater is the strength and the lesser the flexibility. EXAMPLE: Achilles tendon is highly cross-linked. Any factor that causes a decrease in cross-linking will result in weakened collagen fibres leading to a greater chance of fibre breakage.

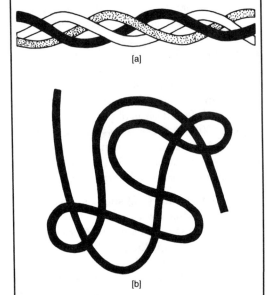

[a]

[b]

Figure 30.5 The general shape of polypeptide chains in: (a) fibrous proteins (triple helix of collagen), and (b) globular proteins.

Quaternary structure

The quaternary structure of proteins exists when polypeptide chains are combined to form a more complex unit (Figure 30.3e). Each chain has its own primary, secondary and tertiary units. EXAMPLE: Haemoglobin consists of two pairs of globin chains. Each chain contains an iron containing structure called a **haem group**, hence the name haemoglobin. Proteins containing a non-amino acid portion are called **conjugated proteins**. The non-amino acid group such as haeme is referred to as the **prosthetic group**.

30.4   Fibrous and globular proteins

Proteins can also be divided into the two groups, fibrous proteins and globular proteins.

Fibrous proteins

Fibrous proteins are composed of long helical chains of entwined amino acids. ANALOGY: The strands in a rope wrap around each other in a similar manner to that of the polypeptide chains. In addition, the polypeptide chains are bound to each other by side chain bonds (Figure 30.5a).

These proteins have great strength, and as the name implies they form the fibres in connective tissue and muscle. EXAMPLES: Collagen, keratin and fibrinogen in connective tissue, and myosin in muscle.

Globular proteins

Globular proteins consist of a folded polypeptide chain which is maintained by the interaction of side chains between nearby parts of the polypeptide chain (Figure 30.5b). ANALOGY: A tangled piece of fishing line has a unique folded shape which usually appears as a mess and any effort to untangle it will alter the shape of the tangle. The function of the protein is directly related to the shape of the tangle.

A large range of different shaped globular proteins exist in the body. EXAMPLES: Enzymes, immunoglobulins and the globin part of haemoglobin. The unique shape of individual enzymes and immunoglobulins enables them to adhere to a complementary shaped structure, that is, a biochemical with enzymes (32.1) and antigens with immunoglobulins (37.2).

30.5 Glycoproteins

These conjugated proteins consist of polypeptide chains covalently linked to carbohydrátes. The relative amount of carbohydrate can vary from a few per cent such as immunoglobulins to 85% in blood group substances. The surface of plasma membranes contain glycoproteins (23.1). These glycoproteins are responsible for the identifying characteristics of a cell that distinguish one cell type from another and provide the unique identity that distinguishes the cells of one person from those of another. Alterations in the shape of a cell-surface protein can lead to the body's immune system no longer recognizing the cells as part of a person thereby resulting the immune system attacking these cells (37.3).

30.6 Lipoproteins

These conjugated proteins contain a lipid bound to the non-polar side chains. The lipoproteins are the main mechanism for the transporting of cholesterol and triglycerides in blood and form the basis of diagnostic tests associated for high blood lipid levels (17.6 — Application: Formation of body emulsions and 26.1). They also form an important part of cell membranes (23.1).

30.7 Denaturation of proteins

Factors that affect cross-linkages such as high temperatures, acidity, alkalinity, detergents and salts will therefore affect the nature of a protein's structure at the secondary, tertiary and quaternary levels. The protein is said to undergo **denaturation**. EXAMPLE: Heating causes a breakage of the cross-linkages between the three polypeptide chains of collagen (Figure 30.5a) resulting in the denatured form of collagen called **gelatin**. Since the unique shape is responsible for the specific actions of many proteins the function of any such protein is altered. EXAMPLE: Enzymes (32.4). Small changes to cross-linkages can be reformed thus reversing the denaturation. However, when the changes are large the denaturation is irreversible. EXAMPLES: Boiling an egg results in the permanent change of egg albumin and sterilizing heat kills bacteria by denaturing the bacterial protein.

30.8 Functional classification of proteins

Proteins can be classified by their function into seven broad groups.

Nutrient proteins

Nutrient proteins or dietary proteins are the body's source of amino acids. Since some amino acids are unable to be formed in the body, these proteins are an essential raw material for the synthesis of other proteins (Table 33.2).

Structural proteins

Structural proteins are fibrous proteins found in connective tissue. EXAMPLE: Collagen. They are used to support body structures, forming a loose mesh in loose connective tissue and a dense framework in dense connective tissue (25.6).

Contractile proteins

Contractile proteins are responsible for muscle contraction. The proteins actin (fibrous) and myosin (globular) effect a contraction by sliding over each other (25.4).

Blood proteins

The four main types of blood proteins are albumin, globulin, fibrinogen and the globin part of haemoglobin. All act as buffers. The specific roles that each of them plays in blood are described in 26.1.

Immunoglobulins

Immunoglobulins or antibodies are globular proteins that are produced by plasma cells. Each specific immunoglobulin acts as a complementary shaped antigen. Antibodies are circulated throughout the cardiovascular and lymphatic systems (37.2).

Hormones

Hormones are regulators of cell function. They play a vital role in the coordination of body function. EXAMPLES: Insulin, antidiuretic hormone. Note that not all hormones are proteins. Some are steroids and others are small amino acid based molecules. A comprehensive description of their actions is given in Chapter 40.

Enzymes

Enzymes are catalysts of chemical reactions, that is, they alter the rate of the chemical reaction without being changed themselves. Without enzymes, most body chemical reactions would proceed at a rate too slow to support life. Enzymes are able to exert their influence in minute concentrations. Enzymes are described in Chapter 32.

30.9 Digestion and absorption of proteins

Because most proteins cannot be absorbed across the intestinal membrane and into the body they must be broken down into a form that can be absorbed.

Digestion

Stomach

Protein digestion begins in the stomach. Under the action of the enzyme pepsin, large protein molecules are broken down to smaller more soluble molecules known as peptides. Pepsin operates most efficiently at a pH of between 1.5 and 2.0 and thus can operate effectively in the highly acidic gastric contents. If gastric hydrochloric acid production is unable to maintain a satisfactory pH, protein digestion in the stomach is minimal.

Small intestine

Pancreatic enzymes split the peptides down to units that contain two or three amino acids. These small peptides are broken down by enzymes secreted by the epithelial cells lining the small intestine.

Absorption

Active transport

Following digestion of the protein into individual amino acids, the amino acids are actively transported (23.5) across the small intestine wall. There are four different carriers present in the membrane for the active transport of amino acids. Each of these carriers transports a specific group of amino acids. EXAMPLE: One carrier is used for the transport of the acidic amino acids while another is used for the basic amino acids.

Most amino acids rely on active transport for their movement across membranes. Without this active transport, an amino acid imbalance will occur in the body.

Application: Cystinuria

Cystinuria is an inherited disorder of membrane transport. It is due to the genetic loss of the mechanism by which cysteine and similar structured amino acids are actively transported across membranes. It appears that the genetic error is a failure to produce the carrier associated with the cysteine group of amino acids in the membranes of the

---

intestine and kidney. The disease is expressed clinically by the formation of calculi in the urinary tract. Calculi result from the elevated levels of urinary amino acid.

Pinocytosis

Small amounts of undigested protein are absorbed by pinocytosis (23.5). The combination of active transport and pinocytosis results in about 90% of ingested protein being absorbed.

Summary

Proteins are molecules consisting of large chains of amino acids. There are twenty common amino acids used to form proteins, of which ten are unable to be synthesized by the body. These latter amino acids are called essential amino acids.

The long chains of amino acids (polypeptides) are organized to provide different levels of structure within a protein. These levels of organization relate to the relative structural complexity of a protein. These levels are:

1. primary; relates to the amino acid sequence;
2. secondary; formation of helixes and pleats;
3. tertiary; folding of polypeptide chains;
4. quaternary; containing several polypeptide chains each acting as a subunit within a protein complex.

Proteins containing prosthetic groups (non-protein groups) are called conjugated proteins. Two of the important conjugated protein forms are glycoproteins and lipoproteins.

Proteins can also be classified as fibrous proteins (rope-like) or globular (considerable folds).

Proteins can be classified according to their function.

1. Nutrient proteins are the body's source of amino acids.
2. Structural proteins are fibrous proteins used to support body structures.
3. Contractile proteins are responsible for muscle contraction.
4. Blood proteins refer to a group of proteins found in blood; the main types are albumin, globulins, fibrinogen and the globin part of haemoglobin.
5. Immunoglobulins or antibodies are proteins capable of neutralizing specific antigens.
6. Hormones are regulators of cell function; note that not all hormones are proteins.
7. Enzymes are catalysts of chemical reactions.

Digestion of protein begins in the stomach where an enzyme breaks the polypeptides down into smaller molecules. In the small intestine, the pancreas and intestine secrete enzymes that complete the digestive process by forming amino acids. The amino acids are then actively transported across the wall of the small intestine. Small amounts of undigested protein are absorbed by pinocytosis.

Chapter 31

Nucleotides and nucleic acids

Objectives

At the completion of this chapter the student should be able to:

1. describe the main structural features of a nucleotide;
2. state the purine and pyrimidine derivatives;
3. explain the main functions of nucleotides and nucleic acid;
4. describe the mechanism of ATP formation;
5. list the products of nucleic acid and nucleotide digestion;
6. state the main differences between DNA and RNA;
7. provide examples of factors that can alter nucleic acid structure.

Nucleotides are an important group of chemicals that participate in nearly all biochemical processes. Nucleotides also form the building blocks for the hereditary molecules DNA and RNA (23.6) that represent the fundamental molecules of life. Nucleotides play an important role in energy production through the nucleotide ATP.

31.1 Nucleotide structure

A nucleotide consists of a heterocyclic amine molecule (8.10), a sugar and one or more phosphate groups. Two different types of heterocyclic amines occur in nucleotides. One type is derived from **purine** and the other from **pyrimidine** (Figure 8.13). The purine derivatives are **adenine** and **guanine** while the three major pyrimidine derivatives are **cytosine**, **uracil** and **thymine** (Figure 31.1). These heterocyclic amines are often referred to as the **bases** or **base units** of nucleotides. The sugar component is a pentose (5-carbon sugar). The two pentose sugars ribose and deoxyribose are involved in forming nucleotides. The base–pentose complex is called a **nucleoside**.

A nucleoside containing pyrimidine is named by removing the -*ine* and replacing it with a **-osine**. EXAMPLE: The combination of adenine and ribose is called **adenosine**. Nucleosides containing pyrimidine are named by replacing the pyrimidine ending and replacing it with **-idine**. EXAMPLE: Uracil forms the nucleoside **uridine**.

The addition of phosphate to a nucleotide results in the formation of a nucleotide. The nucleotide is named by combining the

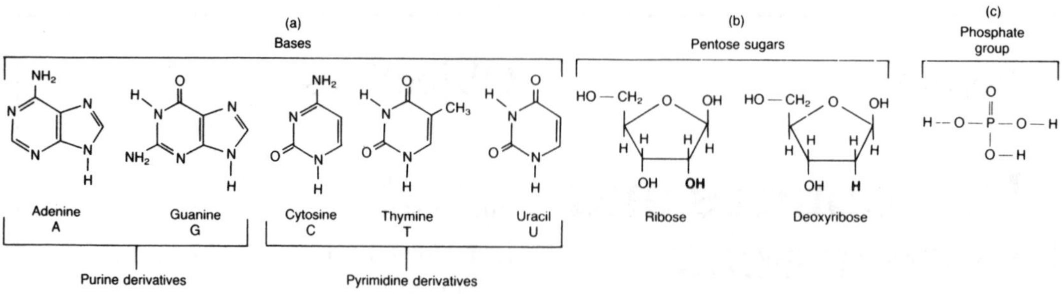

Figure 31.1   Components of nucleosides (a + b) and nucleotides (a + b + c).

nucleoside name with the number of phosphate groups added. EXAMPLE: The energy rich molecule **adenosine triphosphate** (ATP) represents the addition of three phosphate groups to an adenosine nucleoside; addition of two phosphates forms **adenosine diphosphate** (ADP) and one phosphate **adenosine monophosphate (AMP)**.

31.2   Nucleic acid structure

Nucleic acids are formed from long chains of nucleotides which are referred to as polynucleotides. The general structure of **Deoxyribonucleic acid (DNA)** is a double helix and is similar for different animals (Figure 24.9). The composition varies between different animals and is the basis of genetic difference (24.6). Human DNA contains 30% adenine, 30% thymine, 20% guanine and 20% cytosine. The number of nucleotide units varies from about 1000 in viruses to 10^9 in humans.

Ribonucleic acid (RNA) is formed by using the ribose sugar in the nucleoside instead of deoxyribose. Several different forms of RNA are involved in protein synthesis (24.8). In some viruses, RNA is used as the replicating mechanism instead of DNA (35.9). EXAMPLES: Polio virus responsible for polio and the rhinoviruses which are the most common cause of colds. The major differences between DNA and RNA are described in Table 31.1.

31.3   Nucleotide and nucleic acid function

Genetic regulation and protein synthesis

The nucleic acid DNA contains a cell's genetic information, is responsible for the control of cell function and determines the genetic characteristics of an organism. RNA transfers the messages from the DNA to the protein manufacturing centres known as ribosomes as well as assisting the assembling of the proteins (24.10, 24.11).

Energy

The adenine nucleotides ATP and ADP are the main biochemicals responsible for the transfer of energy in the body. The triphosphate molecule ATP, contains large amounts of energy stored in the third phos-

Table 31.1 Comparison of DNA and RNA

Feature	DNA	RNA
Number of polynucleotide strands	Two (double helix)	One (single helix)
Pentose sugar	Deoxyribose	Ribose
Pyrimidine bases	Cytosine, Thymine	Cytosine, Uracil
Purine bases	Guanine, Adenine	Guanine, Adenine
Size	Large	Small
Location in cells	Nucleus	Nucleus and cytoplasm

phate bond. When ATP is broken down to the two phosphate molecule Adenosine DiPhosphate (ADP) and phosphate, large amounts of energy are released:

$$ATP \rightleftharpoons ADP + phosphate + energy$$
Eqn 31.1

This equation is reversible (6.5), that is, the formation of ATP requires ADP, phosphate and energy.

The function of ATP is to provide energy for membrane transport, the synthesis of chemical compounds, and mechanical work. Cells are unable to operate on glucose or fat unless they are converted into ATP. ANALOGY: An electric stove relies on electricity for its supply of energy. The stove is unable to operate on coal, or water in a dam.

Coenzymes

Coenzymes assist the operation of an enzyme (32.3). Adenine nucleotides are components of the three major coenzymes **NAD⁺**, **FAD** and **CoA**. Nicotinamide adenine dinucleotide (NAD⁺) plays an important role in carrying electrons in the process of oxidative phosphorylation. This process is the major source of ATP production in humans (33.7). The other major electron carrier is **flavin adenine dinucleotide (FAD)** and acts in a similar way to NAD.

Coenzyme A (CoA) is a central molecule in metabolism as it acts as a carrier of the 2-C acetyl molecule (33.5) and forms one of the key metabolic interconnecting junctions (33.16).

Hormone mediators

Cyclic nucleotides such as **cyclic AMP (adenosine 3′,5′-monophosphate)** are an important link in hormonal and neuronal homeostatic mechanisms. Cyclic AMP controls cell function by acting as a **second messenger** for certain hormones and neurotransmitters. The main steps in this process are:

1. Cyclic AMP is formed in response to a signal from a hormone or neurotransmitter.
2. The primary messenger locks onto a complementary-shaped receptor which stimulates prostaglandin activity (29.2).
3. Prostaglandins stimulate or inhibit the enzyme adenylate cyclase which converts ATP to cyclic AMP.
4. An increase in adenyl cyclase activity results in an increased quantity of cyclic AMP.
5. Cyclic AMP activates an enzyme within the cell which effects a change in a specific cell function.

31.4 Sources of nucleotides

Foods such as organ meats are rich in nucleic acids. Digestion of nucleic acids, nucleosides and nucleotides occurs in the small intestine as a result of the action of pancreatic enzymes. The end products of digestion are nucleotides, purines, pyrimidines, phosphates and pentoses.

The liver produces most of the purines and pyrimidines required by the body. The nucleotides are formed from a process that combines tetrahydrofolate (substances obtained from diets), the products of certain amino acid reactions, ribose from the pentose phosphate pathway (33.10), ATP and CO_2. Vitamin B_{12} and folic acid are particularly important in the synthesis of nucleic acids (34.1).

Application: Gout

A high dietary intake of nucleotides or a relative inability to recycle the constituents of nucleotides due to a genetic defect, results in the accumulation of the waste product uric acid. The uric acid forms crystals since uric acid is only slightly soluble in water. The crystals are deposited in joints such as the big toe and cause a painful inflammation of the joint concerned. Other sites of crystal formation are soft tissue and the kidneys where stones can be formed.

31.5 Environmental health and safety

The alteration of nucleotide structure can lead to cancer. Factors such as ionizing radiation (11.8), organic solvents (17.6), food additives such as nitrites, chemicals released from cigarette smoking (8.10) and viruses (24.13) can alter nucleic acid structure and therefore function.

Summary

Nucleotides are the building blocks of nucleic acid. Each nucleotide consists of a nucleoside plus phosphate groups. Nucleosides in turn, consist of either ribose or deoxyribose plus a nitrogenous derivative of purine or pyrimidine from which the nucleoside and corresponding nucleotide are named. The major purine derivatives are adenine and guanine. The main pyrimidine derivatives are cytosine, thymine and uracil.

Nucleic acids consist of nucleotide building blocks. DNA consists of two nucleotide chains containing adenine linked to thymine and cytosine linked to guanine RNA consists of a single polynucleotide chain with the same nucleotides as DNA except for thymine which has been replaced by uracil.

The addition of three phosphate groups to the adenine base forms the high energy molecule Adenosine TriPhosphate (ATP). The breaking of the third phosphate bond releases metabolic energy and forms ADP. Adenine nucleotides are also components of the important coenzymes NAD^+, FAD and CoA and the second messenger cyclic AMP.

Digestion of nucleic acids and nucleotides occurs in the small intestine mainly as a result of pancreatic enzymes. An excessive intake of nucleotides or a genetic deficiency affecting the recycling of nucleotides results in the accumulation of the waste product uric acid which results in the deposition of crystals in joints, the kidneys and soft tissues.

Unit Eleven
Human Nutrition II: Regulation of Biochemicals

In this unit of nutrition, the regulation of biochemical processes are related to health care and body function.

Enzymes

Objectives

At the completion of this chapter the student should be able to:

1. explain the mechanism of enzyme function;
2. list the main factors influencing enzyme function;
3. describe the terms active site, substrate, induced fit, enzyme-substrate complex, apoenzyme, coenzyme, isoenzyme, V_{max}, K_m, denaturation, allosteric enzyme;
4. describe the different forms of inhibition;
5. relate environmental health and safety to enzyme function.

Enzymes are the main biological catalysts (6.2) or regulators of biochemical processes in the body. They achieve this action through the alteration of the reaction rates (6.2) to a speed necessary for the maintenance of homeostasis. In this chapter the mechanisms of enzyme action and the factors affecting enzymes action are described.

32.1 Structure and function

The globular structure of enzymes enables an enzyme to act on a specific chemical (30.3). This is achieved through the unique shape of an enzyme locking onto a complementary shaped chemical which is called the substrate (Figure 32.1a). Any factor that alters the shape will alter the relative ability for the enzyme to lock onto the substrate and provide a chemical pathway with a lower activation energy than the uncatalysed reaction (6.1).

Active site

Within an enzyme, a relatively small area has the appropriate shape and charge characteristics to lock onto a specific area of a substrate. The unique shape and charge of the active site confers the property of **specificity** as enzymes are only able to act on molecules that fit into their active sites. ANALOGY: The use of a key is based on the unique shape of the end region of the key (active site) fitting a complementary-shaped lock (substrate). The handle of the key is not directly required for the opening of the lock as is the case with the bulk of an enzyme. The active site of currently known enzymes is a non-polar region which is either a cleft or crevice from which water is usually excluded.

Application: Site of drug action

The specific action of an enzyme provides the mechanism for the selective regulation of chemical reactions within a biochemical pathway. This property of specificity is the basis of the selective action of drugs on body processes. The selective action of a drug results from the drug influencing the function of the active site through either locking onto the active site, locking onto the substrate or altering the shape of the active site. ANALOGY: Blocking a key hole, altering the shape of key or lock, alter the ability of a key to operate a lock.

Weak forces are used to bind a substrate to an enzyme thereby minimizing the energy requirements of the process and providing a relatively easy release of the substrate from the active site following the completion of the reaction. The weak forces of attraction are mainly hydrogen bonds (5.2). An important property of these bonds is the relationship between strength and direction. The greater the angle within the bond, the weaker is the force of the bond (5.2).

The active sites of some enzymes is flexible. The shape or conformation of the active site is only fixed in such enzymes after the substrate is bound. This process is referred to as an **induced fit** (Figure 32.1b).

Enzyme–substrate complex

Following the bonding of an enzyme to a substrate the combined structure is referred to as the enzyme–substrate complex (ES).

While this complex exists, the enzyme assists the breaking of bonds within the substrate to form products. The product results from interactions between the enzymes side chains and the substrate. Stretching of bonds occurs leading to their breakage and the formation of other bonds results in the product being formed. The resulting enzyme-product complex (EP) breaks after a short period as the product breaks free exposing the active site for entry of another substrate molecule.

$$E + S \rightarrow ES \rightarrow EP \rightarrow E + P$$
$$\text{Eqn 32.1}$$

32.2 Classification

The suffix **-ase** indicates an enzyme with the prefix indicating either:

1. the name of the substrate. EXAMPLE: lactase represents an enzyme acting on the sugar lactose; or
2. the type of reaction that the enzyme is involved in. EXAMPLE: lactate dehydrogenase (LDH) is an enzyme that catalyses the reduction of pyruvate to lactate.

Some common enzymes are still described using the old system of ending with **-in**. No relationship existed between the enzymes name and the substrate or reaction. EXAMPLE: Pepsin is an enzyme in the stomach that breaks down protein molecules.

32.3 Apoenzymes, coenzymes and isoenzymes

Some enzymes consist of a protein–nonprotein complex. Both parts are required for the enzyme to function. The protein part is

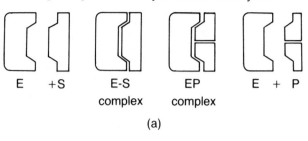

E   +S   E-S   EP   E + P
            complex   complex

(a)

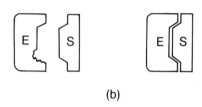

(b)

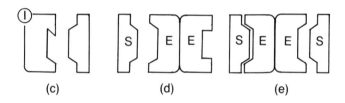

(c)   (d)   (e)

Figure 32.1 Mechanism of enzyme function. (a) Enzyme (E) and substrate (S) combine to form E–S complex followed by enzyme product complex and ultimately enzyme and product. (b) Induced fit. (c) Allosteric inhibition where inhibitor alters the shape of the active site. (d) and (e) Allosteric enzyme action.

called the **apoenzyme** and the non-protein part is referred to as the **coenzyme**.

Coenzymes are essential in the metabolism of carbohydrates, proteins and lipids with Coenzyme A forming a key interconnecting junction in the linking of their metabolic pathways (33.16). An important role of many vitamins is their action as a Coenzyme or as a source for coenzymes. EXAMPLE: Vitamin B_{12} and folic acid (Table 34.1).

Isoenzymes or isozymes are enzymes that have slightly different structural features but have the same function. The relative amounts of each isoenzyme will differ between tissues. These features are used to identify possible damage to a tissue as any alteration in the proportion of the isoenzymes within a tissue reflects an alteration in the biochemical activity of that tissue which is usually a consequence of tissue damage.

Application: Isoenzyme profiles of LDH

The relative amounts of the LDH (Lactate Dehydrogenase) isoenzymes reflect alterations in the production of energy resulting from the manufacture of lactic acid as a result of oxygen insufficiency (33.8). Examples of tissue damage are shown in Table 32.1. Isoenzyme pattens can also be used to detect genetic abnormalities in the foetus. EXAMPLE: Muscular dystrophy.

Table 32.1 Clinical LDH amounts

Body structure	Condition	Isoenzyme pattern
Heart	Myocardial infarction	Moderate increase in LDH_1 Slight increase in LDH_2
Liver	Acute hepatitis	Large increase in LDH_5 Moderate increase in LDH_4
Muscle	Muscular dystrophy	Increase in LDH_1, LDH_2, LDH_3
Blood	Sickle cell anaemia	Moderate rise in LDH_1, LDH_2
Joints	Arthritis with joint effusions	Elevation of LDH_5

32.4 Factors affecting enzyme function

Any factor that alters the shape or bonding ability of the active site will alter the function of an enzyme. Factors such as acidity, temperature and organic solvents can alter enzyme shape and thus hinder enzyme function. EXAMPLE: Enzymes work in a specific pH range. When an enzyme is exposed to an acidity or alkalinity outside that range the enzymes action is diminished. Salivary enzymes operate in a different pH range to that in the stomach (Table 16.3) and are unable to function in this highly acidic area.

The rate of a reaction is increased by temperature (6.1). Enzymes increase the rate of a reaction with increasing temperature until a temperature is reached which alters the enzyme's shape and therefore function. The enzyme has undergone **denaturation**. The temperature at which enzymes activity is greatest is called the **optimum temperature**. Many of the enzymes in the body have optimum temperatures near 40°C and therefore are operating at close to optimum function.

The cooking of food and the sterilization of objects applies this property to destroying enzymes and other proteins in microorganisms in order to prevent contamination (27.2). Storing food at low temperatures slows down the actions of enzymes responsible for food spoilage. It is possible to store an organ for several hours at low temperatures as the low temperature slows down general biochemical processes occurring within the removed organ.

An increase in the concentration of the substrate will increase the rate of the reaction until the available active sites are full. Any further increase in substrate concentration cannot be processed as there are no more available sites and so, the velocity of the reaction cannot proceed any faster a rate. The maximum velocity of a reaction is referred to as the V_{max} while the concentration at which half the active sites are filled for a particular enzyme is constant and is referred to as the **Michaelis constant** which is denoted as K_M (Moles/L). This constant usually indicates the strength of binding between an enzyme and the substrate with a high K_M indicating weak binding. The attraction or **affinity** of an enzyme for a substrate is the inverse of K_M ($1/K_M$).

32.5 Activators and inhibitors

32.6 Allosteric regulation

Activators are substances that increase the activity of an enzyme. EXAMPLE: Zinc ion (Zn^+) increases the activity of the enzyme carbonic anhydrase. Enzyme **inhibitors** are substances that decrease the activity of an enzyme. Altering the levels of either activators or inhibitors is an important medical procedure and is the basis behind the use of drugs to treat medical conditions. Factors that can denature a protein (30.7) have the same inhibitory effect on all enzymes. EXAMPLES: Heat, alcohol and strong acids whereas specific inhibitors affect one enzyme or a group of enzymes.

One group of enzyme inhibitors compete with the substrate by binding onto the active site. These **competitive inhibitors** generally have a similar structure to the substrate which enables these inhibitors to be released resulting in a reversal of the inhibition. As the concentration of substrate increases so does the chance that a substrate will bind to the active site instead of an inhibitor molecule. **Antidotes** act by competing against the inhibitor for the active site.

Another group of inhibitors act by altering the shape of the active site. These enzymes do not compete for the active site but bind to another region of the enzyme that leads to a change in the conformation of the active site. These **non-competitive inhibitors** are usually a different shape to the substrate and cannot be displaced by the substrate (Figure 32.1c). Increasing the concentration of substrate does not alter the extent of the inhibition. These inhibitors are usually irreversibly bound to the enzyme which leads to their accumulation in the body (32.7).

Many compounds regulate the activity of an enzyme by binding onto a complementary-shaped region other than the active site. The binding causes a conformational change which results in either an increased or decreased activity of the enzyme. Enzymes displaying these properties consist of several distinct sections or subunits each with its own active site and are referred to as **allosteric enzymes**. The change in activity results from the conformational change in one subunit being transmitted to another subunit (Figure 32.1d).

Most enzyme interactions take place in several steps which combine together to form a biochemical pathway. The overall result of the steps in a pathway usually results in the formation of products that are substantially different to the original substrate. EXAMPLE: Oxidation of glucose results in the formation of the products CO_2 and H_2O (33.2). In a pathway the product of the first step becomes the substrate of the next step.

$$A \rightarrow B \rightarrow C \rightarrow D \qquad \text{Eqn 32.2}$$

Pathways usually contain a self-regulatory mechanism that prevents the uncontrolled accumulation of a product. The mechanism usually involves the allosteric regulation of an enzyme within the pathway by one of the products further down the pathway. Any accumulation of the product results in inhibition of the enzyme (Figure 32.2) thereby

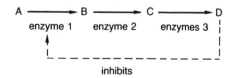

Figure 32.2 Inhibition of a biochemical pathway.

reducing the rate of formation of the product and its further accumulation. This is a negative feedback mechanism (1.2). Where product formation stimulates further product formation the mechanism is referred to as positive feedback. Both these feedback mechanisms require only one enzyme in a pathway to control an entire sequence of biochemical reactions and therefore are an efficient means through which the body can control complex biochemical processes. Drugs involved in regulating a pathway usually affect the enzyme involved in the feedback as it is regulating the pathway.

32.7 Environmental health and safety

The effect of environmental agents on the body involves in many cases the alteration of enzyme function. EXAMPLES: Poisoning, exposure to pollutants such as heavy metals and exposure to organic solvents. Care must be exercised at all times to minimize exposure to these agents as the irreversible binding of agents such as heavy metals can lead to irreversible damage to the body.

Application: Heavy metal poisoning

Heavy metals such as lead (Pb) and mercury (Hg) are poisonous as they change the conformation of an enzyme. The toxic accumulation of these metals results in an alteration to the nervous system which can lead to the irreversible loss of hearing, touch, sight and balance.

Summary

Enzymes are globular structures that contain a specifically shaped region that locks onto a complementary-shaped molecule called the substrate to form the enzyme–substrate complex. Hydrogen bonds are the main forces that link the enzyme to the substrate. The constant K_M is an indicator of strength of binding of a substrate to an enzyme while its inverse reflects the affinity of an enzyme for a substrate. The unique shape of each active site confers the property of specificity that is fundamental to the existence of life. It provides the basis for specific chemical reactions to occur in a regulated manner. The suffix -ase indicates an enzyme although some common enzymes are still described using -in.

Enzymes sometimes consist of a complex consisting of an apoenzyme and a coenzyme with both parts being required for the enzyme to function. Isoenzymes are enzymes that have slightly different structural features but have the same function. They are an important diagnostic tool.

The activity of enzymes is increased with increases in temperature and substrate concentration. Any factor that alters the shape or bonding ability of the active site will alter the activity of an enzyme. These factors may be non-specific and denature the enzyme or specific and only alter the conformation of the active site. Activators increase the activity of an enzyme whereas inhibitors decrease the activity by either directly blocking the active site (competitive inhibition) or by altering the shape from another location on the enzyme (non-competitive inhibition). Competitive inhibition is a reversible process affected by substrate concentration whereas non-competitive inhibition is irreversible and independent of substrate concentration. Allosteric enzymes consist of two or more subunits. The change in activity resulting from the binding of substrate to one active site results in a conformational change on another subunit. This mechanism is particularly important in the feedback control of biochemical pathways. These pathways are the mechanism through which major biochemical changes can be made to a molecule. The irreversible binding of pollutants to enzymes leads to long irreversible changes in body function.

Chapter 33

Metabolism

Objectives

At the completion of this chapter the students should be able to:

1. describe the major metabolic pathways;
2. define absorptive state, post-absorptive state, glysouria, cytochrome nitrogen balance, ketone body, amino acid pool and Cori cycle;
3. list the key interconnecting metabolic junctions;
4. explain the conditions which promote the use of interconnecting pathways;
5. describe the process of oxidative phosphorylation;
6. explain the difference between essential and non-essential amino acids.

33.1 Regulation of metabolism

In this chapter the major biochemical interactions occurring in the body are discussed. Metabolism reflects the overall homeostatic mechanism for regulating chemicals within the body. The previous chapters in this unit have discussed how nutrients are absorbed into the body. The path that these nutrients take following absorption is controlled by enzymes (Chapter 32) and hormones (39.1). The effectiveness of both enzymes and hormones is influenced by certain vitamins and minerals (Chapter 34). The destiny of nutrients can vary according to the homeostatic needs of the body. EXAMPLES: Oxidized for energy, stored in a macro-molecule or converted into another molecule.

The capacity to follow different paths according to need is an important factor in the body maintaining homeostasis in an ever-changing internal environment and provides the body with the flexibility to correct changes resulting from illness.

33.2 Glycogen synthesis and breakdown

Glycogen synthesis

The level of glucose in the blood needs to be maintained in order that a continuous source of energy is provided for tissues such as nervous tissue (28.4). Carbohydrate is stored in the body as the macromolecule glycogen.

The formation of glycogen occurs in the period of absorption following a meal. This period or metabolic state is called the **absorptive state** and usually lasts approximately four hours with an average meal. The synthesis of glycogen is called **glycogenesis** and involves the linking of glucose molecules to form chains and branches (Figure 28.3). This process is achieved through the addition of a phosphate group and the subsequent rearrangement of the molecule into a form that can be added to a molecule within a chain. A special enzyme called branching enzyme is used to form the branches. The addition of a phosphate in a reaction is referred to as **phosphorylation**.

Glycogen breakdown

Following completion of absorption after a meal, the body is in a **post-absorptive (fasting) state**. The energy needs of the body are met through the breakdown of macromolecules. The breakdown of glycogen is similar to a reversal of the synthesis process and is referred to as **glycogenolysis**. A debranching enzyme breaks the branches, an addition of a phosphate follows which is then relocated to form the substance glucose-6-phosphate prior to glucose being formed. Skeletal muscle cells lack the enzyme responsible for forming glucose-6-phosphate and therefore cannot form glucose although the products of the catabolism of glucose-6-phosphate pyruvate (33.5) and lactate (33.8) can be transported to the liver where glucose can be formed. Glucose can also be formed from the breakdown of fat and protein in a process called gluconeogenesis (33.15).

33.3 Production of energy

The production of energy in the body involves the removal of hydrogen atoms during oxidation (6.6), mainly from carbohydrates and fats. The energy released as a result of removing hydrogen from a molecule is not in a form that can be immediately used by the cell. The released energy is mainly used to form the substance ATP (Adenosine Tri-Phosphate) which provides a mechanism for the various body processes to obtain energy (31.3).

33.4 Glycolysis

The chemical pathway of glucose breakdown or catabolism terminates in carbon dioxide plus hydrogen ions. The hydrogen ions combine with oxygen to form the neutral substance water.

Glycolysis or the **Emden-Meyerhof pathway** is a series of ten reversible reactions and represents the first stage in glucose catabolism (Figure 33.1). This stage occurs in the cytoplasmic matrix. The main steps in this stage involve:

1. **addition** of two phosphate ions (phosphorylation) to the glucose from two molecules of ATP;
2. **rearrangement** of the molecule into a symmetrical six-carbon structure called fructose-1,6-diphosphate;
3. **splitting** of this structure into two three-carbon molecules called glyceraldehyde-3-phosphate and dihydroxyacetone phosphate;
4. **removal** of two hydrogen atoms from each molecule resulting in the formation of two molecules of pyruvate (pyruvic acid). The breakage of the hydrogen bonds releases

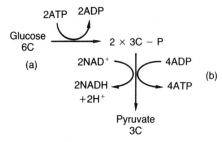

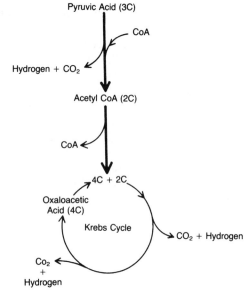

Figure 33.1 Glycolysis. (a) Series of reactions requiring 2 ATP molecules to form Dihydroxyacetone phosphate and Glyceraldehyde-3-phosphate. (b) Removal of phosphate and hydrogen form pyruvate, 4 ATP directly and 4 ATP or 6 ATP indirectly via NADH.

Figure 33.2 The catabolism of pyruvic acid and its relationship to the Krebs cycle.

energy. Most of this energy is ultimately used to:

(a) combine four ADP molecules and phosphate to form four ATP molecules,

(b) combine four NAD^+ molecules with H to form four NADH which in turn form in the presence of oxygen four ATP molecules in skeletal muscle cells and six ATP molecules in the liver and cardiac muscle,

(c) remainder being expended as heat;

5. glycolysis results in the net production of six or eight molecules of ATP as two molecules were required in step 1.

33.5 Breakdown of pyruvate

The pathway for the breakdown of pyruvate varies according to the oxygen environment. In yeast and several other microorganisms **anaerobic conditions** cause the conversion of

pyruvate to ethanol, yielding a net production of two ATP molecules per pyruvate molecule. This process is called **fermentation**. In eucaryotic cells, anaerobic conditions lead to the formation of lactic acid with a net yield of two ATP molecules per pyruvate molecule. In **aerobic conditions** pyruvate is completely catabolized to carbon dioxide and water.

Stage 2 of the breakdown of glucose in aerobic conditions mainly involves the transfer of a two-carbon structure acetyl CoA to the inner mitochondrial membrane (Figure 33.2). This stage involves the following steps.

1. Each pyruvate molecule loses one carbon atom forming a two-carbon acetyl group in the mitochondrial matrix. This step has a net yield of three ATP molecules per pyruvate molecule.

2. The acetyl group attach to a substance referred to as **coenzyme A or CoA** forming the substance **acetyl CoA**. This substance

is at the junction of the major metabolic pathways and will be referred to regularly in the remainder of this chapter. Coenzyme A assists enzyme function and acts as a carrier.

3. Acetyl CoA is transported to the mitochondrial membrane where the complex breaks down. CoA returns to combine with more acetyl while the acetyl group undergoes the final stage of aerobic glucose catabolism.

33.6   Krebs cycle

The catabolism of the acetyl group is referred to as either the **Krebs cycle, citric acid cycle** or the **tricarboxylic cycle** (Figure 33.2). This stage involves the following steps:

1. The acetyl group enters the cycle by combining with a four carbon molecule (oxaloacetic acid) on the inner mitochondrial membrane to form the six-carbon molecule citrate.

2. A series of reactions then occurs which results in the removal of the two carbon atoms from the acetyl group as carbon dioxide and also their associated hydrogen atoms.

3. When the carbon, hydrogen and oxygen are removed from the acetyl group, the original oxaloacetic acid molecule is left. This molecule is then free to combine with another acetyl group and thus oxaloacetic acid in effect acts as a carrier.

33.7   Transfer of energy

The removal of hydrogen in the Krebs cycle releases large amounts of energy. The released energy is used to combine hydrogen with a coenzyme known as NAD. The NAD^+ combines with two hydrogen atoms. This results in the formation of $NADH + H^+$

$$NAD^+ + H_2 \rightarrow NADH + H^+$$
Eqn 33.1

The effect of the formation of NADH is the transfer of the potential energy from a carbon–hydrogen–oxygen molecule to a NADH molecule. At this stage the energy is unable to be used by the cell as cells need the energy to be supplied by ATP molecules.

The NADH is broken down, resulting in the formation of NAD^+ and hydrogen. Some of the released energy is used to form a molecule of ATP. A series of reactions then follows which results in the release of hydrogen ions and the transfer of their electrons and the energy along a chain of substances known as **cytochromes**. As the electrons are passed along the **cytochrome chain** or **electron transport system** the energy required to bind the electrons decreases. This results in a corresponding increase in the amount of energy available for ATP production (Figure 33.3).

The end products of the removal of hydrogen from the Krebs cycle are hydrogen ions (acid), electrons and energy. A substance is required to neutralize the hydrogen ions otherwise the body would be unable to cope with the excessive quantities of acid. These protons are combined with electrons and oxygen to produce the neutral substance water. **The body requires oxygen principally for the neutralization of protons and the removal of electrons formed as a result of energy production**. The energy released during the electron transfer system is used to form ATP.

The transfer of the energy to form ATP is **oxidative phosphorylation** which requires the bonding of a phosphate to ADP. The energy stored in the third phosphate bond is able to be utilized by the cell. Approximately 90% of all ATP is produced by this mechanism.

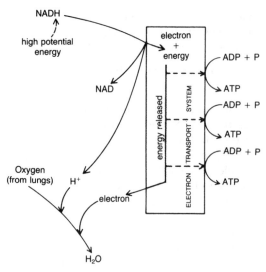

Figure 33.3 The relationship between hydrogen, the electron transport system and ATP formation.

The formation of ATP is dependent upon the release of energy in the electron transport system. If the electron transport system breaks down no ATP is formed by oxidative phosphorylation. EXAMPLE: Cyanide blocks ATP production by preventing the electrons being transferred to oxygen. This leads to a blockage of the electron transport system and thus oxidative phosphorylation.

The functions of hydrogen and oxygen have been shown to be closely related. Without either, homeostasis would be impossible, and therefore death would occur. In the body, the formation of ATP from carbohydrate catabolism is an important mechanism for the functioning of organs such as the brain, which relies upon an adequate supply of glucose and oxygen. Without either, it will fail to function.

The overall ·mechanism of ATP production due to aerobic glucose catabolism is summarized in Figure 33.4. Each turn of the Krebs cycle results in the net production of twelve ATP molecules. Since two acetyl groups are formed from glucose, a net production of twenty-four ATP occurs in the Krebs cycle from one glucose molecule. When combined with the eight ATP produced during glycolysis and the six ATP from pyruvic acid breakdown, a net quantity of thirty-eight ATP molecules results from aerobic catabolism of glucose.

33.8 Lactic acid formation

In the absence of oxygen, that is, anaerobic conditions, pyruvic acid is converted into lactic acid without the formation of any additional ATP molecules. In fact, six ATP molecules are used in this process as a two-carbon compound is converted into a three-carbon compound. The net result of the catabolism of one glucose molecule is the formation of two molecules of the three carbon acid called lactic acid and two molecules of ATP.

Lactic acid formation can occur as a result of oxygen supply not meeting the tissue demands. EXAMPLE: The large increase in oxygen requirements in vigorous exercise can result in insufficient oxygen being supplied to the relevant muscles. Moderate amounts of lactic acid can be buffered by the body preventing acidosis (16.5). In the presence of large amounts of oxygen, lactic acid can be converted in the liver to glycogen which can be utilized at a later time by the body.

33.9 Comparison of energy production

The net total quantity of usable energy produced in the presence of oxygen is eighteen

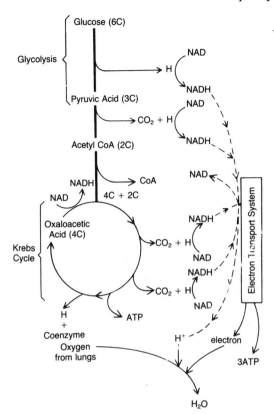

Figure 33.4 Aerobic catabolism of glucose to carbon dioxide, water and ATP.

Table 33.1 Net energy produced during aerobic and anaerobic glucose catabolism in the liver

	Aerobic (no. ATP molecules)	Anaerobic (no. ATP molecules)
Glycolysis	8	2
Lactic acid	—	—
Pyruv	6	—
Krebs cycle	24	—
Total	*38*	*2*

times that produced by anaerobic glucose catabolism (Table 33.1). The supply of oxygen is essential for the efficient use of glucose. Organs such as the brain require large amounts of energy to function. Without oxygen, these organs are unable to produce sufficient energy anaerobically to meet their energy requirements.

33.10 Pentose phosphate pathway

The pentose phosphate pathway or hexose monophosphate pathway represents an alternative oxidative pathway for the catabolism of glucose to lactic acid. This pathway also represents an important path for the synthesis of molecules containing five-carbon sugars such as nucleic acids (31.2) and nucleotides (31.1). The path (Figure 33.5) also is a source of the coenzyme **NADPH** (nicotinamide adenine dinucleotide phosphate). This coenzyme is necessary for the synthesis of fatty acids and steroids. The path is more active in adipose tissue (25.6) than muscle. NOTE: This pathway does not directly involve the production of ATP, however, the ribose can be further broken down to the three-carbon sugar glyceraldehyde

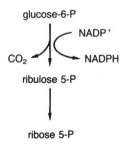

Figure 33.5 The pentose phosphate pathway.

3-phosphate which is an intermediate molecule in glycolysis (33.4) from which ATP is produced.

33.11 Production of energy from fat

The body has a preference for glucose as a source of potential energy. Fat which is more difficult to mobilize is the body's next preference. This order of preference can be altered by hormone action (40.2). Mobilized fat can produce more ATP than glucose since the former contains a greater number of hydrogen atoms.

Fat is the major storage depot of energy in the body. The hydrophobic nature of fat (water repelling) enables fat to be stored free of water. Glycogen is surrounded by large quantities of water and is therefore relatively heavy when compared with fat. Fat can form ATP because its breakdown products can directly enter the Krebs cycle. It can also produce ATP indirectly by being converted to glucose which is subsequently catabolized to produce ATP (Figure 33.6).

The breakdown of fat into its constituent molecules results in the formation of glycerol and three fatty acids (Figure 29.1). Both these substances consist of only carbon, hydrogen and oxygen atoms. The principal of fat energy production is simply the rearrangement of the quantities and proportions of carbon, hydrogen and oxygen into molecules that are found in the previously mentioned pathway used for glucose energy production (33.3).

The three-carbon alcohol, glycerol, is converted in the liver into a three-carbon compound (dihydroxy acetone phosphate) found in the process of glycolysis. This latter substance is in turn converted to the important three-carbon sugar glyceraldehyde-3-phosphate (33.4). This three-carbon sugar can then be converted to glucose by a

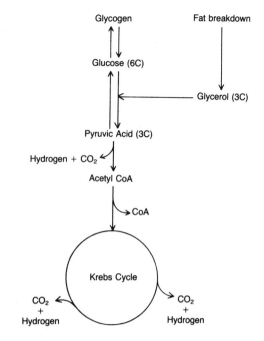

Figure 33.6 The catabolism of glycerol showing its entry into glucose metabolic pathways.

reversal of glycolysis (gluconeogenesis — 33.15), and if necessary glycogen. Alternatively, glyceraldehyde-3-phosphate can be catabolized to produce ATP via pyruvic acid formation (33.5), and if oxygen is present via the Krebs cycle (Figure 33.6).

The catabolism of fatty acids readily takes place in the mitochondrial matrix (22.10) of tissues such as liver and muscle. An enzyme slices off two carbon units of the hydrocarbon fatty acid chain (Figure 33.7). Each two-carbon unit or **acetyl group** is then combined with CoA to form **acetyl CoA**. The acetyl CoA is identical to that formed from glucose catabolism. The acetyl group is transported by the CoA to the site in the mitochondrial membrane where the Krebs cycle breaks down the two-carbon unit to form ATP (33.6).

The action of slicing the fatty acid continues until the fatty acid is completely

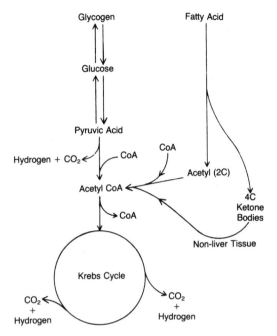

Figure 33.7 The catabolism of fatty acids showing the entry of acetyl CoA into the glucose metabolic pathways.

together to form a four-carbon acid. These acids are called **ketone bodies**. EXAMPLE: Acetoacetic acid.

In humans, the liver is the only organ that produces significant amounts of ketone bodies. However, the liver lacks the enzyme that converts ketone bodies into acetyl CoA. Ketone bodies leave the liver and are transported to most tissues where they are converted into acetyl CoA.

Ketone bodies rely on blood for transport to their breakdown sites, and the acidic nature of these substances can thus influence acid–base balance. During normal metabolism, the quantities of ketone bodies in blood are easily buffered by the various blood buffers. Factors that elevate fat catabolism will increase the concentration of ketones in the blood. Excessive fat catabolism leads to an acidosis of the blood which is referred to as **ketoacidosis**.

broken down. The process of forming acetyl CoA by removing acetyl groups from a fatty acid is referred to as β **oxidation**.

A problem exists with odd numbered hydrocarbon chains since the last carbon atoms in the chain have to form either a three- or one-carbon molecule. In fact, three carbon units are formed. These three-carbon molecules are converted by a series of reactions, and are then able to enter the Krebs cycle.

33.12   Formation of ketone bodies

The breakdown of long chain fatty acids can result in the last four-carbon atoms remaining

---

Application: Ketosis

Ketosis is a form of metabolic acidosis (16.6). The most common causes of ketosis are starvation and diabetes mellitus. In both these conditions a lack of glucose in the body tissues results in large amounts of fat and protein being catabolized. The excessive breakdown of fat and protein results in large quantities of ketone bodies being released into the blood. The abnormally high concentrations of these acids are unable to be successfully buffered and thus acidosis occurs.

The onset of ketosis is associated with malaise, rapid breathing and thirst. If untreated, vomiting, dehydration and finally coma will occur. The large quantities of ketones in the blood also result in ketonuria, that is, the presence of ketone bodies in the urine.

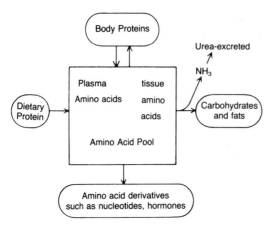

Figure 33.8 The amino acid pool and its relationship with biochemicals.

33.13 Protein anabolism

Amino acid pool

Following their absorption across the small intestine wall, the amino acids enter a common amino acid pool located in the blood and tissues. This pool also contains amino acids that have resulted from the breakdown of tissue proteins during normal metabolism (Figure 33.8). Once the amino acids are in this common metabolic pool the body cannot distinguish from where a particular amino acid has been derived.

The amino acid pool serves as the distribution centre for amino acid based biochemicals such as hormones and nucleotides. The principal site of this amino acid metabolism is the liver. During starvation or when the protein intake is inadequate, the liver loses protein to a greater extent than other tissues. The liver is more susceptible to injury by such agents as alcohol when a situation of depleted protein exists.

Transamination

Within the amino acid pool, some amino acids can be converted into other amino acids. **Transamination** is the process whereby an amine group is transferred from one amino acid to form another amino acid. The chemical that combines with the amine group is usually one formed in the breakdown pathway of carbohydrates and fats. Transamination assists the homeostasis of protein metabolism by being able to alter the concentration of particular amino acids according to the needs of the body.

Not all amino acids can be formed by transamination. Amino acids that are unable to be manufactured by the body have to be supplied by the diet.

Essential and non-essential amino acids

The nutritional value of any protein depends upon the composition and proportion of its constituent amino acids. Approximately half of the amino acids are readily manufactured in the body. These amino acids are therefore not essential in the diet (Table 33.2). The remainder of the amino acids are not readily

Table 33.2 Essential and non-essential amino acids for man

Essential	Non-essential
Arginine	Alanine
Histidine	Asparagine
Isoleucine	Aspartic acid
Leucine	Cysteine
Lysine	Glycine
Methionine	Glutamic acid
Phenylalanine	Hydroxyproline
Threonine	Proline
Tryptophan	Serine
Valine	Tyrosine

made in the body. These **essential amino acids** are either not synthesized at the rate required for normal metabolism or they are not manufactured at all.

Essential amino acids must be supplied in the diet and thus the dietary value of any protein depends upon its content of essential amino acids.

Application: The biological value of proteins

The biological value of a particular protein is determined by its content of essential amino acids. Generally, animal proteins contain all of the essential amino acids and thus have a high biological value. Most plant proteins are of a low biological value because they are deficient in one or more of the essential amino acids. Carefully chosen combinations of plant proteins can have a biological value as high as that of any animal protein.

33.14 Protein catabolism

Deamination

The removal of amine groups from the amino acid pool is termed **deamination**. This process is the main pathway for the removal of nitrogen from the body. On leaving the amino acid pool, the amine forms ammonia. Most of this relatively toxic substance is combined with carbon dioxide to form non-toxic urea which is excreted in the urine. Urea is the main end product of protein catabolism and it accounts for 80–90% of the nitrogen that is excreted in the urine. Some of the am-

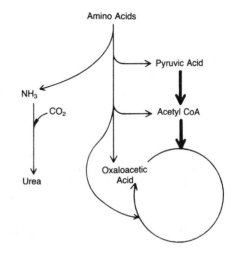

Figure 33.9 Incorporation of the amine-free part of amino acids into the Krebs cycle.

monia is used in the formation of the nucleotides, adenine and guanine. The breakdown of these substances yields the excretory product uric acid.

The fate of the amine-free part of a deaminated amino acid depends on the type of amino acid that has been deaminated. The removal of amine groups from most amino acids means that the remaining part is composed of only carbon, hydrogen and oxygen. These amine-free substances thus contain the essential ingredients for entrance into carbohydrate biochemical pathways.

Formation of carbohydrates and fats from amino acids

Proteins are the last major reserves of energy, since carbohydrates and fats are preferred as energy sources. Proteins can produce energy when the amine-free parts of amino acids are being incorporated into the Krebs cycle (Figure 33.9). Amino acids can be grouped according to the end-products formed as a result of the metabolism of their amine-free part:

1. **Glucogenic** amino acids enter the Krebs cycle as oxaloacetic acid (one of the substances in the cycle). The oxaloacetic acid can then either be catabolized to form ATP, carbon dioxide and water or it is anabolized to form glucose via the process of gluconeogenesis (33.15), and if necessary glycogen or fat. EXAMPLE: Alanine.
2. **Ketogenic** amino acids form the ketone body acetoacetic acid. The ketone bodies leave the liver and are transported to cells where the acetoacetic acid is catabolized to form ATP, carbon dioxide and water. EXAMPLE: Leucine.
3. Deamination of the third group of amino acids results in the formation of glucose and ketone bodies. EXAMPLES: Tyrosine and phenylalanine.

Approximately 60% of the body's protein can be converted in the liver to glucose by gluconeogenesis. The breakdown of this protein is influenced by hormones such as cortisol (Chapter 40).

Nitrogen balance

Nitrogen balance refers to the amount of nitrogen in the urine compared to nitrogen intake over a period of time. When the intake of nitrogen exceeds its excretion, a person has a **positive** nitrogen balance. EXAMPLES: Children, pregnant women, and patients recovering from a prolonged illness. A **negative** nitrogen balance exists when more nitrogen is being excreted than is being taken into the body. This imbalance is due to some factor causing a relative excess of amino acid deamination. EXAMPLES: Starvation, wasting disease and diets lacking sufficient quantities of essential amino acids.

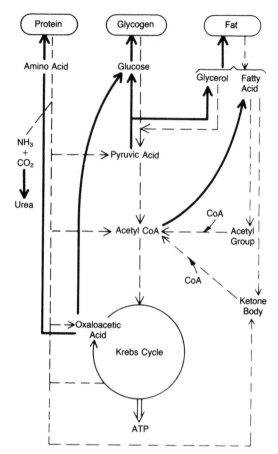

Figure 33.10 The relationship of the Krebs cycle to carbohydrate, lipid and protein catabolism. Note that these biochemicals can be converted into each other by the reversal of catabolic pathways (– – – catabolic pathways, — anabolic pathways).

33.15   Gluconeogenesis

Gluconeogenesis is the formation of glucose from non-carbohydrate substances such as amino acids, glycerol and lactate. This process provides an important backup when

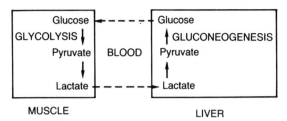

Figure 33.11 The Cori cycle. Lactate formed from muscle activity is converted to glucose by the liver.

a dietary insufficiency of glucose occurs. Gluconeogenesis is essentially a reversal of glycolysis (33.4) as pyruvate is converted into glucose (Figure 33.10). NOTE: Some steps in glycolysis are not reversible reactions and are bypassed through the action of different enzymes.

The main site of gluconeogenesis is the liver and occurs to a small extent in the kidneys. These two organs help maintain the glucose level in the blood thereby providing the brain and muscle as the main users of glucose with sufficient glucose to meet their metabolic needs.

Amino acids are derived from the dietary proteins and during starvation, from the breakdown of proteins in skeletal muscle (33.14). Their main points of entry are oxaloacetic acid and pyruvate. Glycerol can enter this pathway by being converted to pyruvate (Figure 33.6) but fatty acids cannot be converted to glucose in animals (33.11 and Figure 33.10). Lactate is formed in skeletal muscle during anaerobic energy production (33.8). It is a dead end in metabolism and if not reconverted back to pyruvate can cause metabolic acidosis (16.6).

Cori cycle

The relationship between the muscle lactate production and the production of glucose in the liver is referred to as the Cori cycle (Figure 33.11). This cycle provides a release for the accumulation of lactate and in turn provides a replenished supply of glucose for the muscles.

33.16 Interconversion of carbohydrates, lipids and proteins

Carbohydrates, lipids and proteins all have the potential to enter the Krebs cycle in the presence of oxygen, and produce energy in the form of ATP (Figure 33.10). These substances can also be converted into each other. The ability of these important chemicals to form ATP and be interconverted is an important mechanism in the maintenance of body and cell homeostasis. In cases of disease where an imbalance in body metabolism exists, interconversion of body chemicals is essential for a healthy life. EXAMPLE: People with diabetes mellitus convert glycerol and protein into glucose.

Gluconeogenesis is important during periods of starvation when the direct reserves of glucose are only sufficient to last for about a day. Following the depletion of glycogen, the glucose-dependent tissues such as nervous tissue must form glucose from a non-carbohydrate source. The liver is the site of most gluconeogenesis although parts of the kidney also form small quantities of glucose by this process. These two organs help to maintain the blood glucose levels so that the metabolic needs of the brain and muscle can be met.

In addition to gluconeogenesis, the brain can use the substance beta-hydroxybutyrate formed from fatty acids in the liver. Beta-hydroxybutyrate is converted in the brain and other peripheral tissues to acetoacetyl CoA, which is then split to form acetyl CoA and is able to enter the citric acid cycle and produce ATP. This process spares muscle proteins as an energy source in the initial stages of starvation.

Application: Low carbohydrate diets

A person on a low carbohydrate diet converts glycerol and to a limited extent protein into glucose and glycogen. Without this formation of glucose, body function would be severely impaired. The conversion of glycerol to glucose results in decreased levels of body fat and a decrease in body weight. The conversion of glycerol to glucose can be monitored by measuring the concentration of ketones in the urine.

Summary

The major metabolic pathways are:

1. glycogen synthesis and breakdown;
2. glycolysis;
3. Krebs cycle;
4. lactic acid formation;
5. catabolism of fat;
6. protein anabolic pathways;
7. protein catabolic pathways;
8. gluconeogenesis.

These pathways are interconnected (Figure 33.10) to provide the body flexibility in processing and storing the major biochemicals as well as, providing alternative sources for the production of energy. The key interconnecting junctions are: Glucose 6-phosphate, glyceraldehyde-3-phosphate, pyruvate and acetyl CoA.

The production of energy in aerobic conditions provides 38 ATP molecules compared with only two in anaerobic metabolism. Fat contains more energy compared to glucose as fat contains more hydrogen atoms. The oxidation of molecules and the resulting release of energy requires a process whereby the chemical energy can be transferred into a form that can be readily utilized by the body. Oxidative phosphorylation involves the transfer of energy through an electron transfer chain and the subsequent transfer of the energy to form high energy bonds that link a phosphate group to ADP resulting in the formation of ATP. The main vehicle for the supply of energy is the Krebs cycle which undergoes its reactions in the inner membrane of mitochondria.

The monitoring of substances can provide an insight into the relative use of the different pathways. The presence of glucose in the urine indicates a failure to utilize glucose or convert it to fat. Ketone bodies in the urine indicate a relatively high oxidation of fat. A negative nitrogen balance indicates a greater use of amino acids than are being ingested and the possible use of amino acids in gluconeogenesis.

Chapter 34

Vitamins, minerals and water

Objectives

At the completion of this chapter the student should be able to:

1. list the important water soluble and fat soluble vitamins;
2. describe the deficiency effects of each vitamin;
3. list the important minerals and briefly describe their function;
4. describe the role of water in body function.

34.1 Vitamins

Vitamins are organic substances that act in trace amounts to promote enzyme function. They play an important role in regulating biochemical and physiological processes.

Most vitamins cannot be synthesized by the body; they are mainly obtained from food. EXAMPLE: Vitamin C in citrus fruit. No single food can supply all the different forms of vitamins, and thus it is important to have a balanced diet. The daily requirement of each vitamin varies between individuals. Factors such as pregnancy can alter the vitamin requirement within an individual. Abnormally low and high levels of vitamin intake can lead to altered physiological and biochemical function.

Evidence for the actions of vitamins on the body is still conflicting in many cases. The effect of drugs on vitamin absorption and function is little understood at present. In the future, hopefully, a clear picture will emerge as to their precise role in the body and the impact that drugs have on vitamins fulfilling

their role. This book will only attempt to introduce the topic of vitamins to students.

Vitamins are separated into two categories according to their solubility in water.

Water soluble vitamins

These vitamins are dissolved in the gastro-intestinal tract and body fluids. The body has difficulty in storing these vitamins and any excess is excreted in the urine. EXAMPLE: Vitamin C.

The water soluble vitamins consist of the B group of vitamins and vitamin C. The function of each of these vitamins and the effects of their deficiency is summarized in Table 34.1.

Fat soluble vitamins

This group of vitamins are insoluble in water but soluble in fat. Their ability to be stored in cells enables the body to keep an adequate reserve under normal conditions. They

Table 34.1   Water soluble vitamins and their function

Vitamin	Food examples	Function	Deficiency effects
B$_1$ (thiamine)	Most foods except white flour and sugar	Involved in catabolism of pyruvic acid to carbon dioxide and water	Elevated pyruvic acid and lactic acid levels, insufficient energy production, beriberi and polyneuritis
B$_2$ (riboflavin)	Dairy products, eggs, meat, wholemeal bread	Involved in carbohydrate and protein metabolism in tissues such as intestinal wall and skin	Digestive disturbances, dermatitis, eye soreness, cataracts
B$_6$ (pyridoxine)	Unpolished rice, whole-grain cereals, liver, yoghurt	Important in lipid and protein metabolism, maintenance of healthy skin	Dermatitis, nausea
B$_{12}$ (cyanocob-alamin)	Not in vegetables, found in liver, milk, eggs, cheese, meat	Necessary for red blood cell formation, entrance of some amino acids into Krebs cycle and nucleic acid synthesis	Pernicious anaemia, malfunction of nervous system
Nicotinamide (niacin)	Meat, whole-grain cereals, bread and yeast	Important in lipid catabolism for energy release, inhibits cholesterol production	Pellagra
Pantothenic acid	Green vegetables, liver, kidney	Essential in the conversion of lipids and amino acids to glucose, synthesis of cholesterol and steroid hormones	Fatigue, neuromuscular abnormalities, insufficient adrenal hormones
Folic acid	Green leafy vegetables	Important in the Krebs cycle and nucleic acid synthesis	Fatigue, mental depression and nausea
Vitamin C (ascorbic acid)	Citrus fruits, green vegetables, tomatoes	Function is controversial but appears to promote many metabolic reactions, works with immunoglobulins, involved in steroid production and epithelial growth	Slow healing of wounds, anaemia, scurvy

are found in most fatty foods. EXAMPLE: Vitamin A in cod liver oil.

The fat soluble vitamins are vitamins A, D, E and K. A summary of their functions and the effects of deficiencies on the body are listed in Table 34.2.

34.2 Minerals

Minerals are inorganic substances that function in the body in combination with other minerals or with organic substances. The

Table 34.2 Fat soluble vitamins and their function

Vitamin	Food examples	Function	Deficiency effects
A	From carotene in yellow and green vegetables, also directly from fish, liver, oils, and dairy products	Maintains health and vigour of epithelial cells especially mucous membrane cells, important in vision	Night blindness, dry skin and hair, infections of the ear, sinus, respiratory, urinary and digestive tracts
D	Fish, liver, oils, egg yolk, milk, produced in body by exposure to sunlight	Important in calcium and phosphorus absorption and metabolism	Poor muscle tone, retarded skeletal growth leads to rickets
E (tocopherols)	Fresh nuts, wheat germ, green leafy vegetables, seed oils	Suspected of being involved in the formation of DNA, RNA and red blood cells, inhibits membrane lipid catabolism, protects liver and lungs from toxic chemicals	Catabolism of lipids in membranes especially in red blood cells, which leads to haemolytic anaemia
K	Spinach, cauliflower, cabbage, liver and produced in large quantities by intestinal bacteria	Involved in clot formation and probably in the electron transport system	Prolonged bleeding and clotting times

complete function of minerals is still being determined, but the actions of some are already known to be essential for normal metabolism and the maintenance of homeostasis. EXAMPLES: Mineral elements such as calcium are essential for body structure whereas minerals such as sodium play important roles in fluid balance. The body appears to only use the ions of minerals, and thus minerals appear as electrolytes and salts in the body.

The required intake of each varies. Some such as sodium and calcium are needed in relatively large amounts, whereas others such as copper and zinc perform their function from the intake of only trace quantities. A summary of the main mineral elements influencing the body is given in Table 34.3. Additional information relating to electrolytes in blood is given in 26.1.

34.3 Water

Water is the most abundant inorganic compound in the body comprising about 60–70% of the total human body weight. The concentration of water in different tissues varies considerably. EXAMPLES: Fatty tissue and bones contain only minimal quantities of water; brain tissue can contain up to 75%.

The ingestion of food and beverages is the major source of water as in most foods water is the main component by weight. Catabolism of food also provides water for the body. EXAMPLES: Milk 87%, fruits and vegetables 70–90% and rare meat 75%. The oxidation of food in cellular respiration results in the production of water. EXAMPLES: 100 g of fat produces 107.1 mL of water, 100 g of

Table 34.3   The main mineral elements that influence body function

Elements	Food examples	Function
Calcium	Dairy products, egg yolk, green leafy vegetables	Necessary constituents of bone and teeth; essential for hormone manufacture, blood clotting, nerve and muscle activity
Chlorine	Salt in food processing and preparation	Important in fluid balance and hydrochloric acid formation in the stomach
Cobalt	Trace quantities required, sufficient in well-balanced diet	Essential part of vitamin B_{12} and thus plays an important role in red blood cell maturation
Copper	Trace quantities required, sufficient in well-balanced diet	Speeds up haemoglobin formation and is important in the function of some enzymes
Iodine	Trace quantities required, iodized salt, seafoods, vegetables grown in iodine-rich soils	Required for production of thyroid hormones
Iron	Meat, fish, vegetables, fruit, cereals, liver	Essential component of haemoglobin, important in production of ATP
Magnesium	Dairy products, flour, cereals, green leafy vegetables, nuts, soybeans	Required for normal nerve and muscle function
Manganese	Trace quantities required, sufficient in well-balanced diet	Important in the function of some enzymes, haemoglobin synthesis, required for growth
Phosphorus	Meat, fish, dairy products, nuts, maize	Important in acid–base balance, bone and teeth formation, nerve and muscle activity
Potassium	Present in many substances in a normal diet	Important in nerve and muscle function, essential constituent of intracellular fluid
Sodium	Found in all animal foods as salt, present in processed and prepared foods	Essential in blood volume control along with nerve and muscle function
Zinc	Trace quantities required, present in many foods	Constituent of many enzymes

carbohydrate produces 55.5 mL of water and 100 g of protein produces 41.3 g of water.

The polar property of water enables it to form hydrogen bonds and act as a solvent for ions and other polar molecules. Water plays an important role in maintaining the volume of fluid constant within the body. Changes in the volume of any fluid compartment have a significant effect on body function. In dehydration, plasma sodium increases and body weight decreases. EXAMPLE: A small decrease in cell volume is manifested as dehydration. Abnormal water balance is indicated by a change in the concentration of body fluids (plasma sodium changes) and a change in volume of the total body water. A sign of this later change is a change in body weight. The polarity of water molecules causes them to link together to form layers, which are important in maintaining the moistness of membrane surfaces. EXAMPLE: The lung membrane surfaces need to be kept moist for the diffusion of gases.

Water plays an important role in temperature homeostasis as it has the capacity to absorb large quantities of heat without rapidly changing its own temperature. This capacity, along with the large quantities present in the body, enables water to contribute significantly to the maintenance of body temperature. The evaporation of water from the skin is a means of removing large quantities of heat from the body.

Water molecules act as a medium and sometimes as a participant in body chemical reactions. EXAMPLES: The dissociation of salts into ions (17.3) and the formation of water in cellular respiration.

Water is a good tissue lubricant. It is the main ingredient of all body fluids and therefore is important in minimizing friction between adjacent body tissues. It also forms the basis of fluids that are used as protective cushions. EXAMPLE: As the major component of synovial fluid. Water is the main component of the fluid used to protect structures such as the brain and the foetus from physical damage.

34.4 Environmental health and safety

Salt intake

In most Western countries the table salt (NaCl) intake of the general population (about 10 g) is far in excess of that recommended. Excessive intake is due to the addition of salt: at the dinner table;

---

during cooking; and in the commercial processing of food. Excessive salt intake is believed to be responsible for many cases of high blood pressure (hypertension). This condition affects over 20% of the world's population.

Summary

Vitamins are organic substances that play an important role in regulating biochemical and physiological processes. Most vitamins cannot be synthesized in the body. To obtain the correct daily requirement of each vitamin it is important to have a balanced diet. Some vitamins are water soluble while others are fat soluble. The water soluble vitamins are the B complex vitamins and vitamin C. The body has difficulty in storing these vitamins, whereas the fat soluble vitamins are able to be stored in the body. The fat soluble vitamins are vitamin A, D, E and K.

Minerals are inorganic substances that function in the body in combination with other minerals or with organic substances. Some mineral elements such as sodium and calcium are needed in relatively large amounts, whereas others such as copper and zinc are only needed in trace amounts.

Both deficiencies and excesses of minerals and vitamins can produce alterations in body function.

Water is the most abundant inorganic compound in the body. It plays an important role in maintaining the volume of fluid in the body, in assisting in chemical reactions, respiratory function and temperature homeostasis and in minimizing friction between adjacent body tissues.

Unit Twelve
Medical Microbiology

This unit introduces the general features of microorganisms, with particular reference to prevention, control and body response to infectious disease. The different body defence mechanisms are discussed and other factors that initiate immune responses.

The world of microorganisms

Objectives

At the completion of this chapter the student will be able to:

1. list the main groups and subgroups of microorganisms;
2. describe the general distinguishing features of each group;
3. define the terms used to describe microbial groups, interactions and their relationship with the host.

35.1   Introduction

Microbiology involves the study of microorganisms and their effect on living cells. It is a general term encompassing the studies of viruses (virology), bacteria (bacteriology), protozoa (protozoology) and fungi (mycology). Microorganisms (microbes) are generally considered to include: viruses; cells with simple internal structures (procaryotic cells — 22.1); and cells with highly organized structures called eucaryotic cells (22.2). Eucaryotic microbes can consist of individual cells or be simple multicellular organisms. EXAMPLES: Bacteria are procaryotic microorganisms; protozoa and fungi are eucaryotic microbes; the latter group can be single-celled (yeasts) or multicellular (moulds). Medical microbiology also includes the study of the non-microbial group of organisms called helminths, because the prevention and control of diseases caused by both microorganisms and helminths involve the use of similar principles. The study of parasites (parasitology) deals with the parasitic or disease-producing protozoa (EXAMPLE: malaria) and other non-microbial parasitic organisms such as the helminths.

Medical microbiology involves the study of any organisms associated with infectious disease. An **infectious disease** occurs when a noticeable state of abnormality is induced in the body by an organism. Throughout life the body is exposed both internally and externally to a variety of microorganisms. A knowledge of the general characteristics of microorganisms is necessary in the prevention, containment and management of infectious disease.

35.2   Classifying microorganisms

A variety of approaches have been used over the years in classifying different microbes into groups according to their similarities and differences with other microbial groups. Any classification scheme provides a means of identifying a microorganism through a

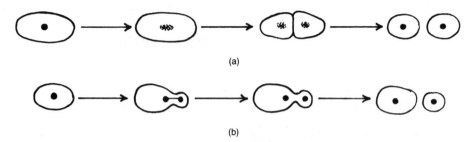

(a)

(b)

Figure 35.1 Asexual reproduction. (a) Bacterium undergoing binary fission. (b) Budding of a yeast cell.

comparative checklist of features. Microorganisms need to be identified in order to treat an infection in an appropriate way. The classification of microbial groups in this book has been based upon the currently accepted one. Because of their individual features, mycoplasma, rickettsiae and chlamydiae are discussed as a separate microbial group, even though they are generally accepted as part of the procaryotic group of microorganisms. Table 35.1 summarizes the similarities and differences of the microbial groups referred to in medical microbiology.

35.3 Sexual and asexual reproduction

One common property of microbes is their ability to reproduce rapidly. Many microbes reproduce by **asexual reproduction**, which usually involves the division of one cell to form two identical daughter cells (**binary fission**): EXAMPLE: Most bacteria (Figure 35.1a). Some microbes undergo a form of asexual cell division called **budding** in which a small new cell is pinched off the parent cell. EXAMPLE: Yeast (Figure 35.1b).

Sexual reproduction involves the combining of two nuclei of different cells in fertilization and the mixing of their genetic material. Microorganisms use several different methods to achieve fertilization. EXAMPLES: In some fungi and protozoa, two cells fuse and the genetic material of one cell is transferred to the other cell. This process is called **conjugation**.

35.4 Cyanobacteria

Cyanobacteria, formerly known as blue–green algae, are procaryotic, single-celled organisms (35.4) widely distributed throughout water and land. They play an important role in the production of oxygen and form supplies of nutrient for fish. Cyanobacteria are more closely related to bacteria than to other algae. The cells can exist singly or in colonies of nearly identical rods or spheres (Figure 35.2). Cells within a colony are held together by a sheath of mucoid membranes. Each cell is surrounded by a stiff cell wall containing mucopeptide. The rigid cell walls and the lack of flagella (tails) or cilia mean that these microbes are virtually non-motile. Cyanobacteria differ from bacteria in their photosynthetic pigments and release of oxygen during photosynthesis. They produce some antibiotic-like substances but are generally of little significance in medical microbiology.

Table 35.1 General features of microbial groups

Feature	Cyanobacteria	Bacteria*	Mycoplasma	Rickettsiae	Chlamydiae	Viruses	Protozoa	Fungi	Helminths
Size	0.5–60 µm	0.2–5.0 µm	0.2–0.3 µm	0.3–3.0 µm	0.2–0.8 µm	0.01–0.3 µm	4 µm–0.1 cm	2 µm–100 cm	1–100 cm
Cell form	Procaryotic	Procaryotic	Procaryotic	Procaryotic	Procaryotic	Acellular	Eucaryotic	Eucaryotic	Eucaryotic
Cell wall	Yes	Yes	No	Yes	Yes	No	No	Yes	No
DNA/RNA	Both	Both	Both	Both	Both	Either	Both	Both	Both
Unicellular/ multicellular	Unicellular	Unicellular	Unicellular	Unicellular	Unicellular	Single particles	Unicellular	Either	Multicellular
Form of reproduction	Asexual	Asexual/DNA exchange	Asexual	Asexual	Asexual	Replication	Asexual/sexual	Asexual/sexual	Sexual
Parasites Internal/ external	Internal	Internal	Internal (intracellular)	Internal (intracellular)	Internal (intracellular)	Internal (intracellular)	Internal (some intracellular)	Either	Internal
Synthesize own ATP	Yes	Yes	Yes	Yes	No	No	Yes	Yes	Yes

*Including filamentous bacteria of up to 100 µm.

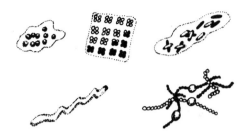

Figure 35.2   Examples of different forms of cyanobacteria.

35.5   Bacteria

Bacteria are similar in cell structure to cyanobacteria but, whereas all cyanobacteria contain photosynthetic pigment, only a few bacterial subgroups do. Figure 35.4 shows typical bacterial cells. The features that distinguish the several thousand bacterial subgroups or species are size, shape, group patterns, and cellular structure. NOTE: A bacterial species is defined as a population of cells with similar characteristics. This differs from the eucaryotic definition described previously (22.2). *Bergey's Manual* is the standard bacterial classification reference used to identify a bacteria. Bacteria can be broadly divided into gram-positive and gram-negative according to their response to the gram stain (22.13 — Application: Gram positive and gram negative bacteria). Some bacteria are capable of living only in the absence of oxygen (**anaerobes**), whereas most bacteria require oxygen to live (**aerobes**). Between these extremes there is a group of bacteria that can adapt to live in either an aerobic or anaerobic environment. They are called **facultative bacteria**. EXAMPLE: *Staphylococcus aureus, Escherichia coli.*

Application: *Escherichia coli*

These bacteria present the typical procaryotic ultrastructure (Figure 35.3a) and usually exist in colonies of rods (Figure 35.3b). *E. coli* is probably the most widely investigated microorganism in microbiology. It is widely used as a model from which are derived a general understanding of bacterial function. *E. coli* are widely used in genetic engineering (35.9 — Application: Genetic engineering) and biotechnology.

E. coli is a common inhabitant of the small intestine. Its presence in food or water is used as an indicator of faecal contamination.

Bacteria are classified according to shape as: **cocci** (spherical), **bacilli** (rod-like) and the **spiral** or **helical** forms (Figure 35.4).

Cocci

Cocci (singular is coccus) can form pairs (diplococci) or chains of variable length (streptococci) by cell division in one plane (Figure 35.4). Diplococci are responsible for bacterial meningitis and gonorrhoea, whereas streptococci are responsible for many upper respiratory tract infections. Cell divisions which alternate in two planes can produce cuboidal groups. Irregular splitting on several planes produces an irregular grape-like cluster (staphyloccoci). EXAMPLE: *Staphylococcus aureus.*

Bacilli

Bacilli (bacillus, singular) are rod-shaped bacteria which can form pairs, (diplobacilli) or chains (streptobacilli) (Figure 35.4d). Many

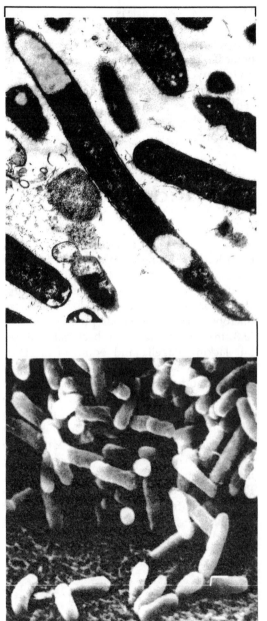

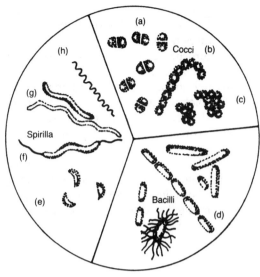

Figure 35.4 Different bacterial forms. Cocci —
(a) diplococci (b) streptococci (c)
staphylococci. Bacilli — (d)
flagellated and non-flagellated
forms. Spiral forms — (e) vibrio (f)
flagellated form (g) non-flagellated
form (h) spirochaeta.

of the bacillus group form large gram-positive
rods containing endospores (Figure 22.5).
EXAMPLE: Clostridia. The clostridia are
responsible for a variety of diseases, botulism
(*Clostridium botulinum*), tetanus (*C. tetans*) and
gas gangrene (several clostridia species).

Spiral forms

The **spiral** forms occur mainly as unattached
individual cells. The length and number of
spirals varies in different species. **Vibrio**, or
comma-shaped bacteria, are short and contain incomplete spirals (Figure 35.4e).
EXAMPLE: *Vibrio cholerae* causes cholera.
Spirilla (spirillum, singular) are rigid spiral-
shaped bacteria that either have no flagella
and are therefore non-motile (Figure 35.4f,g)

Figure 35.3 *E. coli*. (a) Ultrastructure (×20 000)
and (b) external appearance
(×10 000).

or else can move with the aid of flagella (22.13) (Figure 35.4f, g). EXAMPLES: *Spirillum minor* causes rat-bite fever.

The **spirochaetes** are a large diverse group of spiral-shaped microbes which, although possessing no flagella, propel themselves by the flexible motion of structures wrapped around the cell called axial filaments (Figure 35.4h). Three of the important groups are Treponema, Borrelia and Leptospira. EXAMPLES: *Treponema pallidum* causes syphilis; *Borellia recurrentis* causes relapsing fever or borreliosis, a leptospira is responsible for Weil's disease or leptospirosis, and *Leptospira interrogans* causes infective jaundice.

35.6 Mycoplasma

The **mycoplasmas** were previously called pleuropneumonia-like organisms or PPLO. They are often classified as belonging to the bacterial group, but some of their properties are different from those of the other major forms of bacteria. Mycoplasma are considered to be the smallest free-living self-replicating units of life. They are capable of independent growth and metabolism, and because they are similar in size to the larger viruses they can act as intracellular parasites. Since they lack a bacterial cell wall, they can assume various shapes and alter their size. They are bounded by a unit membrane which is gram negative (22.13). A tip structure enables mycoplasmas to anchor themselves to epithelial cells and thus resist the cleaning action of mucus and cilia.

Mycoplasmas are widely distributed in nature. They form part of the normal microbial population in the mouth, respiratory and urogenital membranes of humans. They can cause inflammatory conditions of the respiratory and urogenital tracts.

Mycoplasma pneumoniae is one of the causative agents of primary atypical pneumonia. Mycoplasmas are completely resistant to penicillin but are inhibited by tetracycline or erythromycin. They can grow on appropriate cell-free media. When grown on agar the centre of the whole colony is embedded beneath the surface giving a 'fried egg' appearance.

35.7 Rickettsiae

These procaryotic microbes were often regarded as being intermediate between bacteria and viruses but are usually now classified as part of the bacterial group. **Rickettsiae** comprise about a dozen different microbes. They are small procaryotic cells (0.3 μm) containing most bacterial features but lacking flagella and endospores. They exist as very short rods which can be paired or form short chains; they divide like bacteria and are sensitive to antibiotics. Rickettsiae differ from mycoplasma in being unable to survive outside a host cell. Once inside a living cell they grow and divide within the cytoplasm. They are spread by blood-sucking insects such as lice, fleas, ticks and mites. Rickettsial diseases in humans are characterized by fever and rash. EXAMPLES: Typhus fever, Q. fever and Rocky Mountain spotted fever.

35.8 Chlamydiae

Chlamydiae or **Bedosoniae** are small-celled intracellular parasites which lack certain mechanisms for the production of energy which they have to acquire from the biochemicals around them in the host cell.

This total intracellular dependence led to their classification as viruses, but it is now recognized that they have features that are distinct from those of viruses. They show some similarities to bacteria, e.g. both chlamydiae and bacteria contain DNA and RNA, multiply by binary fission, possess ribosomes and respond to antimicrobial drugs whereas viruses lack these features. The cell wall of chylamydiae is similar in structure to that of gram negative bacteria and is inhibited by penicillins. Chlamydiae are similar to rickettsiae and are currently placed within this group.

Chlamydiae have a complex and unique life cycle which begins when the small thick-walled infectious form binds onto the surface of a potential host cell following transmission from a host such as birds. The chlamydiae is phagocytosed (Figure 23.10) and incorporated into a vacuole within the host cell. In the next 24–48 hours the thick wall becomes thinner and the chlamydiae undergoes rapid binary fission until the host's vacuole is completely filled with a microcolony of chlamydiae. The walls of the cells in the colony thicken in preparation for release from the host cell and attachment to other cells. EXAMPLE: *Chlamydia trachomatis* is a major cause of urogenital tract infections in humans and the eye disease, trachoma.

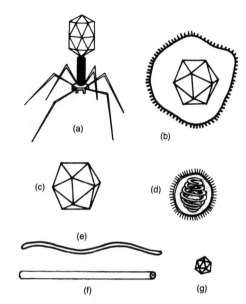

Figure 35.5 The relative size and diversity of viruses: (a) T-even bacteriophage, (b) herpes virus, (c) adenovirus, (d) influenza virus, (e) filamentous virus, (f) rodlike virus, (g) poliovirus.

35.9 Viruses

Viruses are the smallest living infectious agents (Figures 35.5 and 35.6). Because they lack cellular structure (acellular) viruses have to use the biochemical machinery and raw materials of a host cell for 'reproduction' or replication.

A virus particle consists of the reproductive material DNA or RNA in a 'core' surrounded by a protective protein coat (or **capsid**) and enzymes used for entry into a host cell (Figure 35.5). The capsid protects the inner hereditary material containing genes and also helps the virus particle to attach to the host cell. An additional layer containing a mixture of organic material sometimes overlays the capsid. The entire virus particle, with or without the additional layer, is called a **virion**. The virion is the extracellular infectious form capable of surviving in the extracellular environment. The virion is able to attach to a specific site on the surface of a potential host cell and either the whole virion or part of it enters the cell by methods such as phagocytosis, pinocytosis or injection. It is not essential for a virion to enter a cell. EXAMPLE: In some bacterial viruses only the genetic material (**genome**) is injected into

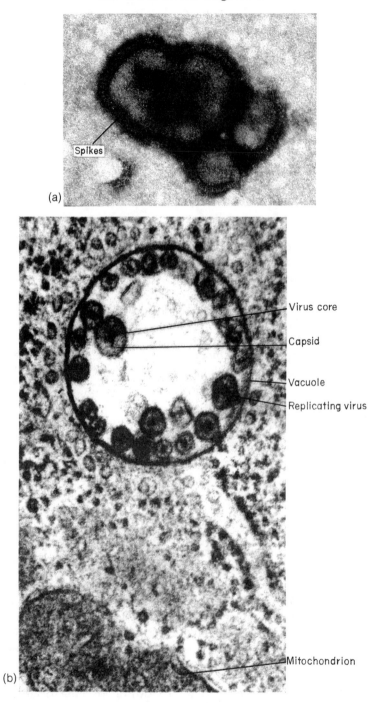

Figure 35.6 Virus structure (a) flu virus showing spikes (×156 000) (b) Dengue virus located within a vacuole (×130 000).

the bacterium while the capsid remains on the cell's surface.

A virus follows one of two pathways after entering the cell. Firstly, the genome, consisting of several genes, can redirect the host's genetic machinery to produce new virus particles using the raw materials within the cell. EXAMPLE: A cell infected with a poliomyelitis virus can produce 10 000 new virions. The second pathway involves an initial latent period when the virus remains inactive. Such viruses can remain inactive for long periods without interfering with the activities of the cell or the well-being of the host organism. EXAMPLE: The herpes virus remains latent within nerve cells until a stress factor activates it.

The effect of virus production on host cells varies according to the virus. The cell either dies, survives or is transformed. When the cells die they release their contents of virions to the extracellular fluid. EXAMPLE: Poliomyelitis. In some instances, the host cell is able to satisfy the biochemical requirements of both the virus and itself and the virus is subsequently extruded through the cell wall without killing the host. EXAMPLE: Filamentous DNA bacteriophages. Virus forms with similar genetic structures to their host are able to integrate with the chromosomal DNA of the host cells causing an increase in the rate of cellular metabolism and multiplication of the host cell. The host cell has been transformed into a potential tumour-forming cell. A virus with the potential for forming a tumour is called an **oncogenic virus**. EXAMPLE: Papovaviruses possess oncogenic potential for the formation of a papilloma tumour.

Viruses usually infect specific types of cells. EXAMPLE: A virus that invades bacteria will not invade human cells. Viruses can be broadly classified according to the host organism which they normally infect; animal, bacterial, plant and insect viruses. EXAMPLE: Viruses that invade bacteria are called **bacteriophages** or **phages**. Figure 35.7 shows a typical bacteriophage life cycle. A more specific classification of viruses is based on their DNA or RNA content or on their general chemical composition, size, structural features and other measurable features.

Application: Genetic engineering

The ability of viruses to invade bacteria and alter a host's manufacturing capacity is made use of in genetic engineering. A gene representing the manufacture of a desired polypeptide is inserted into the DNA of bacteria, such as *Escherichia coli*. The *E. coli* then produce the desired protein in a similar fashion to the proteins required for a virion. Human hormones such as insulin and enzymes can therefore be manufactured by the biochemical machinery of bacteria. Genetic engineering is expected to play an ever increasing role in diagnostic and therapeutic aspects of health care in the future.

35.10   Protozoa

Protozoa are single-celled eucaryotic organisms which ingest their food materials as particles. The food is usually digested in a vacuole. They are the largest unicellular organisms.

When protozoa are exposed to adverse conditions they generally have the capacity to form a cuticle (not a true cell wall) and become inactive. The resulting **cyst** can resist adverse conditions. When conditions become favourable the protozoa return to their active state. The formation of a cyst sometimes precedes reproduction. Some protozoa are

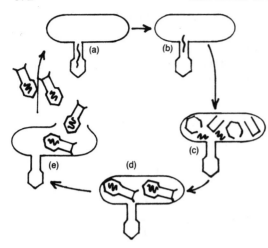

Figure 35.7   The typical bacteriophage life cycle.
(a) Virus attaches to bacterium.
(b) Viral DNA hereditary material
(genome) is injected into bacterium.
(c) Synthesis of new viral DNA and
proteins. (d) Assembly of virus.
(e) Release of viruses.

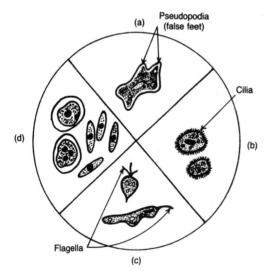

Figure 35.8   The protozoa subgroups (a)
Sarcodina, (b) Ciliophora, (c)
Mastigophora, (d) Sporozoa.

able to reproduce sexually. EXAMPLE: The malaria-causing plasmodium. Amoeba and the flagellates simply reproduce asexually by dividing into two or more parts to form new organisms.

Protozoa are divided into groups according to their means of locomotion (Figure 35.8). The following groups contain organisms associated with disease in humans. The **Sarcodina** or **Rhizopodea** group move by bulging and retracting their protoplasm in the form of a false foot or pseudopod. EXAMPLE: *Entamoeba histolytica* which causes amoebic dysentery. The entamoeba can be transferred as cysts in faeces or contaminated food and water. The **Ciliophora** or **Ciliata** move by the rapid rhythmic beating of cilia. EXAMPLE: *Balantidium coli* can cause chronic recurrent dysentery. The **Mastigophora** group or flagellates use the whiplike actions of flagella. EXAMPLE: *Trichomonas vaginalis* causes trichomoniasis, a widespread infection of the urogenital tract. **Giardiasis** is one of the most common parasitic diseases of the gastrointestinal tract. The **Sporozoa** have no external means of locomotion and are amongst the most important of the disease-producing protozoa. Their complex life cycle includes a spore stage. Blood-sucking insects are a common vehicle for the transmission of this protozoan group. EXAMPLE: Some types of plasmodia are capable of causing malaria when transmitted by certain types of mosquito.

35.11   Fungi

Fungi are a large diverse group of eucaryotic organisms. Only about one hundred of the many thousands of fungi types cause disease in humans. These non-photosynthetic organisms range from relatively simple unicellular organisms such as yeast, to multicellular

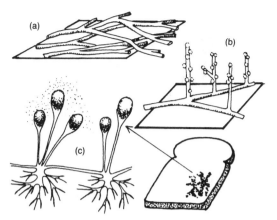

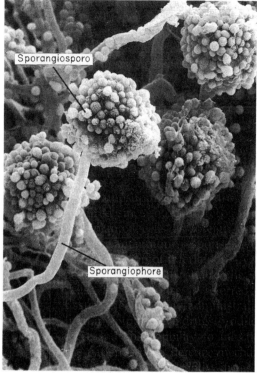

Figure 35.9 Fungi showing (a) vegetative mycelium, (b) hyphae with spores and (c) sporangia.

Figure 35.10 Fungi from bread showing sporangium containing many sporangiospores (×500).

structures such as mushrooms and moulds. Fungi, like plants, contain a cell wall for rigidity and shape (22.12). Multicellular fungi consist of a mass called a **mycelium** (Figure 35.9a), which consists of a network of threadlike structures called **hyphae** (Figure 35.9b). Adjacent cells within hyphae may be separated by cross walls or may be perforated thereby allowing the free movement of nuclei and cytoplasm within the hyphae. The final size of a mycelium depends on the availability of nutrients and a satisfactory environment for growth. The portion of the mycelium penetrating into the nutrient medium is called the **vegetative mycelium**, while the part projecting above the surface of the medium is called the **aerial or reproductive mycelium**.

Hyphae are formed from the elongation of reproductive cells called **spores**. Fungi are mainly classified into groups according to their method of asexual or sexual spore formation. Some fungi form sexual spores when the nuclei of two hyphae make contact with each other and fuse. Other fungi form asexual spores by either pinching off swollen bodies in the reproductive mycelium or

by forming spores in internal sacs. Spores are often concentrated in aerial sacs called **sporangia** (Figure 35.9c). A sporangium can contain hundreds of spores called sporangiospores (Figure 35.10). Spores are used as a vehicle for spreading fungi as they are easily transported to new environments. If the new environment is favourable the spores germinate and produce new hyphae.

Fungal or mycotic infections can be divided into superficial, subcutaneous and deep (systemic) mycoses. The general health of patients is usually not affected by superficial fungal infections of the skin, hair and nails. The dermatophytes are an important group of similar fungi that only invade superficial tissue. EXAMPLES: Two forms of ringworm are *Tinea glabrosa*, which is tinea of the skin, and *Tinea cruris*, which is tinea of the groin. *Tinea pedis* or athletes foot is caused by either trichophyton fungi or *Epidermophyton floccosum*. Treatment involves the thorough removal of infected and dead epithelial structures followed by the application of a topical antifungal agent. Fungi involved in subcutaneous mycoses grow in soil and on decaying vegetation and may enter the subcutaneous tissue through damaged skin. EXAMPLE: *Sporothrix schenckii* causes the chronic condition sporotrichosis. Systemic mycoses are usually acquired by inhaling certain soil fungi. EXAMPLE: Histoplasmosis is caused by *Histoplasma capsulatum*. Some mycoses are initiated when the normal bacterial population has been subjected to an extended period of broad spectrum antibiotics. EXAMPLE: Thrush is caused by a large increase in the natural population of the yeast, *Candida albicans*.

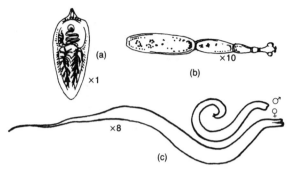

Figure 35.11 General features of helminths. (a) The fluke, *Fasciola hepatica*. (b) The tapeworm, *Echinococcus granulosus*. (c) The roundworm, *Enterobius vermicularis*.

35.12   Helminths

Medical microbiology usually includes a study of the parasitic worms or helminths. The vast majority of health-related helminths are represented by the flatworms (platyhelminths) and the roundworms (nematoda or Aschelminths) (Figure 35.11). Both groups contain specific structures such as nervous, excretory and reproductive systems. The helminths vary in size from nearly microscopic to over one metre in length. Diagnosis of these worms usually requires the recognition of the immature microscopic sized stages (larvae and eggs) in the faeces. The prevention and control of helminths require the use of microbiological principles.

Flatworms

There are two medically important groups of flatworms: **flukes** (Trematoda) and **tapeworms** (Cestoda). The flukes are flat leaflike worms lacking segmentation and with suckers for attachment to the host. Flukes often have a complicated life cycle involving several intermediate hosts. After entry into the body they inhabit specific sites where they develop into adults. The common sites for flukes include the intestine (*Fasciolopsis buski*), lung (*Paragonimus westermannii*), liver (*Fasciola hepatica*) (Figure 35.11a) and blood (Shistosomas). Flukes can be divided into two groups according to their sexual characteristics: a group containing both male and female sex organs (hermaphroditic), and a group containing only one sex organ (bisexual). The fertilized eggs of all flukes can be found in faeces.

Tapeworms are elongated ribbonlike segmented worms which cause chronic digestive disorders. They contain a head with muscular suckers and sometimes hooks for attaching themselves to the intestinal wall (Figure 35.11). Below the head is a growth area from which arises a series of mature segments containing both male and female sex organs. Individual segments containing eggs can break off and be removed in the faeces while the head is still attached to the intestinal wall and still able to produce new segments, thus enabling the worm to continue growing. The eggs released in the faeces must undergo stages of larval development in intermediate hosts such as fish, pigs or cattle before the adult form inhabits humans. EXAMPLE: Pig tapeworm (*Taenia solium*) undergoes stages of larval development within the pig and is transferred to humans who eat the improperly cooked meat.

Roundworms

Roundworms lack segments but contain a complete digestive tract. They have a long elongated body which tapers at both ends (Figure 35.11c). A few members of this group have hooks or cutting plates around the mouth for attaching to intestinal walls. EXAMPLE: Hookworms. There are two different sexes in most roundworms, and they reproduce sexually, whereas the flatworms are bisexual or hermaphroditic.

Roundworms exist in all types of habitat and each type has a distinct life cycle. EXAMPLES: Pinworms (*Enterobius vermicularis*) have no intermediate hosts in their life cycle and they have the capacity for reinfection within the gastrointestinal tract. After the eggs have been ingested, the larvae hatch and develop directly into adults within the intestine. Ascariasis (*Ascaris lumbricoides*) has no intermediate hosts but only becomes infective when it matures, after two to three weeks incubation in the soil. After being ingested, they penetrate the intestinal walls, enter the circulation and travel to the lungs and thence to the trachea. They are then coughed up and swallowed. On re-arrival in the small intestine they develop into adults.

35.13 Microbial ecology

Ecology is the study of the relationship of organisms to their environment. Humans and other animals live in a microbial environment. Microbes are found within our body, on the body's surface, in the air we breathe, in the water, in the soil, in many foods we eat and on most objects that we touch. Microorganisms usually exist in an environment consisting of different microbial groups. These microbial groups may or may not influence each other. The interrelationships between microorganisms and their host may be harmless, beneficial or harmful. A study of microbial group interactions and their relationship with the host is necessary in order to understand the impact of microbes on body homeostasis. General ecological terms are used to describe these interrelationships.

Neutralism or **independence** refers to a completely independent association where neither organism affects the existence of the other. It can occur between two microbial populations when no competition exists between each population for any nutrient present in limited quantities.

Symbiosis is a collective term used to describe any dependent association between two different populations. This term is often used interchangeably with mutualism although mutualism refers to only one form of symbiosis.

Mutualism refers to a co-existence in which each organism benefits from the association. EXAMPLE: In humans and many animals bacteria in the intestinal tract depend upon the human's ingested food for nutrients. Some of these bacteria produce vitamin K which can be absorbed into the body for the benefit of the host although the host is not dependent on this supply of vitamin K.

Commensalism occurs when only one

organism benefits from the association while the other is not affected. Commensalism is a very common form of interrelationship between humans and microbes, as humans can supply an environment favourable to the growth of particular microbes. EXAMPLES: Microbes living off non-living organic substances on body surfaces and within the gastrointestinal tract. The commensal microbes can be arranged into two groups: microbes regularly occupying a region (resident flora) and those nonpermanent microorganisms inhabiting a region (transient flora). The transient flora are derived from the environment and inhabit the skin and mucous membranes for a limited time.

Antagonism refers to a relationship in which one microbial population adversely affects the growth of another. This can be due to one population secreting a substance that either inhibits the growth of or kills the other group. EXAMPLE: Strains of the mould Penicillium produce the antibacterial substance penicillin. One microbe may produce five or six different antimicrobial agents (antibiotics) to ensure success in a competitive environment. Another possible mechanism of antagonism is the initiation of a host defence mechanism by one group to be used against the other. The presence of microbial antagonism is sometimes detected when antibiotics are administered to a patient for a specific microbe. The appearance of another infection can indicate an antagonistic relationship, the microbe responsible for the second infection being now able to grow in the absence of the suppressing action of the treated microbe. Some diseases therefore require the administration of a combination of antibiotics.

Parasitism is a relationship between organisms in which one organism derives some degree of support from another at the latter's expense. The parasite feeds on the cells, tissues, or fluids of another organism.

A **saprophyte** obtains nutrients from non-living organic material produced by or derived from other organisms. A saprophyte can become a parasite if it derives its support at the expense of the host. Parasitism is most successful when the host is able to supply the required nutritional support while continuing to function within reasonably normal limits. This relationship ensures the survival and growth of both the host and parasite. Parasites living within tissues or cells of the host are called **internal parasites** or **endoparasites**. EXAMPLES: Hookworm in the gastrointestinal tract. Parasites living on the skin or outer mucousal surfaces of the host are called **external parasites** or **ectoparasites**. These parasites utilize living host tissue or blood. The presence of ectoparasites on a host is called an **infestation**. The entry of parasites into an organism can result in an infection.

Summary

Medical microbiology involves the study of the prevention, containment and management of infectious disease. The areas of study in medical microbiology are bacteriology, virology, protozoology, mycology and parasitology.

The preceding topics of this chapter have discussed the diversity in microbial life and the mechanisms that microbes use for surviving in their environment. Associated with this capacity to survive is their relative ability to be transmitted to new environments. The prevention and control of diseases relate to the characteristics of each microbial group and the ability of each group to survive, grow and reproduce in a particular environment. The methods of transmission of a particular group to new environments must be understood if the most effective approach to limiting the spread of a microbe is to be applied. The procaryotic microbial groups are:

1. Cyanobacteria are procaryotic cells containing photosynthetic pigments and a cell wall. These microbes are of little significance in medical microbiology.
2. The bacterial group contains many similar structures to the cyanobacteria. There are several thousand bacterial subgroups, distinguished by features such as size (mycoplasma), shape (cocci, bacilli and spiral), group patterns (diplo-, strepto- and staphylo-), cellular structure (spores, flagellum, gram-positive and gram–negative) and biochemical function (aerobic and anaerobic).

The small sizes of mycoplasma, rickettsiae and chlamydiae enable these microbial subgroups to act as intracellular parasites.

The viruses are acellular structures that act as intracellular parasites by utilizing the host cell's biochemical machinery. The extracellular infectious form or virion has a protective protein which coats the hereditary material. The virus host cell either dies, transforms or survives. Oncogenic viruses are able to transform a host cell into a tumour-forming cell.

Protozoa are single-celled eucaryotic organisms. Many of these organisms can form inactive cysts during adverse conditions. Protozoa are divided into the subgroups sarcodina, ciliophora, mastigophora and sporozoa.

Fungi are a large diverse group of eucaryotic plants that range from unicellular organisms such as yeast to multicellular structures such as moulds. The multicellular fungi are made up of hyphae which form a branching interlacing network called the mycelium. Fungi are classified into subgroups according to their method of spore formation.

The platyhelminths and nematoda represent the majority of health related helminths. These multicellular eucaryotic organisms are usually diagnosed by the presence of microscopic sized stages of these organisms in the faeces. The two medically important groups of flatworms are trematoda and cestoda. Most of the helminths are gastrointestinal parasites.

Microorganisms are found in the following ecological interrelationships: neutralism, symbiosis, mutualism, commensalism, antagonism and parasitism.

Chapter 36

Microorganisms and disease

Objectives

At the completion of this chapter the student will be able to:

1. describe the factors involved in the infection process;
2. describe the ways in which common diseases are spread;
3. describe the methods used to prevent and control infectious disease;
4. define the terms used to describe the destroying or suppressing of microbes;
5. explain the mechanisms of action of antimicrobial agents.

36.1 The infective process

The process of infection involves the microbes' points of entry into the body, establishment and multiplication within the host and the point of discharge from the body. It also involves the microbes' capacity to cause disease and the host's capacity to resist infection.

The capacity to cause disease is called **pathogenicity**. A non-pathogen is a non-disease producing microbe. Many non-pathogens such as resident flora have the capacity to produce infection and disease when the host's environment is altered or when there is a decrease in body defence mechanisms due to a factor such as stress, age or organic disease. The distinction between pathogen and non-pathogen is dependent upon individual host responses to a particular microbe.

Virulence is a term which describes the relative ability of a pathogen to produce a disease. EXAMPLE: A strain of bacteria that requires fewer microbes to produce infection than another strain under particular conditions, is considered to be more virulent than the latter. Virulence depends on invasiveness and toxigenicity. **Invasiveness** is the ability to infect hosts, survive and multiply; **toxigenicity** is the ability to produce substances that are toxic to the host. Microbes are generally most virulent when freshly dispersed by an infected person and are usually less virulent in a carrier. The fewer the microbes entering the body, the lower their chance of overcoming body defence mechanisms.

When a population is infected by an endoparasite a percentage of the population displays no symptoms of the disease. An individual containing the microbe but lacking symptoms is termed a **carrier**. The presence of carriers indicates that an infection may occur without disease. The carrier can still spread the infectious agent, which she or he temporarily harbours for varying periods of time. EXAMPLE: In typhoid fever there can be long-term carriers.

To minimize the risk of or prevent the transmission of an infectious disease one must have a knowledge of the entry, exit and transmission routes of the microbe. Infection commences at the site of entry of an endoparasite into a host. The major sites in humans are: respiratory tract, gastrointestinal tract, urogenital tract, skin and superficial mucous membranes. The point of entry also presents the last opportunity to prevent an infection and therefore understanding microbial modes of entry is important in the prevention and control of infectious diseases.

The points of entry or portal of entry vary for different microbes. EXAMPLES: Dermatophytes such as ringworm infect the skin whereas the influenza virus enters by the inhalation of droplets. The respiratory tract is the easiest portal of entry and the most difficult to control. Microbes in inhaled air are subjected to nasal hair filtration, mechanical removal and re-routing by mucus into the throat. Body defence mechanisms are described in Chapter 37. The gastrointestinal route offers an easy entry point for microbial groups as any microorganism in contact with the hands, food or drink can enter the mouth.

The skin, mucous membranes and urogenital tract offer more limited access to microbes than the respiratory tract and gastrointestinal tract. When microbes are deposited directly into deeper tissues as a result of factors such as trauma and injection the route is called the **parenteral route**. Any factor that alters the normal external defence mechanisms protecting the various portals of entry will allow easier access to microbes with an increased likelihood of infection. EXAMPLE: Tissue trauma. The relative ability of a particular microbial group to enter

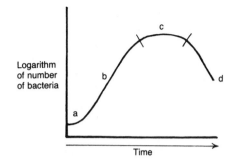

Figure 36.1 The growth stages of microbes. (a) Lag phase, (b) growth (or log) phase, (c) stationary phase and (d) death phase.

the body will affect the establishment and survival of the microbe within the host.

The **incubation period** is the time interval between the infection and the appearance of the first symptoms of the disease. **The ability of a microbe to establish itself and multiply within the host following entry into the body depends on the supply of nutrients from the host, the defence mechanisms of the microbe, its ability to spread throughout tissues, and the defence mechanisms of the host.** The environmental conditions near the entry site play an important role in the invasiveness of a microbe. A lack of oxygen will inhibit the growth of oxygen-dependent (aerobic) microbes but have no effect on anaerobic microbes. Other factors such as acidity and relative availability of nutrients also play a key role.

In a favourable environment microbes will grow and reproduce rapidly. The development of a microbial population and the establishment of infection in the body follow four distinct phases (Figure 36.1).

The first, or **lag**, phase represents a period of no growth in which the microbes adapt to their new environment. This period corresponds to the incubation period of some diseases. The **log** or **exponential** phase is the growth phase of the population. It represents the period of greatest rise in cell population when there is a plentiful supply of nutrients. This phase corresponds to the appearance and spread of the symptoms of disease. The **stationary** phase is characterized by a levelling off in cell division (Figure 36.1). The rate of reproduction is now approximately equal to the rate of microbial death, owing to a slow depletion of nutrients and the accumulation of toxic waste products. This phase often corresponds to the period of maximum impact of the disease (acute period). The **decline** or **death** phase occurs when a greater number of microbes are dying than are being produced, probably because of the accumulation of toxic substances, a depletion of available nutrients or the effects of the host's defence mechanisms. In this phase, which corresponds to the recovery phase of the body in fighting an infection, the disease symptoms are subsiding and a feeling of well-being develops. Spore-forming bacteria may not demonstrate a death phase. The duration and slope of each phase will vary to some extent according to the type of microbe and the effectiveness of the host's defence mechanisms.

Microbes have a variety of **defence mechanisms** which can be used to defend themselves against host defence mechanisms. EXAMPLE: Bacterial cells can contain capsules or surface coatings that resist phagocytosis. Some microbes release toxins to destroy the phagocytic cells. An increase in the effectiveness of a microbe's defence mechanism can result in an increase in virulence.

The relative ability of the host's defence mechanisms to destroy a pathogenic microbe depends on previous exposure to the microbe, extent of trauma at site of entry, health of patient and the state of the body's defence mechanisms.

Once a colony has been established a pathogen may remain confined to a particular location (localized infection). EXAMPLE: Abscesses and boils. Other microbes may spread throughout the body in a generalized infection. The spread is assisted by the lymphatic system and bloodstream. **Bacteraemia** occurs when bacteria are found in the bloodstream but do not multiply. **Septicaemia** occurs when bacteria multiply in the bloodstream causing an infection of the bloodstream. **Viraemia** refers to the presence of viruses in the blood. Viruses can spread by releasing toxins that destroy surrounding tissue while some bacteria release enzymes that increase the permeability of the gel in the tissue spaces. EXAMPLE: Enzyme hyaluronidase. When toxins enter the bloodstream and cause disease the condition is called **toxaemia**.

Pathogenic microbes also have routes of discharge called portals of exit. The important portals of exit are: faeces; urine; mouth; nose and respiratory passage discharges; saliva and blood. Contact with these exit points or excretions from that region will result in the contamination of objects and the spreading of the microbe. Any measures aimed at containment of a particular infection require a knowledge of the exit point of the microbe. EXAMPLE: Faeces may contain the salmonella bacterium and discharges from the respiratory tract may contain the bacterium causing whooping cough or the influenza virus.

36.2   Spread of infection

An understanding of the ways in which common diseases are spread is important in minimizing the spread of infection and preventing future outbreaks of the disease.

The ability of a pathogen to spread disease

is dependent on: its ease of access to the diseased host's excretions; its ability to survive in a possibly harmful environment between the two hosts and its ability to infect a susceptible host.

Communicability refers to the ability of a microbe to be communicated to another person from an infected individual. Pathogens vary in communicability, which is dependent upon the host that supports survival and multiplication of the pathogen and its relative ease of transmission. The term 'a reservoir of infection' refers to the source where the microbe has survived and multiplied. The period of communicability is the time or times during which the pathogen may be transferred directly or indirectly from a source of infection. EXAMPLE: Measles is a highly communicable disease for a period of about nine days, i.e. from four days before the rash appears to about five days afterwards.

The main modes of transmission are direct and indirect contact. Direct contact involves close physical encounters, though not necessarily actual bodily contact, between the susceptible and the infected persons. EXAMPLES: Handshaking and sexual intercourse. Some of the diseases transmitted by direct contact are: measles, sexually transmitted disease, staphylococcal diseases and tinea. **Indirect contact** refers to the spread of the microbe to a susceptible person via an intermediate contaminated object called a **fomite**. The object and even food items have the capacity to harbour the microbes which are transferred to a susceptible person who handles the object or places food in the mouth. EXAMPLES: Water, foods, air, toilet articles, doorhandles, toys, bedding, glasses and instruments may all transmit infection by indirect contact.

Airborne or **droplet infection** is a common method of spreading respiratory tract infections. The larger droplets of mucus containing pathogens can settle and contaminate dust on the floor, equipment and furniture. Pathogens on the smaller droplets (droplet nuclei) can remain alive suspended in air for long periods.

Ingestion of contaminated food enables particular microbes to enter the intestine and cause diseases such as gastroenteritis. Flies, cockroaches and vermin can convey pathogens to food, though these are not the main sources of contamination. The cooking of foods prior to eating decreases the likelihood of food-borne diseases, providing correct temperature storage of the food is maintained after cooking. The ingestion of improperly cooked pork can result in Trichinosis and tapeworm infections. Attention to personal hygiene and clean food preparation areas are essential for minimizing food contamination, and preventing spread of such diseases as Hepatitis A, Shigellosis.

Insects such as flies can convey disease by mechanically transferring it on parts of their body such as feet. Sometimes an insect transfers the infection by biting. EXAMPLES: Mosquitoes transfer malaria, dengue fever (36.7 — Application: Mosquito-borne diseases) yellow fever (Figure 36.2), eastern and western encephalitis; the rat flea transfers the bubonic plague bacterium.

Fomites are objects that spread infection, such as handkerchiefs, bedding, glasses, towels and money. To prevent the spread of the disease by indirect contact all articles used by an infectious patient should be regarded as contaminated. The articles should be carefully disinfected or destroyed. (8.2 — Application: Antiseptics and disinfectants and 36.5).

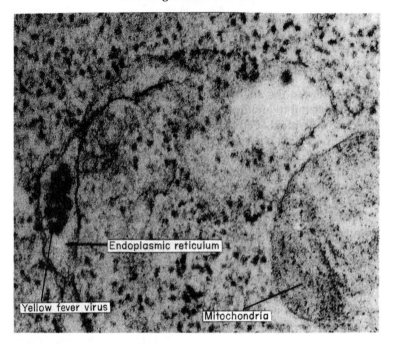

Figure 36.2   Yellow fever virus inside endoplasmic reticulum (×90 000).

36.3   Transmission of infectious disease by health care personnel

The prevention and control of disease is based upon the microbial characteristics introduced in the preceding topics of this unit. Any health care person is a potential carrier and transmitter of a disease, and should know the means of prevention and control of infectious disease to limit its spread. The main factors involved in prevention and control of disease are: destruction or control of pathogens by hygiene, chemical or physical means; removal of potential transmission routes by hygiene, chemical or physical means; and improved human resist-ance to the disease by artificially stimulated immune responses and specific treatment of infections.

36.4   Anti-microbial terms

The following terms are used in health care to describe the destruction or suppression of microbes:

1. **Sterilization**: the complete destruction of all forms of microbial life. An object is either sterile or non-sterile. This is an absolute term as nothing can ever be partly sterile.
2. **Asepsis**: absence of pathogenic microbes. Techniques that prevent entry of living microorganisms or contact with them. Medical asepsis is a condition excluding

the infectious agents of a communicable disease, whereas surgical asepsis refers to the exclusion of all microbes.

3. **Disinfection**: the process of destroying pathogens or rendering them inert on inanimate objects by chemical (disinfectants) or physical agents. Disinfectants are usually not active against bacterial spores and are too toxic to be applied directly to tissues.

4. **Antiseptic**: a substance applied to tissue that will inhibit the growing and multiplication of microbes without necessarily destroying them. An agent that prevents the growth of microbes causing sepsis in wounds.

5. **Germicide**: an agent that kills the growing microbial forms but not necessarily the resistant spore forms.

6. **Bactericides**: an agent that kills bacteria. Similar terms are fungicide for fungi, virucide for viruses and sporicide for spores.

7. **Sanitization**: the removal of pathogens to an acceptable safe level from inanimate objects by mechanical or chemical cleaning. EXAMPLE: The everyday control of microbial populations on utensils involved in food and drink distribution.

8. **Cleaning**: this refers to the removal of dust and dead organic matter and not microbial populations. Decontamination: the process of removing all microbes from an object containing a heavy growth of microorganisms.

9. **Antibiotic**: a chemical produced by microorganisms which has the capacity in dilute solutions to kill or inhibit the growth of other microbes.

10. **Antimicrobial**: general term referring to the suppression or destruction of any microorganism.

11. **Bacteriostasis**: the growth and multiplication of bacteria are temporarily suppressed during the presence of the bacteriostatic agent. Removal of the

agent results in a resumption of growth and multiplication of the bacteria. Similarly fungistasis refers to fungi and virustasis refers to viruses.

36.5 Control of infectious diseases

The control of infectious diseases depends upon the integration of disinfection and sterilization agents with correct aseptic techniques. In any environment involving patients a minimum goal should be cleanliness. Without cleanliness it is difficult to establish and maintain aseptic conditions.

Asepsis

Asepsis should be the goal of all members of a health team. Without a conscientious approach by the whole team the goal of asepsis will not be realized.

Medical asepsis involves general housekeeping cleanliness measures. EXAMPLES: Dust removal, laundering, disinfecting and scrubbing. Some additional techniques are also required for infectious diseases. EXAMPLES: Hygienic approaches towards body functions and excretions such as hand washing, adequate disposal of facial tissues and covering the mouth when coughing; precautionary measures taken to prevent direct person to person transmission of disease. Surgical asepsis involves additional techniques aimed at preventing the introduction of any pathogens into an area such as disinfecting and sterilizing the environment to the maximum possible extent combined with the use of protective clothing and techniques aimed at minimizing the transmission of disease. EXAMPLES: Sterilizing surgical instruments, dressings and sutures; use of sterile gloves, gowns, masks and caps. Surgical asepsis should be applied to any situation where a patient is at a high risk of being infected. EXAMPLES: Surgery, post-operative surgical wounds and in nurseries.

Isolation

Control of any infectious disease is based upon its communicability and the means by which it is transmitted. Where necessary, the initial step in control is the isolation of an infectious patient, their excretions and possibly their clothing. EXAMPLES: Patients with chickenpox or varicella should be isolated until all lesions have crusted; patients with diseases such as AIDS or hepatitis B require careful handling and blood, saliva, sweat, breast milk, semen, syringes, needles, wound discharges and excreta should be disposed of carefully. The need to re-use contaminated items and areas requires a knowledge of the general limitations of disinfecting contaminated materials.

Sterilization and disinfection

The most common agent used in sterilization and disinfection is heat, which has the potential to kill all microbes. The effectiveness of using heat as a sterilizing agent is determined by the temperature and the duration of exposure (Figure 36.3). The temperature at which all particular pathogens are killed in ten minutes is called the thermal death point. The time taken for killing one-tenth of the population (decimal reduction time) is often used to describe the rate of killing. The thermal death time is the time it takes at a certain temperature to kill a stated number of organisms (or spores) under specified conditions. Most vegetative cells will be destroyed between 50°C and 70°C

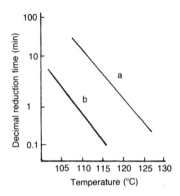

Figure 36.3 The difference in the temperatures and the rate of killing with time for (a) typical heat-resistant microbes and (b) typical non-heat-resistant microbes.

with ten minutes' exposure. Detergent plus hot water from 60°C to 100°C is used for sanitization purposes. Water boiled for ten to thirty minutes kills all microbes except heat-resistant bacterial endospores. Temperatures greater than 100°C are achieved by autoclaves.

Application: Autoclaves

An autoclave is a closed chamber which acts in a similar manner to an every-day household pressure cooker. As the pressure is increased within the chamber the temperature rises proportionately according to Charles' Law (19.2). The greater the temperature and pressure, the shorter the time required for killing the heat-resistant bacterial spores and viruses. At 121°C of moist heat exposed heat resistant bacterial spores will be killed in 15–20 minutes. (Note that the use of dry heat requires a higher temperature and longer time.) The timing must take into account the relative accessibility of the steam to the microbes within a material.

Pathogens on inanimate objects can often be destroyed by chemical disinfectants, but these are usually toxic to human tissues, which limits their usefulness. Another factor that needs to be considered when applying disinfectants is the concentration of disinfectant required to kill a particular density of pathogens without damaging the environment. Thorough cleaning prior to the application of a disinfectant lowers the microbial density. The lower the density of microbes the greater is the efficiency of a disinfectant. When applying a disinfectant to an object it is important to consider the physical properties of that object as these influence the effectiveness of the disinfectant. EXAMPLE: Hard, smooth surfaces are relatively easy to disinfect whereas surfaces containing cracks, porous materials or grooves are difficult to disinfect. Some common chemical agents are formalin or aldehydes, halogens, phenol and alcohols, and quarternary ammonium compounds.

Ultraviolet light is used to sterilize air and exposed areas. The most effective wavelength is 260 nm. Because u.v. light has a low penetration capacity, its action is only effective if the exposed surface is clean. The effectiveness of u.v. is determined by the intensity of the source and its distance from the area to be sterilized (11.2).

Personal hygiene

Personal hygiene is important in limiting the transmission of disease. One of the most common means of transmitting microbes is by unwashed or insufficiently washed hands, as hands always carry microbial flora. Hands should be freshly washed with antiseptic soaps or detergents when patients and any related objects are to be handled. Hands should also be washed after a patient or their objects have been handled. Particular attention should be paid to the back of the hands,

each side of the fingers, the finger-nails, wrists and palms. The hands should be positioned so that contaminated water will not run up the arms. Wherever possible use dry paper towel as wet; used towels can retain pathogens.

Hair should be shampooed frequently and if long it should be constrained by a hairnet to prevent it coming in contact with contaminated surfaces. The skin should also be kept clean to minimize accumulation of pathogens.

Antimicrobial agent mechanisms of action

An infected person should be treated with an antimicrobial agent or a combination of agents. Agents that effectively injure or destroy the pathogens without substantially altering human tissues, should be used. Most antimicrobial agents function in one or more of the following ways.

1. They inhibit the production of a cell wall or alter a cell wall's effectiveness. Removal of or injury to the cell wall leaves the relatively fragile plasma membrane vulnerable to rupture and cell lysis. All penicillins and cephalosporins are selective inhibitors of bacterial cell wall manufacture (22.13 — Application: Gram positive and gram negative bacteria). Griseofulvin inhibits the development of fungal cell walls.

2. They alter membrane permeability or inhibit active transport across cell membranes. The plasma membrane of bacteria and fungi are structurally different from animal cells. This difference enables bacterial and fungal membranes to be broken or destroyed by selective agents. The leaking of the intracellular contents leads to the death of cells. EXAMPLES: Polymyxins such as Neosporin and Neotracin act on gram-negative bacteria,

and polyenes such as Nystatin and Amphotericin B act on fungi. The antibacterial action of detergents is partly due to their ability to lower the surface tension on the bacterial membrane. These surface active agents can alter the selective permeability of membranes (23.2) resulting in a loss of useful metabolic compounds. EXAMPLES: Cationic detergents such as certain quarternary ammonium compounds.

3. They inhibit the manufacture of proteins by preventing the translation and transcription of genetic information. Bacterial and eucaryotic cells differ in a few essential steps in the manufacture of proteins. Specific antibacterial drugs have been developed to act upon bacteria at these steps. EXAMPLE: The aminoglycosides such as Streptomycin and Neomycin are believed to have a similar action in altering the actions of RNA. Other drugs involved in the inhibition of protein manufacture include the tetracyclines and chloramphenicol. The tetracyclines are active against bacteria, mycoplasmas and rickettsiae.

4. They inhibit DNA replication. The mitomycins form strong chemical bonds between the two complementary DNA strands which prevents them from separating during replication (24.7). DNA replication is similar in animal and bacterial cells. The inability of the mitomycins to discriminate between animal and bacterial cells limits their use as anti-microbial agents. Certain antiviral agents act by blocking the incorporation of chemicals into DNA. EXAMPLE: Halogenated pyrimidines such as idoxuridine compete with thymidine to form non-functional DNA. These agents are toxic to human cells which limits their use in topical applications against viruses such as herpes simplex. Other antiviral agents act by inhibiting specific viral enzymes responsible for DNA replication. EXAMPLE: Acyclovir inhibits a specific enzyme in the herpes virus. Ultraviolet light damages bonds between adjacent thymine molecules, leading to incorrect replication.

5. They inhibit the production of nucleic acids thereby inhibiting the formation of DNA and RNA. EXAMPLES: Sulphonamides block the formation of DNA in some bacteria, chlamydiae and some protozoa.

6. They inhibit penetration of viruses into cells. EXAMPLE: Amantadine prevents the entry of certain viruses, especially influenza A, into susceptible cells.

7. They alter enzyme structure by chemicals or heat. Substances such as chlorine, iodine, strong acids and strong alkalis bring about structural changes in enzymes and other proteins, i.e. they denature them (30.7). Moist heat also denatures proteins. The alteration in their protein structure results in death or inhibits the growth of the microbes.

8. They coagulate microbial proteins. Certain chemicals have the capacity to inactivate or destroy enzymes by coagulating these colloidal particles (17.6). EXAMPLES: Alcohol, phenol and formalin.

9. They oxidize proteins. Chemical agents which readily release oxygen can be lethal to cells if key enzymes are inactivated by the removal of hydrogen or electrons in the process of oxidation (ketones — 8.1). EXAMPLES: Oxidizing agents such as hydrogen peroxide, sodium perborate, potassium permanganate and the halogens (6.6).

10. They inhibit enzyme activity by interfering with the reaction between an enzyme and the cell chemicals (32.4). EXAMPLES: Heavy metal compounds such as mercury, copper and silver and zinc.

11. They ionize molecules. When ionizing radiation (11.8) is applied to microbial cells and viruses in sufficient quantities, key cell structures such as DNA and lysosomal membranes are ionized and microbial death results.

12. They cause mechanical disruption of microbial structures. The application of ultrasonic sound at frequencies greater than 100 000 Hertz causes bacterial membranes to disintegrate and proteins to coagulate.

36.6 Body defence mechanisms

Certain infectious diseases in man can be prevented if the body defence mechanisms are enhanced by immunization. It is important for health team members and/or persons at risk to be protected from infectious disease by fully immunizing themselves against diseases for which effective vaccines have been developed. The mechanisms for increasing human resistance to disease are described in the next chapter.

36.7 Environmental health and safety

The environment harbours a wide range of pathogens. The means of transmission also varies from air droplets to other animals such as mosquitoes. Appropriate precautions must be taken at all times to minimize the risk of infection and transmitting infections. The preventative measures range from the taking of anti-malarial tablets and screening against mosquitoes to using condoms for sexually transmitted diseases such as AIDS. Where patients with an infectious disease present a potential hazard to staff, other patients and visitors, the correct procedures as identified for a specific disease must be strictly adhered to as the consequences of transmission can be long-term illness and possibly death.

Application 1: Hepatitis-B

Hepatitis B (HBV) is a major concern to health-care workers who are in daily contact with blood. They have a considerably higher incidence of this disease than the general population. HBV can be transmitted through blood associated contact such as needle-stick injuries as well as body fluid secretions. EXAMPLE: Saliva and breast milk. Symptoms of the disease vary from asymptomatic through to loss of appetite, low-grade fever, joint pains and later jaundice. A strong relationship exists between liver cancer and the HBV virus.

Prevention of hepatitis B can be achieved through vaccination and using the correct procedures to eliminate direct contact with blood and body secretions.

Application 2: Mosquito-borne diseases

Many millions of people die throughout the world each year as a result of vectors transmitting diseases. One of the most common vectors is the mosquito.

Mosquitoes are responsible for the transmission of a wide range of diseases. Two of these diseases are malaria and dengue fever.

Malaria is due to an infection of the red blood cells by *plasmodium* protozoans (35.10) which have been in-jected into the blood by the mosquito *Anopheles*. The disease annually kills 1.5 million people and is currently increas-ing throughout the world. The disease is now increasing in areas where it was almost eliminated. Each year about 300 million people in 102 countries are infected by mosquitoes. The main signs and symptoms of the disease are periodic chills, fever that leaves a per-son drenched in sweat and exhausted, vomiting and severe headaches. These appear for one- to three-day periods followed by asymptomatic periods. The development of super-resistant strains to the traditional drugs such as chloroquine and the development of mosquitoes resistant to the pesticides is viewed with concern as an increasing number of persons are now presenting with the disease in Europe and other regions of the world following trips to areas previously considered as low risk.

Dengue fever results from the injection in a person of the *arbovirus* dengue fever virus (Figure 35.6) by the mosquitoes *Aedes albopictus* and *Aedes aegypti*. This disease was once a benign flu-like illness but is now one of the leading causes of morbidity and mor-tality among Southeast Asian chil-dren. Persons with the disease present with a fever, joint pain, skin rash and mental depression. The more serious form of the disease involves severe haemorrhaging and is referred to as dengue haemorrhagic fever.

Summary

The prevention and control of diseases relate to the characteristics of each microbial group and the ability of each group to survive, grow and reproduce in a particular environment. The methods of transmission of a particular group to new environments must be under-stood if the most effective approach to limiting the spread of a microbe is to be applied.

The process of infection involves a microbe's capacity to cause disease, its entry into the body, its establishment and multiplication within the host and its point of discharge from the body. The growth and death of a microbial population involve the following phases: lag, growth, stationary phase and decline. Pathogenicity is the capacity to cause disease; virulence refers to the relative ability of a pathogen to produce a disease. Virulence depends on invasiveness and toxigenicity of the pathogen. Carriers have the capacity to harbour a microbe and spread the disease. The main points of entry vary for different microbes. In humans they are: respiratory tract, urogenital tract, skin, gastrointestinal tract and superficial mucous membranes.

Incubation time is the interval between infection and the appearance of the disease. The body defence mechanisms, microbial defence mechanisms, supply of nutrients and the pathogen's ability to spread through-out tissues will determine the extent of the infection. The results can be localized or generalized such as bacteraemia, septicaemia and viraemia. The release of toxins into the bloodstream is called toxaemia.

The main portals of exit are: faeces, urine, mouth, nose and respiratory discharges and saliva.

Communicability is dependent upon: the microbe's ease of access to the host's excre-tions, the reservoir of infection and the ability to infect a susceptible host. The transmission of disease can be either by direct or indirect contact. Diseases can be spread by airborne droplets, ingestion of contaminated food or water, vermin, insects and fomites.

The main factors involved in the prevention and control of disease are:

1. Destruction and control of pathogens by chemical-physical means and hygiene.
2. Improved human resistance to disease.

The following terms are used to describe the various means of destruction, suppression or removal of microbes: sterilization, asepsis, disinfection, antiseptic, germicide, bactericide, sanitization, cleaning, decontamination, antibiotic, antimicrobial and bacteriostasis. The control of infectious diseases depends upon:

1. The integration of disinfection and sterilization agents with isolation and correct aseptic techniques.

2. Preventive measures aimed at increasing the resistance of individuals and communities by immunization, optimal nutrition and general community awareness of hygiene principles.

Most antimicrobial agents function in one or more of the following ways: they alter cell walls, alter membrane function, inhibit the translation and transcription of genetic information, inhibit DNA replication, inhibit the production of nucleic acids, inhibit the penetration of viruses into cells, alter the structure of microbial enzymes, coagulate microbial proteins, oxidize proteins, inhibit the reaction between enzyme and its substrate, ionize molecules and mechanically disrupt microbial structures.

Chapter 37

Body defence mechanisms

Objectives

At the completion of this chapter the student will be able to:

1. describe the different body defence mechanisms;
2. describe the stage of an immune response;
3. explain the differences between humoral and cell-mediated immunity;
4. explain the mechanisms of actively acquired immunity;
5. explain how allergies, autoimmune diseases, cell surface antigens, immunosuppressive drugs, and tissue rejection relate to body defence mechanisms;
6. describe monoclonal antibodies.

An important feature of body homeostasis is the need for homeostatic mechanisms to protect the internal environment from harmful foreign matter. Several homeostatic mechanisms known as immune systems serve the function of body defence, that is they attempt to give the body immunity against harmful foreign matter.

The harmful foreign material can be one of the following: chemical, EXAMPLE: Foreign proteins; bacteria, EXAMPLE: *Staphylococci*; viruses, EXAMPLE: *Herpes*; other micro-organisms, EXAMPLE: *Rickettsia*.

There are several homeostatic mechanisms involved in the protection and removal of harmful foreign matter. These mechanisms involve the epithelial tissue, blood, reticulo-endothelial system and the lymphatic system.

The body's defence mechanisms can be separated into those restricting the entrance of foreign particles into the body, that is, external defence mechanisms, and mechanisms that neutralize and remove foreign particles that have entered the body, that is, internal defence mechanisms.

37.1 External defence mechanisms

The tissues and fluid of the body are surrounded by a wall of epithelial cells. These cells form the basis of the external defence mechanism.

Epithelial tissue

The epithelial tissue lines the skin, respiratory tract, gastrointestinal tract and urogenital tract. This wall acts as the first line of defence. Breaking the skin surface often results in an invasion of microorganisms into the body. The epithelial cells form part of the body's non-specific defence mechanism which is unable to differentiate between different types of foreign matter.

There are several ways that epithelial tissue prevents foreign organisms from entering the extracellular regions of the body: arrangement of epithelial cells, secretions from epithelial cells, surface structures of epithelial cells.

Arrangement of epithelial tissue

Epithelial tissue consists of cells that are closely packed together. The tight packing results in little intercellular material between the cells (Figure 25.2). No intercellular material is present at the surface of these cells since the plasma membranes of adjacent cells are joined together. This joining of membranes effectively seals the surface of epithelial tissue. Patients suffering from burns are extremely susceptible to infection since the damaged epithelial barrier can no longer perform its protective function.

Secretions from epithelial cells

Some epithelial cells have the ability to secrete substances, that is, they act as glands. The type of secretion varies according to the location of the epithelial tissue.

The epithelial cells of the skin produce keratin which confers a tough and waterproof property to the surface of the skin. In addition, the skin contains sweat glands that secrete substances that are capable of killing bacteria. In the ear, some epithelial cells produce the protective substance, wax.

Some of the epithelial cells lining the respiratory tract, gastrointestinal tract, urogenital tract and conjuctivae secrete mucus. The mucus traps any foreign matter that has entered these regions of the body. The trapped material is retained by the mucus until the material is mechanically removed.

The enzyme lysozyme is secreted from epithelial cells that produce nasal mucus, tears, saliva and skin secretions. This enzyme is able to break down the cell walls of many bacteria.

A large proportion of foreign material that enters the stomach is destroyed by the highly acidic nature of the stomach's hydrochloric acid. This acid is secreted by epithelial cells lining the stomach wall.

Surface structures of epithelial cells

Nasal hairs prevent the entry of large particles into the respiratory tract. The smaller particles that pass through the hairs are entrapped by the mucus and moved towards the exterior by ciliated cells. The foreign material can be removed from the respiratory tract by the mechanical action of coughing and sneezing. Foreign material that enters the gastrointestinal tract is entrapped by mucus and moved to the highly acidic stomach by the action of epithelial cells containing cilia.

37.2 Internal defence mechanisms

The internal defence mechanism is brought into action when the first line of defence has been penetrated by foreign particles. Internal defence mechanisms can be divided into specific and non-specific.

Non-specific defence mechanisms

Non-specific defence mechanisms can be thought of as the second line of defence. These defence mechanisms are unable to differentiate between different foreign objects.

Blood

Blood plays an important role in the defence of our body against foreign particles. The white blood cells, and in particular the neutrophils, have the ability to phagocytose foreign matter. The presence of foreign particles provides a stimulus which attracts white blood cells to the area of invasion. Phagocytosis of the foreign matter ensues, with the likely result being rapid removal and destruction of the foreign object (23.5).

The fibrous nature of fibrin enables it to assist white blood cells by entangling the foreign material for sufficient time to enable the phagocytes to act.

Reticuloendothelial system

The reticuloendothelial system is a functional system that consists of highly phagocytic cells broadly distributed throughout the body. These cells are located in such tissues as bone marrow, lymphoid tissue, loose connective tissue, spleen, lung and nervous tissue. The majority of these cells appear to originate from monocytes. The reticuloendothelial cells have the ability to engulf and then digest foreign material. The ability to digest this material is due to the large array of powerful enzymes located in their lysosomes (22.10).

Lymphatic system

The lymphatic system is composed of the spleen, tonsils and thymus, tissue called lymph nodes, and a network of lymphatic vessels. These vessels drain fluid from the interstitial regions and return it to the vascular system. This fluid is referred to as lymph.

The lymph passes through lymph nodes on its journey from the interstitial regions to the vascular system.

Lymph nodes contain phagocytic cells of the reticuloendothelial system located in a mesh of fibrous tissue. The lymph nodes function as filters of unwanted particles. The fibrous mesh traps or slows down particles, after which the phagocytic cells engulf and break down the unwanted particle.

The nodes are strategically located so as to pick up microorganisms that get past the main entry barriers such as the respiratory tract.

Inflammatory response

The inflammatory response to harmful foreign material involves the combined action of non-specific defence mechanisms and the repair of any damaged regions. Generally **inflammation** is the response of tissues to infection or injury. It involves the destruction and walling-off of the injurious agent along with any cells that the agent may have destroyed. Following neutralization of the agent, a complex series of events is initiated which results in the healing of any damaged tissue.

The symptoms of inflammation are heat, redness, swelling and pain. Loss of function may occur but it is dependent upon the magnitude and site of inflammation.

The process of inflammation can be summarized in stages:

1. Stage 1 — the small blood vessels at the site of infection or injury dilate which results in an increased flow of blood carrying white blood cells to the area. The dilation is probably due to histamine. The increased blood flow is observed as a redness. Histamine also increases the permeability of blood vessels which leads to the movement of fluid and phagocytic white blood cells into the interstitial fluid. The increased flow of fluid into the inter-

stitial region results in a localized oedema.

2. Stage 2 — the accumulated white blood cells, principally neutrophils and monocytes, phagocytose the deleterious agent, resulting in the destruction or weakening of the foreign intruders. The end-product of this action is the formation of a fluid containing cell debris which is known as **pus**.

3. Stage 3 — the increased permeability of small blood vessels results in the leakage of fibrinogen to the interstitial fluid. Conversion of the fibrinogen into fibrin results in the formation of a clot (26.2). The clot isolates the infected area thus helping prevent the spread of the infection.

In recent years, a group of substances known as prostaglandins have been found to be released in inflammation.

Prostaglandins are a group of lipid substances that are extremely potent physiological agents (29.2). It appears that prostaglandins contribute to the genesis of fever, pain, vasodilation and increased permeability of blood vessels. The production of many prostaglandins is inhibited by aspirin-like drugs. These drugs reduce the signs and symptoms of inflammation.

Specific defence mechanisms

The entry of a foreign particle into the circulation or tissues is usually successfully countered by the non-specific defence mechanism. A backup defence mechanism or third line of defence is sometimes necessary to overcome the foreign invasion. EXAMPLE: Some microorganisms have the capacity to multiply inside phagocytes and also destroy phagocytes. This third line of defence involves mechanisms that can recognize and overcome specific foreign particles. These mechanisms are thus referred to as specific defence mechanisms.

Foreign particles can be toxins, foreign proteins, microorganisms or tissue cells from another organism. All of these particles contain a region that will react with the specific defence mechanisms, that is, they contain a region which is known as an antigen. The antigen evokes an immune response which involves the production of special lymphocytes. Each different form of antigen has its own unique shape. This property is used by the body to identify and combat a particular type of antigen.

The basis of specific defence mechanisms is the ability of special cells to form moulds of the shape of the active part of the antigen. This is followed by the production of cells and gamma globulin proteins that contain the mould of the antigen's active region. These moulds can combine with the antigen, effectively deactivating the antigen's effect on the body. The deactivated antigen is then destroyed by phagocytic activity.

The first step in specific defence mechanisms is the processing of an antigen by a macrophage. The macrophage phagocytoses the antigen (Figure 37.1) and then the active part of the antigen is 'processed' into a form that will be recognized by certain lymphocytes. The processed antigen is moved to the surface of the macrophage where contact with recognition lymphocytes occurs. These recognition lymphocytes respond to the processed antigen by initiating either of the following two mechanisms (Figure 37.2):

1. **humoral** immunity involving the production of antibodies;
2. **cell mediated** immunity involving the production of specialized lymphocytes that contain antigen receptors on their plasma membranes.

Humoral immunity

In humoral immunity, the contact of a recognition lymphocyte with its specific antigen results in the following process (Figure 37.2).

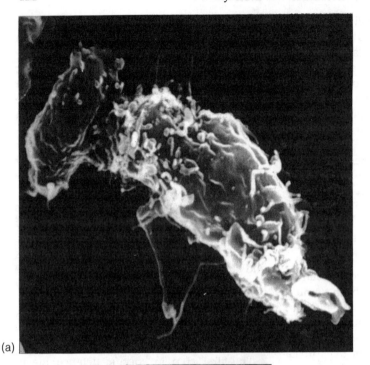

(a)

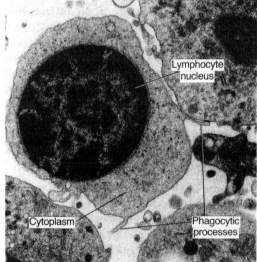

Lymphocyte
nucleus

Cytoplasm

Phagocytic
processes

(b)

Figure 37.1 Phagocytosis. (a) External view of a
macrophage phagocytosing a
blood cell. (b) Typical lymphocyte,
showing few organelles and long
phagocytic processes (×18 000).

The recognition lymphocyte rapidly divides
resulting in the formation of large numbers
of cells known as B-lymphocytes or B-cells.
This process of B-cell proliferation usually
occurs in the lymph nodes near the site of
antigen entry. This rapid increase in cells
results in the lymph node becoming grossly
enlarged. The enlarged lymph node may become tender due to pressure and stretching
on the surrounding tissue.

After five to seven days, some of the
B-lymphocytes have been transformed into
plasma cells. These latter cells increase in
number and remain in the lymph nodes
secreting gamma globulin proteins that have
a complementary shape to the specific antigen. These proteins are called **antibodies** or
immunoglobulins (Ig) and they are secreted
into the lymph fluid. These immunoglobulins
circulate throughout the body and combine
with their complementary antigen thereby
deactivating the antigen.

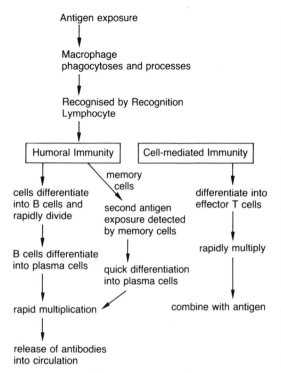

Antigen exposure

↓

Macrophage
phagocytoses and processes

↓

Recognised by Recognition
Lymphocyte

↓

| Humoral Immunity | Cell-mediated Immunity |

cells differentiate
into B cells and
rapidly divide

memory
cells

second antigen
exposure detected
by memory cells

differentiate into
effector T cells

↓

B cells differentiate
into plasma cells

quick differentiation
into plasma cells

rapidly multiply

↓

rapid multiplication

combine with antigen

↓

release of antibodies
into circulation

Figure 37.2 Specific immunological response to an antigen.

The different forms of immunoglobulin are identified by an alphabetic letter. Presently, there are five different forms or classes of immunoglobulins which are represented as IgA, IgD, IgE, IgG and IgM. All immuno-globulins of a particular class contain the same basic structure apart from the terminal region of the polypeptide. This variable terminal region is the site where an immuno-globulin binds with an antigen. A special antigen called T-dependent antigen requires the B cells to work with macrophages and helper T cells. All immune responses that produce IgG, IgA and IgE involve helper T cells.

During the stage of transformation of B-lymphocytes into plasma cells some of the B-lymphocytes remain unchanged, that is, they

remain as recognition lymphocytes for that particular antigen. These cells act as **memory cells** for any subsequent invasion of the antigen. These memory cells continually circulate throughout the lymphatic and cardio-vascular systems in search of their specific antigen. They tend to accumulate in the spleen and peripheral lymph nodes.

Following the first encounter with an antigen, an individual is said to be sensitized to that antigen. The individual possesses a certain quantity of circulating immuno-globulin along with a reserve of memory cells. These cells are able to rapidly multiply and be converted into plasma cells in a short period of time. The individual is thus able to fight the antigen soon after it enters into the tissues and blood.

The immunity acquired as a result of exposure to an antigen can be acquired in several different ways:

1. When a person is exposed to the antigen through some natural process such as infection, the individual is said to have **actively acquired immunity**.
2. If a small sample of an antigen is introduced by artificial means into a person, the result is also actively acquired immunity. This preparation of antigen is known as a **vaccine**. The result of vaccination is a small initial response to the antigen, and more importantly the production of antibodies and recognition lymphocytes which immunize the individual against any subsequent natural invasion of the antigen.
3. When an individual acquires antibodies and recognition lymphocytes without any exposure to the antigen the immunity is called **passively acquired immunity**. This form of immunity can also be acquired by either natural or artificial means. A foetus acquires immunity by obtaining the mother's antibodies through the placenta. These maternal antibodies provide a tem-

porary immunity for the first few months of the life of the newborn infant. This natural passive immunity can be mimicked by injecting serum containing antibodies. These immunoglobulins offer a temporary immunity against the antigens of diseases such as hepatitis and measles.

Cell-mediated immunity

Cell-mediated immunity involves the production of specialized lymphocytes that mature in the thymus. These cells are called effector T-cells and they interact with antigens by means of specific structures on the surface of the cell referred to as receptors. There are three main types of effector T-cells: **Helper T-cells (T$_H$)**, **suppressor T-cells (T$_S$)** and **cytotoxic T-cells (T$_c$)**. Helper T-cells help other T-cells and present antigens to B-cells. Suppressor T-cells appear to turn off immune responses while cytotoxic T-cells destroy target cells such as cancer and transplant tissue upon contact. Since T-cells combine directly with the antigen, the immune response is referred to as **cell-mediated immunity** (Figure 37.2).

The T-cells perform their function at the lymph nodes, spleen, tonsils and blood where they constitute 70–80% of all lymphocytes. The ability of T-lymphocytes to recirculate throughout the body enables these cells to recognize and bind with antigens shortly after infection.

When a specific shaped antigen encounters a recognition T-cell with a complementary shaped receptor, it binds to that T-cell. The T-cell is now activated or sensitized. Following sensitization, the T-cell rapidly divides to form enormous numbers of identical T-cells that circulate in the blood and lymph and lodge in the lymph nodes. The receptors on these cells combine with the complementary-shaped antigen thus deactivating the antigen. The T-cell then secretes substances such as the antiviral protein gamma interferon. This substance enhances the production of enzymes that digest the antigen.

Following either active or passive exposure to an antigen, the body acquires immunity by retaining an increased number of specific recognition and sensitized T-cells for very long periods of time. These cells are quick to respond to any further exposure to the antigen.

Cell surface antigens

All nucleated cells contain multiple antigens on their surface. An individual's immune system normally 'recognizes' its own unique surface antigens and distinguishes between these antigens and those of foreign cells. These antigens are called **histocompatability antigens** or **'self' antigens**. These antigens are components of the major histocompatability complex (MHC) which are unique to an individual. Only identical twins have exactly the same histocompatability antigens. If the surface antigens are 'recognized' as foreign, T-cells are produced to destroy the foreign cells.

Some of the most important antigens appear to be the HLA (Human Leucocyte Antigen) group. There are thirty possible histocompatability antigens. Each individual has five of the thirty antigens, which are determined by five genes. Because histocompatability antigens occur throughout the body, tissue from one region may be grafted in another without the body recognizing the grafted tissue as foreign. Prior to transplanting organs, the tissue of the donor and recipient is checked for HLA compatability. The greater the similarities between the donor and recipient HLA group the greater is the likelihood that the recipient immune system will accept the donor tissue.

Some cell surface antigens are different in different cell types within an individual and therefore act as identification markers for different cell types. This latter feature plays an important role in immune related diseases involving specific cells. EXAMPLES: Cancer and autoimmune disease.

Application: Immunosuppressive drugs

Transplantation of an organ or tissue requires the suppression of the immune response.

Immunosuppressive drugs are required since the body recognizes the transplanted cells as foreign and will produce an immune response involving the production of Interleukin-4A which activates T-cells to attack the donor cells. This response is referred to as **tissue rejection**. The administration of immunosuppressive drugs produces an increased susceptibility to infection as the patient's body defence mechanisms are suppressed. Recently drugs have been introduced which appear to suppress the T-cells and not the B-cells so that part of the function of the immune system is retained. EXAMPLE: Cyclosporin.

37.3 Disorders of the immune system

Disorders of the immune system vary from slight discomfort to life threatening situations.

Allergy

Allergy or hypersensitivity results from a person being oversensitive to a particular antigen which is referred to as the **allergen**. A wide range of allergens have been found to cause oversensitive responses in individuals. EXAMPLES: Penicillins, foods, dust, pollen and cosmetics.

The first exposure to the allergen results in the production of antibodies. Unlike a normal humoral response, in some individuals these antibodies attach to granular cells known as **mast cells** located in connective tissue (25.6).

The second exposure to the allergen results in the antibodies combining with the antigens. This reaction causes the breakdown of the granules in the mast cells which results in the release of large quantities of histamine.

The release of histamine results in inflammation, constriction of vessels with smooth muscle walls such as the respiratory and blood vessels, oedema due to histamine causing an increase in blood vessel permeability.

Application: Anaphylactic shock

Anaphylactic shock is a rapidly developed allergic reaction which may result from either a systemic or local reaction. The excessive release of histamine can result in difficulty of breathing due to the constricted air passages. In addition, the increased blood vessel permeability results in widespread oedema which leads to a lowered blood volume. Failure to reverse the histamine effect by administering antihistamines or epinephrine (adrenaline) can result in death.

Aids

Acquired Immune Deficiency Syndrome (AIDS) is a viral disease which kills T-cells. The virus retrovirus Human immunodeficiency virus (HIV) is believed to be responsible for destroying the T-cells of humans which decreases the ability of the body to defend itself against disease and leaves victims vulnerable to fatal infections and cancers. The actual cause of death is often either pneumonia or a rare skin cancer called Kaposi's sarcoma. The main modes of transmission appear to be sexual intercourse and direct contact with contaminated blood. The community groups most vulnerable are homosexual men, bisexual men, intravenous drug users and partners of the above.

Autoimmunity

The immune system normally differentiates between foreign particles and its own particles. **Autoimmunity** is the formation of an antigen within the body and the subsequent formation and reaction of antibodies to that antigen. The antigen can be formed as a result of a non-antigenic foreign particle or altered cell function producing abnormal proteins and cells. A wide range of diseases have been attributed to autoimmunity. EXAMPLES: Addison's disease, rheumatoid arthritis, pernicious anaemia and myasthenia gravis.

37.4 Monoclonal antibodies

A procedure has been developed in recent years for producing large quantities of a specific antibody. These homogeneous preparations are called monoclonal antibodies. Each batch of monoclonal antibody will combine only with a specific complementary antigen. Monoclonal antibodies are now being produced for diagnostic use. EXAMPLES: Monoclonal antibodies directed

against a particular hormone, protein or drug can be used to determine very small amounts of such a molecule in body fluids.

Monoclonal antibodies are now being used to direct specific chemicals to particular cell groups. The injected monoclonal antibodies are able to act as 'magic bullets' because the monoclonal antibody is complementary to the surface antigens of the target cells. Since antibody–antigen reactions are specific, administered monoclonal antibodies will only attach to cells containing the appropriate surface antigen. This process has recently been used to diagnose and treat cancer. Tumours can be detected by combining a gamma-emitting radioisotope to a monoclonal antibody for that tumour. A gamma camera (12.7) can then detect the gamma emissions, emanating from both primary and secondary tumours, as these cells combine with the specific monoclonal antibody–radioisotope complex. Recent clinical trials indicate that tumours such as melanoma can be destroyed by injecting either a greater quantity of a monoclonal antibody–radioisotope complex than is used for diagnostic purposes, or by injecting a monoclonal antibody–cytotoxic drug complex.

Summary

The defence of the body against harmful foreign matter involves the following mechanisms:

1. External defence mechanisms which rely on the arrangement, secretions or specialized surface structures of epithelial cells. The function of epithelial tissue in defence mechanisms is to restrict the entrance of harmful substances. It is regarded as the first line of defence and is non-specific,

that is, it does not differentiate between different invaders.

2. Internal defence mechanisms exist in two forms, those that are non-specific and those that attach to a particular invader.

The internal non-specific defence mechanism involves white blood cells that phagocytose foreign matter. The series of steps in a non-specific response of tissues to an invasion is referred to as inflammation. An inflammatory response involves inflammation and the repair of any damaged region.

Specific defence mechanisms can be subdivided into humoral immunity involving the production of immunoglobulins (antibodies) and cell-mediated immunity which involves the production of specialized lymphocytes that selectively attack different forms of foreign matter. Specific defence mechanisms rely on the recognition of a particular antigen (toxins, foreign proteins, microorganisms, and cells from other organisms) and the subsequent immune response. The immune response involves the formation of large numbers of B-lymphocytes (B-cells) and T-lymphocytes (T-cells) from recognition lymphocytes.

The B-cells are transformed into plasma cells. The plasma cells produce large quantities of specific complementary immunoglobulin (antibody) which circulates throughout the body and neutralizes the antigen. The T-cells contain a specific receptor that combines with, and neutralizes, its complementary antigen.

Following the immune response, recognition B- and T-cells multiply rapidly in the body after contact with their specific antigen. These sensitized cells enable the body to rapidly counter any further invasions of a particular antigen. The individual is said to have acquired an immunity to that antigen.

Actively acquired immunity can result from a natural process such as infection. It can also be artificially acquired by using a vaccine that initiates a small immune response to that particular antigen.

Passively acquired immunity involves the acquisition of immunoglobulins and recognition lymphocytes by natural or artificial means. EXAMPLE: The foetus acquires immunity naturally, whereas injecting serum containing immunoglobulins is an artificial acquisition. The recognition of transplanted material as foreign, initiates an immune response referred to as tissue rejection.

All nucleated cells contain multiple antigens on their surface, some of which are known as histocompatability antigens. The most important antigens are the HLA group, which is determined by five genes. HLA compatability is used as an important criterion in determining donor–recipient tissue compatability. Recent medical advances have produced immunosuppressive drugs that act selectively on the T-cells. This means that only part of the immune system is suppressed.

Disorders of the immune system account for a wide range of health problems that vary from slight discomfort to life-threatening situations. An allergy results from a person being oversensitive to a particular antigen. The result of this hypersensitivity is the release of large quantities of histamine. In severe allergic reactions anaphylactic shock can occur. Another disorder is the misrecognition of some of the body's own cells as foreign. This results in autoimmune diseases.

Monoclonal antibodies are homogeneous preparations of a specific antibody, used to detect minute quantities of body chemicals. They can be combined with radioisotopes for diagnosing primary and secondary tumours. Monoclonal antibodies combined with either radioisotopes or cytotoxic drugs can be used to selectively destroy tumours.

Unit Thirteen
Control and Regulation of Body
Function: Neuroendocrine Systems

This unit introduces the organization and
function of the nervous and endocrine
systems. The interrelationship between these
systems is related to homeostatic
mechanisms.

Chapter 38

General organization and function of the nervous system

Objectives

At the completion of this chapter the student should be able to:

1. describe the general organization and function of the nervous system;
2. list the principal components of the central nervous system;
3. explain the difference between white and grey matter;
4. describe where spinal nerves and sympathetic nerves connect with the spinal cord;
5. compare the organization and actions of sympathetic nerves with parasympathetic nerves;
6. describe the process of biofeedback.

38.1 Body communication systems

To coordinate body homeostatic mechanisms it is necessary to have a communication network that can detect, integrate and adjust the actions of each homeostatic mechanism. The ability of nerves to conduct impulses rapidly along their axons gives them the potential to fulfil the role of rapid conveyers of information in the body. The extensive network of nerves throughout the body enables nerves to realize their potential. The network of nerves is known as the **nervous system**. Any factor that interferes with their ability to conduct impulses or removes part of the nerve network will result in the potential function of nerves not being realized.

Other forms of communication play an important role in body homeostasis. A mechanism exists whereby information is transferred by regulatory couriers through the blood system from an integrating centre to a region which responds to the courier. This system is called the **endocrine system** and the couriers are known as hormones. This system requires less energy to function than the high energy demanding nerves. The endocrine system is generally involved in the co-ordination of the body's metabolic activity.

A third form of communication is the slow flow of substances down the axons of nerves. These substances are referred to as **trophic factors** and the movement of substances is called **axoplasmic flow**. This communication path is used to maintain the homeostasis of tissues with which nerves connect. It plays an important role in the development, maintenance and regeneration of the nerve network. EXAMPLE: Individuals who have their vagus nerve severed in an attempt to combat peptic ulcers will have regrowth of the nerve to its original connection site over a period of time. The trophic factors guide the nerve back to the original tissue. Axoplasmic flow also serves the purpose of connecting the nervous and endocrine systems in the region of the brain known as the hypothalamus.

38.2 General organization of the nervous system

This chapter is an overview of the nervous system for the purpose of familiarizing the student with the major pathways and commonly referred to structures. A general knowledge of the nervous system is essential for understanding how the body coordinates homeostatic mechanisms in response to altered internal and external environments.

There are several ways of classifying the various networks in the nervous system. The following is one of the most popular classifications (Figure 38.1):

1. **Central nervous system** (CNS) — consists of the brain and spinal cord. The CNS integrates incoming information and relays responses to the peripheral nervous system.
2. **Peripheral nervous system** — consists of the spinal nerves, cranial nerves and the autonomic nervous system (ANS). The spinal nerves convey information to the CNS from receptors and relay the messages from the CNS to the effectors via the somatic nervous system, thus eliciting a response. The autonomic nervous system

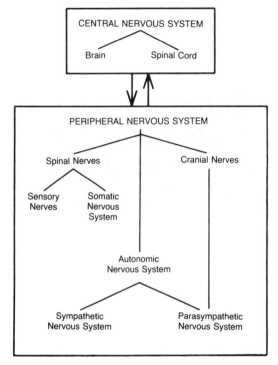

Figure 38.1 General organization of the nervous system. Note that some cranial nerves form part of the parasympathetic nervous system.

carries information to and from the CNS that involves smooth muscle, cardiac muscle and glands. The ANS can be subdivided into the sympathetic nervous system and the parasympathetic nervous system. These two systems have opposite actions on smooth muscle, cardiac muscle and glands. The sympathetic nervous system has a stimulatory action whereas the parasympathetic has an inhibitory action.

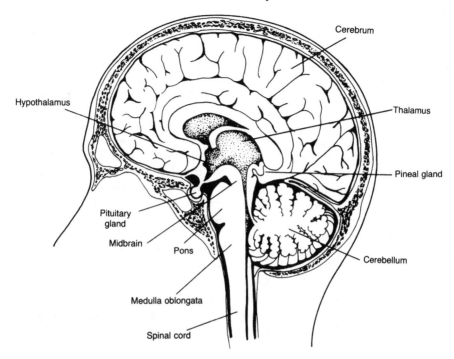

Figure 38.2 General organization of the central nervous system.

38.3   Central nervous system

The brain and spinal cord constitute the nerve network referred to as the CNS. The brain has the ability to regulate and co-ordinate homeostatic mechanisms. It can perform this action by responding directly to incoming information or by initiating an action according to previous experience. In addition, it can initiate learning, exploratory behaviour and exercise.

The spinal cord is a continuation of the brain. It acts as a distributor of information for the brain to the various regions of the body where it connects with the regional peripheral nervous system.

The CNS can be divided for convenience into the following four divisions according to its anatomical arrangement (Figure 38.2).

1. forebrain;
2. midbrain;
3. hindbrain;
4. spinal cord.

Forebrain

The **forebrain** or **cerebrum** is the anterior region of the brain which contains the large lobes referred to as the **cerebral hemispheres** or telencephalon. It also contains a region known as the **diencephalon** which consists of the thalamus, hypothalamus and pineal gland.

Cerebral hemispheres (telencephalon)

The cerebral hemispheres are two lobes that are identical in shape and size. They are the site of conscious thought and are referred to as the higher centres. The higher centres are located in the outer region consisting of grey matter which is called the **cerebral cortex**. The cerebral cortex is the principal control centre for the body. It receives information, integrates and compares it with relevant past information and sends out decisions that control a great proportion of body function.

White matter, that is, myelinated nerve tracts, are located beneath the cerebral cortex. They convey information to and from the various regions of the cerebral cortex. Located within the cerebral hemispheres are aggregations of grey matter known as **basal ganglia**. The basal ganglia or cerebral nuclei assist the cerebral cortex in maintaining smooth purposeful skeletal muscle contractions. Damage to nerves in this region results in shaking of the hands and loss of discrete movements of the body. EXAMPLE: Parkinson's disease.

Thalamus

The thalamus acts as a giant relay centre that distributes sensory information to the cerebral cortex. A particular piece of sensory information, such as a signal indicating pain, is distributed to the relevant regions of the cerebral cortex that deal with pain.

The thalamus has extensive connections with the cerebral cortex and the hypothalamus. Since the hypothalamus connects the endocrine system to the CNS, the thalamus acts as a relay centre for the transmission of endocrine actions to the cerebral cortex.

Hypothalamus

The hypothalamus links the endocrine and nervous systems. It has connections with the cerebral cortex, thalamus, retina, posterior part of the pituitary gland and the sympathetic nervous system. It also contains aggregations of grey matter or nuclei that are involved in the control of thirst, appetite and temperature. The hypothalamus also coordinates hindbrain homeostatic centres such as the cardiovascular and respiratory centres. Receptors in the hypothalamus monitor the level of individual substances in the blood and the osmotic balance.

The hypothalamus appears to be the central integrating area for initiating homeostatic mechanisms in response to stress.

The relationship between the hypothalamus and the endocrine system is described in 39.4.

Pineal gland

The pineal gland is a tiny gland about 0.5 cm long that has recently been found to be an important link between the nervous and endocrine systems. This gland is linked to CNS via the sympathetic nervous system. A description of its nervous connection and the actions of this gland occurs in 39.3.

Midbrain

The midbrain or mesencephalon portion of the brain connects the forebrain to the hindbrain. Briefly, this segment of the brain contains conduction pathways for both sensory and motor messages between the forebrain and the hindbrain. An additional function of this region is the coordination of visual and auditory reflexes.

Hindbrain

The hindbrain or rhombencephalon contains three principal structures known as the cerebellum, pons and medulla oblongata.

Cerebellum

The cerebellum is the second largest region of the brain. It is situated over the medulla and pons. It is a highly specialized part of the CNS, being involved in the subconscious coordination of movements of skeletal muscle such as those required for the maintenance of posture and balance. This function of the cerebellum is shown by the effect of damage to the cerebellum. Damage results in a lack of skeletal muscle coordination.

Pons

The pons links the nerve pathways from the medulla oblongata and cerebellum with the midbrain. It contains a respiratory centre that works in conjunction with a respiratory centre in the medulla oblongata to regulate the rate of breathing.

Medulla oblongata

The medulla oblongata acts as a link between the spinal cord and the remainder of the brain. It also plays an important role in homeostasis by containing coordinating centres for the following homeostatic mechanisms:

1. cardiac centre — regulates heart rate;
2. vasomotor centre — regulates blood vessel diameter and thus blood pressure;
3. respiratory centre — acts with the pons respiratory centre to regulate the rate of breathing.

Most motor nerve pathways originating from each cerebral hemisphere cross in the medulla, resulting in the right side of brain controlling the left side of the body.

Spinal cord

The spinal cord is a long rod of nervous tissue that connects the medulla with the body. It is located in a canal that is found near the centre

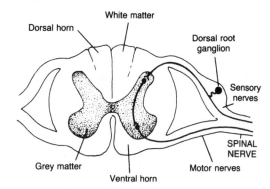

Figure 38.3 Cross-section of the spinal cord showing the point of entry and exit of spinal nerves.

of the vertebral column. Figure 38.3 shows a typical cross-section through the spinal cord. Note that the relative position of the white and grey matter is reversed when compared with cerebral hemispheres, that is, the white matter now surrounds the grey matter.

The white matter contains groups of long nerve fibres called tracts. These tracts either carry information to the brain (ascending) or transmit messages from the brain to segments of the spinal cord (descending). The ascending and descending tracts originate and terminate respectively at specific points along the cord in the grey matter.

The **grey matter** is essentially a region consisting of nerve connections or synapses (25.5) and short neurons that link other neurons originating or terminating within the grey matter.

At thirty-one points along the cord, spinal nerves enter and leave the spinal cord and pass through natural holes in the vertebral column to the body. These nerves are either **sensory (afferent) nerves** conveying information from a particular segment of the body or they are **motor (efferent) nerves** that carry messages to skeletal muscles (effectors). The spinal efferent nerves form the **somatic nervous system**. The spinal cord is effectively divided into functional segments for different regions of the body.

The point of entry of sensory neurons at a particular segment is located at the dorsal (posterior) horn of the spinal cord (Figure 38.3). These neurons form synapses in the grey matter with either motor neurons, ascending neurons or short interconnecting neurons. Motor nerves form a synapse in the ventral (anterior) horn of the grey matter and leave the spinal cord. The cell bodies of those neurons occur near the cord in a region called the dorsal root ganglion. The sensory and motor nerves form a common group of fibres known as the **spinal nerve**. Each spinal cord segment consists of a pair of spinal nerves, one of which communicates with a segment of the left side of the body and the other the corresponding segment on the right side of the body.

Connections exist within the spinal cord between the sensory and motor neurons of the same segment. This results in the formation of a localized communication system. This enables rapid local responses to changes in the environment that are referred to as spinal reflexes.

Application: Stretch reflexes

Tapping the knee elicits a knee jerk reflex response. Sensory neurons detect the tap and stimulate the motor neurons with which they synapse. The motor neurons stimulate a contraction in the muscle that extends the lower leg (Figure 38.4). This reflex has not required any action by the brain and is thus a rapid acting homeostatic mechanism.

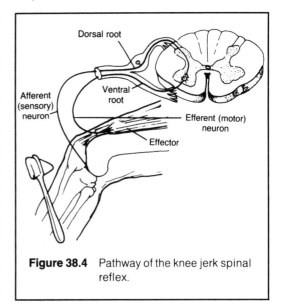

Figure 38.4   Pathway of the knee jerk spinal reflex.

38.4 Peripheral nervous system

The peripheral nervous system (PNS) consists of the spinal nerves, cranial nerves and the autonomic nervous system. The nerves of the PNS conduct information from the body to the CNS where it is analysed and effector messages are delivered to the relevant region of the body. The PNS is an important part of many homeostatic mechanisms since it acts as the afferent and efferent pathways (1.2).

Spinal nerves

A spinal nerve enters and leaves a particular segment of the spinal cord. Each spinal nerve is composed of an afferent or sensory neuron and an efferent or motor neuron.

The afferent neurons contain sensory nerve endings or receptors. EXAMPLES: Tempera-

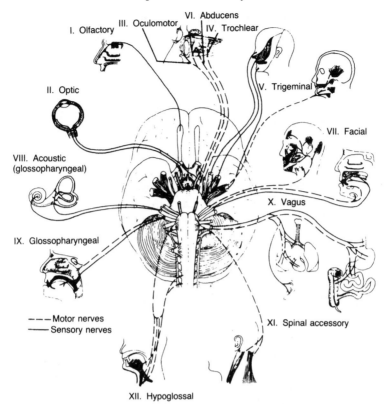

I. Olfactory

III. Oculomotor

VI. Abducens

IV. Trochlear

V. Trigeminal

II. Optic

VII. Facial

VIII. Acoustic
(glossopharyngeal)

X. Vagus

IX. Glossopharyngeal

— — — Motor nerves
——— Sensory nerves

XI. Spinal accessory

XII. Hypoglossal

Figure 38.5 The twelve cranial nerves and the structures with which they connect. (Lankford, *Integrated Science* for *Health Students*, p. 221, 1979, reprinted with permission of Reston Publishing Co., a Prentice Hall Co., 11480 Sunset Hills Road, Reston Virginia 22090).

ture, stretch. **Receptors** play an essential part in body homeostasis as they detect alterations in the body's internal and external environments. EXAMPLES: Chemical receptors, stretch receptors. When stimulated, these receptors send impulses along the axon entering a spinal cord segment at the dorsal (posterior) horn and are then transmitted via a synapse to either its complementary motor neuron or to nerves of the CNS.

The efferent neurons leave the spinal cord at the ventral (anterior) horn and then connect with muscle or glands. These neurons influence many body homeostatic mechanism responses.

Cranial nerves

There are twelve pairs of nerves that are directly connected with the brain (Figure 38.5). They are associated with functions such as sight (optic nerve), hearing (auditory nerve), smell (olfactory nerve), facial expression (facial nerve) taste (facial, glossopharyngeal nerves) and many other sensory and motor functions related to the head.

The cranial nerve known as the vagus leaves the head and innervates many organs.

It plays a major role in the autonomic nervous system.

Autonomic nervous system

The autonomic nervous system is a nervous system that connects the CNS to smooth muscle, cardiac muscle and glands. It is composed of two separate systems that exert opposite effects on effector tissue. The **sympathetic nervous system** is an excitatory or stimulatory system whereas the **parasympathetic system** is generally considered to be an inhibiting system. The sympathetic system is a highly energy demanding system that enables the body to overcome imbalances within itself. The parasympathetic is generally a deactivating system that requires less energy.

The autonomic nervous system was considered to be independent of conscious control. An increased understanding of the autonomic system has led to the ability to train people to consciously influence homeostatic mechanisms that maintain the body's internal environment. This process is known as **biofeedback** (1.4) and will be referred to later in this chapter.

Sympathetic nervous system

The sympathetic nervous system originates from the thoracic and lumbar regions of the spinal cord. The neurons enter one of two chains of ganglia that run parallel to the spinal cord (Figure 38.6). The cell bodies of these sympathetic nerves are located in the grey matter of the spinal cord. These neurons form synapses with the cell bodies of post-ganglionic nerves in the ganglia.

Ganglia are merely junction regions between the neurons that synapse with the CNS and those that innervate the internal muscles and glands. Some of the ganglia occur near the organs with which they connect. Others such as the superior cervical ganglion is an extension of the ganglionic chain. This latter ganglion is the junction box for the sympathetic nerves located in the upper regions of the body.

The general effect of the sympathetic nervous system is constriction of smooth muscle tubes, increased rates of muscle contraction, elevated breathing rates and increased secretions from glands. These effects result from the use of the stimulatory neurotransmitter norepinephrine (noradrenaline). The neurons are thus sometimes referred to as adrenergic nerves.

Parasympathetic nervous system

The parasympathetic nervous system connects with the CNS via some of the cranial nerves and a group of nerves leaving the spinal cord in the sacral region (Figure 38.7). These nerves form synapses in ganglia close to or in the organs that they are innervating. The post-ganglionic neurons are thus short. There appears to be no direct connection between the cranial and sacral parts of the parasympathetic nervous system. Not all organs and internal muscles are connected with the parasympathetic system.

The principal nerve involved in parasympathetic function is the vagus. This nerve innervates a large number of organs including the heart, kidneys and liver, along with the respiratory and digestive systems.

The parasympathetic nerves generally exert an inhibitory action on tissue. The neurons use the neuro-transmitter acetylcholine and are thus often referred to as cholinergic nerves.

Summary

The nervous system can be divided into the:

1. Central nervous system which contains the brain and spinal cord.

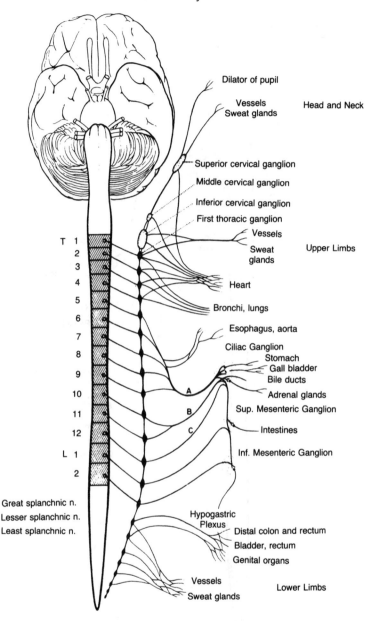

Dilator of pupil

Vessels
Sweat glands   Head and Neck

Superior cervical ganglion
Middle cervical ganglion
Inferior cervical ganglion
First thoracic ganglion
Vessels
Sweat
glands   Upper Limbs

Heart

Bronchi, lungs

Esophagus, aorta

Ciliac Ganglion
Stomach
Gall bladder
Bile ducts
Adrenal glands
Sup. Mesenteric Ganglion

Intestines

Inf. Mesenteric Ganglion

Hypogastric
Plexus
Distal colon and rectum
Bladder, rectum
Genital organs

Vessels   Lower Limbs
Sweat glands

T 1
2
3
4
5
6
7
8
9
10
11
12
L 1
2

A
B
C

Great splanchnic n.
Lesser splanchnic n.
Least splanchnic n.

Figure 38.6 Organization of the sympathetic nervous system. (Reprinted with permission of Macmillan Publishing Co., Inc. from *The Human Body: Its Structure and Physiology*, 4th edition, copyright © 1978 by Sigmund Grollman.)

2. Peripheral nervous system which contains the spinal nerves, cranial nerves and the autonomic nervous system. The efferent spinal nerves represent the somatic nervous system, that is, the nerves going from the CNS to skeletal muscle.

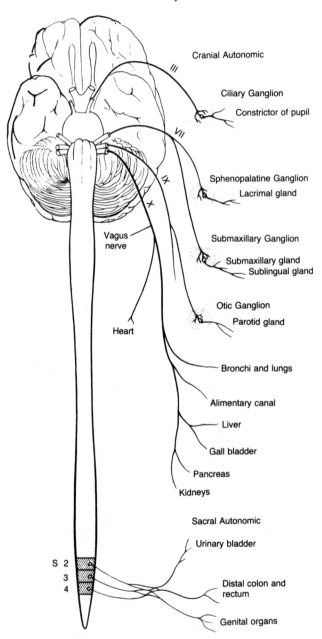

Figure 38.7 Organization of the parasympathetic nervous system. (Reprinted with permission of Macmillan Publishing Cl., Inc. from *The Human Body: Its Structure and Physiology*, 4th edition, copyright © 1978 by Sigmund Grollman.)

The brain consists of the:

1. forebrain which contains the cerebral hemispheres, basal ganglia, thalamus, hypothalamus and pineal gland;

2. midbrain which connects the forebrain to the hindbrain;
3. hindbrain which contains the cerebellum, pons and medulla oblongata;

Some of the functions of the brain are:

1. Brain generally acts as an integrating centre for many homeostatic mechanisms.
2. Hypothalamus and pineal gland connect the nervous system to the endocrine system.
3. Thalamus and cerebellum play an important part in the coordination of skeletal muscle movements.
4. Medulla oblongata acts as a coordinating centre for cardiovascular and respiratory homeostatic mechanisms.

The spinal cord connects the medulla with the body. It contains ascending and descending tracts which carry information to and from the brain.

Spinal nerves form part of the peripheral nervous system. A pair of spinal nerves enters each of the thirty-one spinal cord segments. These nerves carry sensory information to the spinal cord and instructions from the spinal cord to the effector tissue.

Cranial nerves connect directly with the brain. The twelve pairs are mainly responsible for sensory and motor functions in the head, except for the vagus which has a wide body distribution.

The autonomic nervous system is subdivided into the sympathetic and parasympathetic nervous systems. The sympathetic nervous system generally has a stimulatory action whereas the parasympathetic nervous system is usually an inhibiting system. Sympathetic nerves originate from the thoracic and lumbar spinal cord segments. Parasympathetic nerves consist of several cranial nerves, and a group of nerves leaving the spinal cord in the sacral region. The vagus is the principal parasympathetic nerve.

Chapter 39

Neuroendocrine connections

Objectives

At the completion of this chapter the student should be able to:

1. define the terms hormone, target tissue, target gland and tropic hormone;
2. describe the relationship between the nervous system and the endocrine system;
3. describe how the adrenal medulla, pineal gland, hypothalamus and posterior pituitary act as neuroendocrine connections.

The endocrine system is composed of a series of glands that secrete substances called hormones directly into the bloodstream. This system plays a vital role in the maintenance of homeostasis. An **endocrine gland** performs the function of secreting substances into the bloodstream. Other secretory organs, known as **exocrine glands**, secrete substances into ducts for transmission to their site of action.

The endocrine system contains a variety of homeostatic mechanisms. These mechanisms rely upon hormones to relay messages from the integrating centres to the effector sites in order to elicit the desired response. The action of a particular hormone is often supported or inhibited by other hormones. The interaction of hormones in the body results in a coordinated body response to any imbalance in the internal environment.

39.1 Terms associated with the endocrine system

The following terms are frequently used in any discussion of the endocrine system.

Hormones

A **hormone** is any substance that is released into the blood in small amounts and which on arrival at a particular tissue elicits a response. Each hormone regulates specific cell reactions by increasing or decreasing particular cellular processes. They never initiate actions and their regulatory action on a cell is based on either altering enzyme activity or membrane transport.

Hormones are either derivatives of lipid or amino acid metabolism.

Lipid hormones

Lipid hormones occur as steroids secreted from either the adrenal cortex or gonads. EXAMPLES: Cortisol and aldosterone from the adrenal cortex; oestrogen and testosterone from gonads. The prostaglandins are considered to be tissue hormones by some physiologists. An overview of their actions in the body is described in 29.2.

Amino acid based hormones

Hormones derived from amino acids can either exist as peptides or modifications of amino acids. The peptide hormones range in size from small peptide molecules to large polypeptides. Examples of peptide hormones are insulin and antidiuretic hormone. Hormones such as thyroxin and adrenaline are modifications of an amino acid.

Target tissue

Target tissue refers to the tissue that is acted upon by a hormone. This tissue exhibits a specific physiological response to the hormone. When the tissue is another endocrine gland, the gland is referred to as a **target gland**. EXAMPLES: The adrenal cortex, thyroid and gonads are target glands that respond to hormones secreted from the anterior pituitary gland.

Tropic hormones

Tropic hormones regulate the release of hormones from a target gland. EXAMPLE: Adrenocorticotropic hormone (ACTH) is secreted from the anterior pituitary and influences the secretion of hormones from the adrenal cortex.

39.2 Endocrine dependence on the nervous system

The endocrine system plays a major role in body homeostasis, most of its actions being involved in the control of metabolism. For the endocrine system to function in a co-ordinated manner, it requires an integrating centre and receptors. These receptors inform the integrating centre of how effectively it is functioning (1.2). In most endocrine homeostatic mechanisms the brain plays a direct or indirect role as the integrating centre.

The body's metabolism needs to be adjusted according to both the internal and external environment. The nervous system is used to detect changes in the environment. It also forms the afferent part of the communication network.

Connections exist between the nervous system and the endocrine system, that is, **neuroendocrine connections** occur. It is important to realize that most endocrine actions are influenced by the nervous system, which is why psychological stress can influence normal body metabolism.

39.3 Neuroendocrine connections

The following five pathways show how the nervous and endocrine systems are connected.

Hypothalamus–adrenal medulla

The hypothalamus and the endocrine gland known as the adrenal medulla are connected

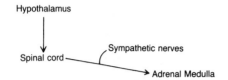

Figure 39.1 The neuronal connection of the hypothalamus and adrenal medulla.

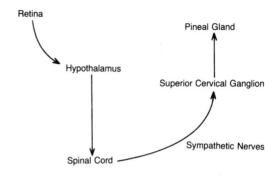

Figure 39.2 The neuronal connection of the retina and hypothalamus with the pineal gland.

by a nerve pathway (Figure 39.1). This pathway consists of a nerve tract in the spinal cord which connects with sympathetic nerves that innervate the adrenal medulla. Remember that the hypothalamus is connected to the thalamus which in turn is linked to the cerebrum. Command signals can thus also pass from the cerebrum or forebrain to the adrenal medulla.

Stimulation of the adrenal medulla by nerve impulses results in the release of the potent stimulatory hormones epinephrine (adrenaline) and norepinephrine (noradrenaline). These hormones are responsible for increasing the ability of the body to cope with stress (1.3). This is achieved by increasing the performance of the heart and lungs and increasing blood sugar levels and the breakdown of glucose. The combined effect of these actions is an increased quantity of adenosine triphosphate (ATP).

The connection of the adrenal medulla via a nerve pathway to the cerebral cortex enables the adrenal medulla to respond to stress rapidly and effectively. The cerebrum receives information from the external environment through receptors in the eye, ear, nose, mouth and skin. Through these receptors, the body is able to detect potential stressful situations and prepare itself almost immediately for the stress.

Retina–hypothalamus–pineal gland

A pathway of nerves connects the pineal gland with the retina via the hypothalamus (Figure 39.2). This pathway originates at the retina where light/dark stimuli are converted into nerve impulses. Some of these nerve impulses travel via a nerve tract to the lateral regions of the hypothalamus. Nerve fibres then pass down the spinal cord and synapse with sympathetic nerves that connect with the pineal gland via the superior cervical ganglion.

The pineal gland appears to be involved with, or may even be the site of, the biological clock, since hormones secreted by the pineal gland are influenced by the presence of light.

Until recently, this gland was thought to only function in children as it calcifies before puberty. Presently, evidence suggests that it functions throughout life and that calcification of the gland does not interfere with its function.

The neuroendocrine connection involving the pineal gland appears to play a major role in endocrinology since the pineal gland is now considered to be the 'master' endocrine gland. It is involved in the regulation of body metabolism on a twenty-four hour cycle. This cycle is called the circadian rhythm.

The influence of the nervous system on the pineal gland is shown when the pineal gland secretes the hormones melatonin and

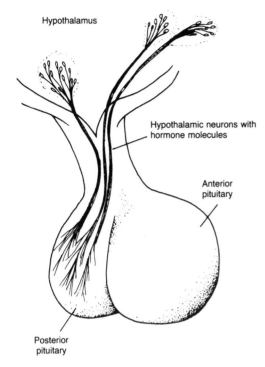

Hypothalamus

Hypothalamic neurons with hormone molecules

Anterior pituitary

Posterior pituitary

Figure 39.3 Neuronal connection of the hypothalamus with the posterior pituitary gland.

pituitary gland or neurohypophysis (Figure 39.3). Nerves originating from the hypothalamus terminate in the posterior pituitary. These nerves produce the hormones oxytocin and anti-diuretic hormone (vasopressin) in response to neural and hormonal information. Following production in the cell body of these neurons, the hormones travel via axoplasmic flow to the posterior pituitary gland (38.1). This journey takes between one and two hours. The hormones are stored in the posterior pituitary and released in response to stimulation of the hypothalamic nerves.

This neuroendocrine pathway plays an important role in the homeostasis of body fluid concentration.

Hypothalamus

All of the above neuroendocrine connections involve the hypothalamus. The hypothalamus influences the release of hormones from the major endocrine gland known as the anterior pituitary or adenohypophysis.

The hypothalamus secretes a group of regulating hormones that travel via a localized vascular network to the anterior pituitary gland (Figure 39.4). Each particular hormone has the property of stimulating or inhibiting the release of a hormone with a similar structure from the anterior pituitary.

Stimulation of particular neurosecretory cells in the hypothalamus results in the release of a specific regulating hormone. This substance then travels via the blood to the anterior pituitary where it regulates the release of its complementary hormone. A description of this mechanism and the hormones released from the anterior pituitary is described in 40.2.

In the case of the anterior pituitary, the hypothalamus contains the neuroendocrine connection within it, since regulating hormones are secreted directly into the blood

arginine-vasotocin (AVT) in response to darkness. Their levels of secretion are five times that found at noon. This suggests that light stimuli being detected by the retina are inhibiting the production and release of hormones in the pineal gland.

Hormones from the gland such as melatonin and arginine-vasotocin influence the endocrine function of the hypothalamus, pituitary and various other endocrine glands. The relationship between the pineal gland and the endocrine system is discussed in 40.2.

Hypothalamus–pituitary gland

The hypothalamus forms a neuroendocrine connection with the posterior region of the

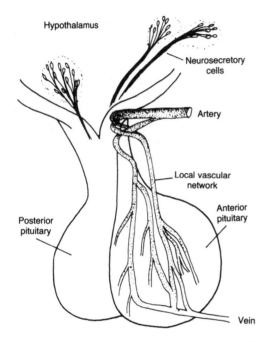

Hypothalamus

Neurosecretory cells

Artery

Local vascular network

Anterior pituitary

Posterior pituitary

Vein

Figure 39.4 Connection of the hypothalamus with the anterior pituitary gland.

cells are specialized neuroendocrine cells which convert substances to amine and polypeptide hormones. Some of these cells are capable of producing more than one hormone. The functions of this system are still unknown, although its malfunction has led to an understanding of the system's diversity throughout the body. APUD cells are altered under certain conditions to produce hormone-secreting tumours, called APUDomas or neuroendocrinomas. These tumours occur in a variety of forms and are identified by the APUD cell enzyme D.D.C. (L. Dopa Decarboxylase). APUDomas are often named according to the hormone produced by the APUD cancer cells. EXAMPLES: Insulin-secreting APUDomas are called insulinomas; gastrin hormone secreting cells from the gastrointestinal tract are called gastrinomas.

stream. The anterior pituitary is indirectly connected to the nervous system via the controlled release of regulating hormones from the hypothalamus.

APUD system

APUD or the Amine Precursor Uptake and Decarboxylation neuroendocrine system consists of easily identifiable groups of cells widely dispersed throughout the body and is probably connected to the sympathetic nervous system. All APUD cells, which are located in a variety of tissues and organs, have common cell characteristics. EXAMPLES: Both endocrine and non-endocrine tissue of the gastrointestinal tract, lungs, pancreas and pineal gland. The APUD

Summary

The endocrine system consists of an inter-related system of glands. Endocrine glands secrete hormones directly into the blood whereas exocrine glands secrete substances such as enzymes into ducts. A hormone is any substance that is released into the blood in small amounts and elicits a response on its target tissue. If the target tissue is another endocrine gland the hormone is referred to as a tropic hormone. Nerve receptors are used to detect alterations in the environment. Information of any alterations is conveyed to the integrating centre (usually the brain). The instruction is then conducted via nerve pathways to neuroendocrine connections where the impulses are converted into the secretion of the relevant hormone.

The important neuroendocrine connections are the adrenal medulla, pineal gland, hypothalamus, posterior pituitary and APUD system.

Chapter 40

General organization and function of the endocrine system

Objectives

At the completion of this chapter the student should be able to:

1. describe the general functions of the endocrine system;
2. describe the vertical and horizontal hierarchies of endocrine organization;
3. describe the endocrine functions of the hypothalamus and pineal gland;
4. describe how the hypothalamus regulates the secretion of hormones from the anterior pituitary;
5. explain how feedback influences hormonal secretion;
6. describe how stress influences the endocrine system, and in particular the adrenal glands.

40.1 General organization and function of the endocrine system

The endocrine system is organized as a highly integrated network where the actions of one gland can greatly influence the function of other glands.

The endocrine system performs the following functions:

1. regulation of the composition and volume of extracellular fluid by altering the ionic composition and volume of extracellular fluid;
2. regulation of ATP production by promoting metabolic activity;
3. regulation of digestion and absorption;
4. adapting the body to changes in the external environment;
5. adjusting the body's defence mechanisms to cope with the penetration of harmful foreign substances into the body;
6. control of growth and development;
7. development of sperm and the maturation and release of ovum for reproduction;
8. development of the embryo, foetus and newborn baby.

The major endocrine glands and their principal actions are listed in Table 40.1. These glands can be arranged into two hierarchies or levels of organization which can be referred to as the vertical and horizontal hierarchies.

Table 40.1   The major endocrine glands, their hormones and the principal actions of the hormones

Gland	Hormone	Actions
Adrenal cortex	Glucocorticoids	Cortisol and corticosterone inhibit the inflammatory response, maintain blood glucose levels during starvation by increasing protein catabolism and decreasing glucose catabolism
	Mineralocorticoids	Aldosterone stimulates the reabsorption of sodium ions in the kidney and the elimination of potassium ions
	Gonadocorticoids	Male androgens and female oestrogens play a role in secondary sexual characteristics particularly the androgens
Adrenal medulla	Epinephrine or adrenaline	Reinforces actions of sympathetic nervous system; increases cardiac output, blood sugar level and metabolic rate
	Norepinephrine or noradrenaline	Constricts blood vessels, increases systolic and diastolic pressure
Gonads	Oestrogen	Secreted by the ovaries, growth and maintenance of female reproductive organs, breasts and secondary sex characteristics, initiates the preparation of the uterus for embryo implantation
	Progesterone	Secreted by the corpus luteum, essential for completion of the uterus lining in preparation for embryo implantation
	Testosterone	Secreted by the testes, promotes the development of male secondary sex characteristics and development of sex organs
Pancreas (islets of Langerhans)	Insulin	Increases glucose transport into cells and accelerates the conversion of glucose into glycogen, the net effect is a lowered blood glucose level
	Glucagon	Raises blood sugar level by increasing glycogen breakdown
Parathyroid	PTH (parathyroid hormone) or parathormone	Elevates blood calcium concentration by increasing its absorption from the small intestine and its breakdown in bone; it decreases blood phosphate concentration
Pineal gland	Melatonin	Inhibits hypothalamus and the pituitary gland
	AVT (arginine vasotocin)	As above but more potent
Pituitary–anterior	ACTH (adrenocorticotropic hormone)	Stimulates the secretion of hormones from the adrenal cortex
	TSH (thyroid-stimulating hormone)	Stimulates the secretion of hormones from the thyroid gland

Table 40.1 *Continued*

Gland	Hormone	Actions
	FSH (follicle-stimulating hormone)	Stimulates the maturation of follicles in the ovaries, the secretion of oestrogen from the follicles and the formation and maturation of sperm
	LH (luteinizing hormone) or ICSH (interstitial cell-stimulating hormone)	Stimulates the maturation and release of follicles, the development of the corpus luteum, the secretion of testosterone in males
	HGH (human growth hormone) or somatotropin	Acts on tissues to promote growth by increasing the rate of amino acid transport in cells, stimulates the preferential breakdown of fat instead of glucose
	Prolactin	Acts on the mammary gland to stimulate milk secretion
	MSH (melanocyte-stimulating hormone)	Increases skin pigmentation
Pituitary–posterior	ADH (antidiuretic hormone)	Maintains or expands blood volume by increasing water reabsorption from the kidneys, maintains blood osmolality
	Oxytocin	Stimulates muscular contraction in the pregnant uterus and the ejection of milk
Thyroid	Thyroxin	Regulates catabolism and anabolism, accelerates body growth, glucose absorption from the small intestine
	Triiodothyronine	Same actions as thyroxin but is three to five times more potent
	Calcitonin (thyrocalcitonin)	Inhibits breakdown of calcium from bone and accelerates calcium absorption by bone

40.2   Vertical hierarchy

The **vertical hierarchy** consists of a chain of target glands and tropic hormones. Each gland regulates the release of hormones from the next gland in the hierarchy. ANALOGY: In a series of waterfalls, the water from the top waterfall causes water to flow out of the next waterfall and so on in a 'cascade effect'. The hypothalamus and pineal gland appear to be at the top of the hierarchy.

Endocrine functions of the hypothalamus

The **hypothalamus** performs the vital task of being the receptor or detector for many endocrine homeostatic mechanisms. The hypothalamus is able to detect chemical variations in the blood since it is not protected by the blood-brain barrier (18.1).

Information from the higher centres of the brain can influence the response that the hypothalamus may make. EXAMPLE: Anxiety, emotional disturbances can influence the hypothalamus and alter the expected homeostatic response. EXAMPLE: Elevated blood cortisol levels would normally result in the hypothalamus initiating a series of endocrine steps that lead to a decreased blood cortisol concentration. However, a patient under stress stimulates the release of cortisol. Since higher centres have the ultimate authority, this can result in either the cortisol level being maintained or increased. The normal homeostatic response of a decreased blood cortisol concentration has been overriden and has resulted in an abnormal blood cortisol level.

Hypothalamus–anterior pituitary

The influence that the hypothalamus exerts over the anterior pituitary is of particular importance since the latter gland acts as an intermediary gland between the hypothalamus and several peripheral glands. The tropic hormones secreted by the anterior pituitary and the glands that they influence are listed in Table 40.2. An additional hormone known as human growth hormone or somatotropin is secreted by the anterior pituitary. This hormone influences a variety of metabolic effects (Table 40.1).

The hypothalamus secretes specific **regulating hormones** for each of the anterior pituitary hormones. These regulating hormones are referred to as either releasing

Table 40.2 Anterior pituitary tropic hormones and their respective target glands

Tropic hormone	Target gland
ACTH	Adrenal cortex
FSH	Ovaries and testes
LH	Ovaries
ICSH	Testes
TSH	Thyroid

hormones or inhibiting hormones according to their actions on the anterior pituitary. These hormones elicit a specific action by only influencing the release of their complementary anterior pituitary hormone.

The hypothalamic hormones are secreted from the hypothalamus in response to nerve activity. They then flow to the anterior pituitary via a localized vascular network (39.4 and Figure 39.4). At the anterior pituitary gland, **releasing hormones** stimulate the release of their corresponding pituitary hormone. EXAMPLE: Corticotropic-releasing hormone stimulates the secretion of ACTH. A **release-inhibiting hormone** restrains the release of its corresponding anterior pituitary hormone. EXAMPLE: Prolactin release-inhibiting hormone (PIH) prevents the release of prolactin from the anterior pituitary. Absence of PIH results in the release of prolactin since the restraint on the secretion of prolactin has been removed.

Pineal gland

In humans, the pineal gland functions throughout life. Calcification of the gland is probably an indicator of the secretory activity of the gland. Calcification appears to have little effect on the endocrine secretory cells. These cells are called **pinealocytes**.

An indication of the function of the pineal gland is its extensive vascular network. Endocrine glands require a highly vascular network for the efficient release of their hormones into the body's bloodstream. The pineal gland's importance in the endocrine system can be gauged by the observation that it is the second-most vascular organ in the human body (the kidney is first).

The pineal gland has been referred to as the 'regulator of regulators', that is, it regulates the endocrine system. It appears that the pineal gland is involved in the regulation of the hypothalamus, pituitary, parathyroid and pancreas. The pineal gland exerts an inhibitory effect on the hypothalamus via the hormones melatonin and arginine vasotocin and thus opposes the actions that the hypothalamus elicits on the endocrine system.

An important aspect of pineal gland function is its neuronal connection with the retina. The pineal gland responds to increases in light intensity by decreasing the secretion of its hormones. Therefore, during the day minimal inhibition of the secretion of hypothalamic regulating hormones exists. At night, elevated levels of melatonin and arginine vasotocin decrease hypothalamic secretion. The pineal gland thus initiates a **circadian rhythm**, that is, a twenty-four hour cycle system. This action suggests that the pineal gland plays an important role in the functioning of the 'biological clock'.

The function of the pineal gland in the body homeostasis is only beginning to be unravelled. In the near future it is hoped that a greater knowledge of the gland's actions on the body will enhance the understanding of body homeostatic mechanisms, and in particular the function of the biological clock in these mechanisms.

Hypothalamus–anterior pituitary–target glands

The control of peripheral endocrine glands by the hypothalamus and anterior pituitary gland is summarized in Figure 40.1. The following steps are involved in these hormonal pathways:

1. the hypothalamus secretes a regulating hormone that travels via a short localized vascular system to the anterior pituitary gland;
2. the anterior pituitary responds to a releasing hormone by secreting a corresponding tropic hormone; if the regulating hormone is a release-inhibiting hormone

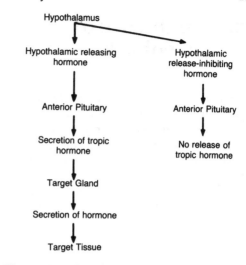

Figure 40.1 Control of peripheral endocrine glands by the hypothalamus and anterior pituitary gland showing a vertical hierarchy.

the result is a decreased secretion of the corresponding tropic hormone;
3. the tropic hormone travels via the vascular system and stimulates the secretion of a hormone from the target gland;
4. the target gland's hormone then travels via the vascular system to the target tissue where a response occurs.

Application: Control of adrenal cortex

The hypothalamus secretes corticotropic-releasing hormone (CRH) which stimulates the anterior pituitary to secrete adrenocorticotropic hormone (ACTH). The ACTH travels via the vascular system to the adrenal cortex where it elicits the release of a variety of hormones such as cortisol and aldosterone.

40.3 Influence of feedback

In homeostatic mechanisms, a feedback loop is necessary to inform the integrating centre of the effect of its actions on the body. This enables the integrating centre to make further fine adjustments in an attempt to correct any remaining imbalance (1.2).

In the hypothalamus–anterior pituitary–target gland endocrine pathway, two negative feedback loops usually exist. These loops are shown by using the example of ACTH and the adrenal cortex.

When the adrenal cortex hormones reach a critical level in the blood, hypothalamic receptors detect this level and suppress the release of CRH. The inhibition of CRH results in no stimulus reaching the anterior pituitary for the release of ACTH. The failure of ACTH to be released results in the adrenal cortex failing to release further quantities of its hormones. As these hormones are utilized, the blood levels decrease until the initial inhibition of CRH is removed. Once this inhibition is removed CRH, ACTH and the adrenal cortex hormones are in turn secreted (Figure 40.2).

A second shorter feedback loop also functions. This loop involves the adrenal cortex hormones directly inhibiting the secretion of ACTH from the pituitary.

40.4 Horizontal hierarchy

The endocrine system also functions in a **horizontal hierarchy**, that is, a variety of hormones may influence the levels of a particular substance. EXAMPLE: Blood glucose levels can be altered by the actions of insulin,

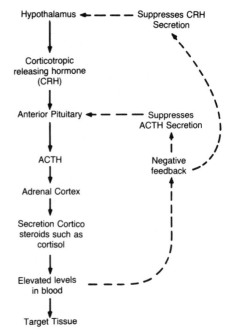

Figure 40.2 Relationship of adrenal cortex secretion to hypothalamic and anterior pituitary gland function.

glucagon, adrenaline, human growth hormone, thyroxin and cortisol.

The effect of a particular hormone in altering the level of a substance in the blood will therefore influence the secretion of other hormones involved in the regulation of that substance. EXAMPLE: A decreased blood sugar due to the action of insulin stimulates the release of glucagon.

The action of many hormones is considered to be interrelated with other hormones. It is therefore necessary for the integrating centre to take into account the levels of other hormones when responding to an altered chemical level.

Application: Hormonal influence on blood glucose levels

Insulin promotes increased movement of glucose across cell membranes along with increased utilization of glucose within the cell. The net effect of these actions is a decreased blood glucose level.

Glucagon acts in the liver to increase the quantities of glucose in the blood by increasing glycogen breakdown in the liver. Glucagon and insulin act together to regulate the storage of incoming glucose and the release of glucose between meals. Other hormones can also influence blood glucose levels in certain circumstances.

Epinephrine (adrenaline) is released in response to stress. This hormone elevates blood glucose levels by increasing the breakdown of muscle and liver glycogen. The increased quantities of glucose enhance energy production in time of need.

Thyroxine increases blood glucose levels by facilitating glucose absorption in the same intestine.

Cortisol and ACTH maintain blood glucose levels for the brain during starvation by decreasing glycogen and glucose catabolism, and increasing protein catabolism for energy production.

Somatotropin (human growth hormone) elevates blood glucose levels by accelerating fat catabolism and inhibiting non-essential use of glucose.

40.5 Stress and the endocrine system

Stress is a condition of the body produced by a variety of injurious agents called stressors (1.3). The stress may result from such things as injury, starvation, emotional disturbance and excessive noise. Any factor that causes stress will initiate a homeostatic response. Most of these homeostatic responses will exert either a direct or indirect stimulation of hormones in the endocrine system. The hypothalamus appears to be involved in the integration of the nervous and endocrine responses to stress. The effect of this integration is shown in the 'fight or flight' response (Table 1.1). This response involves the action of the hypothalamus on sympathetic nerves. The effect of this action is increased heart rate, constriction of blood vessels in the skin and abdomen, dilation of blood vessels in skeletal muscle and dilation of bronchioles. The rapid action of these nerves prepares the body for fight or flight.

A slower sustained and more generalized effect is achieved by releasing epinephrine (adrenaline) and norepinephrine (noradrenaline) from the adrenal medulla. The release of these hormones is due to the action of the hypothalamus on sympathetic nerves that connect with the adrenal medulla. The release of hormones from the adrenal medulla as a consequence of a stressor, is thus due to a direct stimulation of this peripheral gland by the hypothalamus.

Stress can also influence the secretion of hormones from the peripheral endocrine glands by exerting an influence on the secretion of regulating hormones from the hypothalamus. The result of stress on the hypothalamus is the altered secretion of tropic hormones and subsequently altered target gland function. Note that stress can override the feedback loop which can result in a resetting of the homeostatic mechanism. If the stress remains, the resetting will lead to an altered level of circulating hormone.

Application: Stress and the adrenal cortex

Stress exerts an indirect effect on the adrenal cortex via the vertical hierarchy of the hypothalamus–anterior pituitary (Figure 40.3). Stress stimulates the release of corticotropin-releasing hormone (CRH) from the hypothalamus. The CRH stimulates the release of ACTH from the anterior pituitary. The ACTH then travels via the blood stream to the adrenal cortex where it stimulates the release of cortisol. The stimulation of ACTH release may even occur when an elevated blood ACTH level exists, that is, stress overrides the normal homeostatic mechanisms.

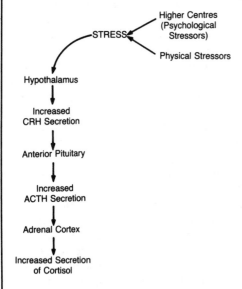

Figure 40.3 Effect of stress on cortisol secretion.

40.6 Diabetes mellitus: an example of endocrine malfunction

Diabetes mellitus is the most prevalent endocrine malfunction. It can be described as a chronic disorder due to a relative or absolute deficiency of insulin. Symptoms include the presence of glucose in the urine (glycosuria) and elevated blood glucose levels. These symptoms usually result from a malfunction in the secretion of insulin from the beta cells of the pancreas. The relative lack of insulin results in an inability of glucose to enter most cells and, as a consequence, blood glucose levels remain elevated for an abnormally long time after a meal. When the blood glucose levels exceed the T_m for kidney reabsorption, glucose appears in the urine (23.5).

The high blood glucose levels stimulate the hypothalamic blood glucose receptors to initiate the normal homeostatic mechanism for decreasing blood glucose, that is, pancreatic secretion of insulin. In patients where the pancreatic beta cells are destroyed, a failure of the homeostatic mechanism occurs.

The relative intracellular deficiency of glucose can cause an acid/base imbalance as a result of an elevated breakdown of fats and protein. This catabolism occurs in an attempt to supply sufficient energy for cell function.

Excessive catabolism of fats and protein can lead to metabolic acidosis (16.6). The acidosis results from the abnormally high levels of ketone bodies produced as a consequence of fat and protein catabolism.

Summary

The endocrine system is involved in the homeostatic control of many important body functions including:

1. regulation of the composition and volume of extracellular fluid,
2. regulation of ATP production;
3. regulation of digestion and absorption;
4. adapting the body to changes in the external environment;
5. adjusting the body's defence mechanisms;
6. control of growth and development;
7. development of mature sperm and ovum;
8. development of the embryo and foetus.

The endocrine system is arranged into two hierarchies known as the vertical and horizontal hierarchies.

The vertical hierarchy usually involves a neuroendocrine connection that controls the release of a series of tropic hormones. The end result of a vertical hierarchy is the secretion of hormones from a peripheral endocrine gland. Feedback and higher centres can influence the secretion of tropic hormones.

The horizontal hierarchy involves the secretion of several hormones for a particular substance. The effect of one hormone usually influences the secretion of other hormones. The interrelationship of hormone actions necessitates an integrating centre to take into account the levels of other hormones when responding to an altered chemical level.

The pineal gland appears to play an important role in the control of the endocrine system. It secretes hormones in response to changes in light intensity. These hormones are involved in the regulation of hypothalamic function.

Stress is a condition of the body produced by a variety of injurious agents called stressors. The hypothalamus appears to play a major part in the integration of the nervous and endocrine responses to stress. The feedback loop in homeostatic mechanisms can be overridden by stress originating from the higher centres, for example psychological stressors.

Alterations in the function of part of a homeostatic mechanism results in the inability of the mechanism to perform its normal regulatory role. In diabetes mellitus the relative or absolute deficiency of insulin results in glycosuria and elevated blood sugar levels.

Appendix A

Normal values in frequently used blood and plasma pathology tests

	SI unit	Old unit
BLOOD		
Haemoglobin		
Males	7.4–11.2 mmol/L or 12.0–18.0 g/dL	12–18 mg/100 mL
Females	7.14–10.00 mmol/L or 11.5–16.0 g/dL	11.5–16.0 mg/100 mL
Red blood cells		
Females	$3.9–5.6 \times 10^{12}$/L	$3.9–5.6 \times 10^6$/μL or mm^3
Males	$4.5–6.5 \times 10^{12}$/L	$4.5–6.5 \times 10^6$/μL or mm^3
White blood cells	$4.0–11.0 \times 10^9$/L	4000–11 000/mm^3
Platelets	$150–400 \times 10^9$/L	150 000–400 000/mm^3
PLASMA		
Bicarbonate (HCO_3^-)	21–32 mmol/L	21–32 meq/L
Calcium (Ca^{2+})	2.25–2.60 mmol/L	4.5–5.2 meq/L or 9.0–10.4 mg/100 mL
Chloride (Cl^-)	95–105 mmol/L	95–105 meq/L
Cholesterol	2.6–6.5 mmol/L	100–250 mg/100 mL
Creatinine		
Females	0.04–0.10 mmol/L	0.45–1.10 mg/100 mL
Males	0.06–0.12 mmol/L	0.68–1.40 mg/100 mL
Glucose	5.0–6.6 mmol/L	80–120 mg/100 mL
Magnesium (Mg^{2+})	0.80–1.05 mmol/L	1.6–2.1 meq/L or 1.95–2.55 mg/100 mL
Phosphate (inorganic)	0.8–1.5 mmol/L	2.5–4.6 mg/100 mL
Potassium	3.8–5.0 mmol/L	3.8–5.0 meq/L
Sodium	137–149 mmol/L	137–149 meq/L
Urea	3.2–7.5 mmol/L	19–45 mg/100 mL
Uric acid	0.18–0.47 mmol/L	3–8 mg/100 mL

Common SI unit conversions

Physical property	Non-SI unit	SI unit	Conversion to SI unit	Conversion from SI unit
Density	pounds per cubic ft	grams per cubic cm	× 0.016	× 62.43
Energy	calorie	kilojoule	× 4.18	× 0.24
Illumination	foot-candles	lux (lx)	× 10.76	× 0.093
Length	inch	centimetre (cm)	× 2.54	× 0.39
Length	feet	centimetre (cm)	× 30.48	× 0.033
Length	yard	metre (m)	× 0.91	× 1.094
Mass	pound	kilogram (kg)	× 0.45	× 2.22
Mass	ounce	gram (g)	× 28.35	× 0.035
Pressure	millimetres of mercury (mmHg)	kilopascal (kPa)	× 0.133	× 7.52
Pressure	pounds per square inch (psi)	kilopascal (kPa)	× 6.88	× 0.145
Pressure	centimetres of water	kilopascal (kPa)	× 0.098	× 10.23
Radioactive source	curie	bequerel (Bq)	× 3.7 × 10^{10}	× 0.27 × 10^{-10}
activity	curie	G bequerel	× 37	× 0.027
Radiation dose	rad	gray (Gy)	× 0.01	× 100
Radiation dose — human	rem	sievert (Sv)	× 0.01	× 100
Volume	gallon (UK)	litre (L)	× 4.5	× 0.22
Volume	gallon (US)	litre (L)	× 3.8	× 0.26
Volume	pint (UK)	litre (L)	× 0.57	× 1.75
Volume	pint (US)	litre (L)	× 0.47	× 2.13

Temperature

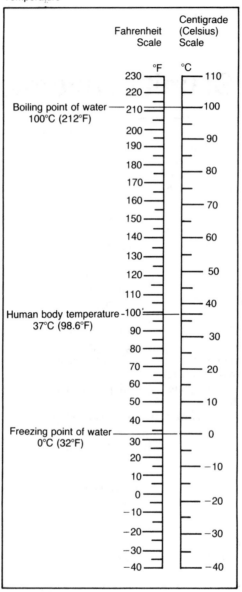

Temperature Conversions

$$°C = \frac{(°F - 32) \times 5}{9}$$

$$°F = \frac{°C \times 9}{5} + 32$$

Appendix C

A guide to group names, generic drug names and proprietary names

Group/Compound	Generic Name	United Kingdom	USA/Canada	Australia
			Examples of Proprietary Names	
Adrenergic Stimulant/ Adrenaline/Epinephrine (USA)	Adrenaline Epinephrine	Eprifin	Adrenaline	Eprifin
Adrenergic Stimulant/ Noradrenaline (Norepinephrine USA)	Noradrenaline Norepinephrine	Levophed	Levophed	Levophed
Analgesic/Acetylsalicylic Acid)	Aspirin	Aspro, Disprin	Bayer Aspirin	Aspro, Disprin
" /Codeine	Codeine	Codis, Panadeine	Codalan No 1	Codis, Panadeine
Analgesic/Morphine sulphate	Morphine	Nepenthe	Morphine	Morphine Sulphate injection
Antiangina/Glyceryl Trinitrate Nitroglycerin (USA)	Glyceryl Trinitrate Nitroglycerin (US)	Nitrocine	Transiderm-nitro	Transiderm-nitro
Antiarrhythmias/Lignocaine Hydrochloride	Lignocaine Lidocaine (US)	Xylocardz	Xylocard	Xylocard
Antibiotic/Aminoglycosides	Streptomycin	Streptomycin	Streptomycin	Streptomycin
Antibiotic/ "	Neomycin	Neomin	Neomycin	Neomycin
" /Anthracycline	Mitomycin	Mitomycin C	Mitomycin C	Mutamycin
" /Benzathine Penicillin	Benzathine Penicillin	B-Pen	Bicillin	Bicillin
" /Bacitracin	Bacitracin	Neobacrin	Mycitracin	Topisporin
" /Polymyxin sulphate	Polymyxin	Neosporin	Neosporin	Neosporin
" /Tetracyclines	Tetracycline	Tetrex	Tetracyn	Tetrex
" "	Doxycycline	Vibramycin	Vibramycin	Vibramycin
" /Vancomycin Hydrochloride	Vancomycin	Vancocin	Vancocin	Vancocin
Antifungal/Polyenes (Ampotericin)	Ampotericin	Ampotericin	Fungilin	Fungizone
" /Sulphonamide (Nystatin)	Nystatin	Nystan	Nilstat	Nilstat
Antifungal Antibiotic/Griseofulvin	Griseofulvin	Grisovin	Grisactin	Grisovin
Antiviral/Acyclovir (Halogenated pyrimidine)	Acyclovir	Zovirax	Zovirax	Zovirax
" /Idoxuridine	Idoxuridine		Stoxil	Stoxil
Antidiarrheal/Aluminium Hydroxide	Aluminium Hydroxide		Alu-Tab	Alu-Tab
" /Kaolin	Kaolin		Kapectolin PG	Kaopectate

Appendix C *Continued*

Group/Compound	Generic Name	Examples of Proprietary Names		
		United Kingdom	USA/Canada	Australia
Antihypertensive/Methyldopa	Methyldopa	Aldomet	Aldomet	Aldomet
" /Reserpine	Reserpine	Seraspil	Seraspil	Seraspil
Antimetics-Antinauseants/ Hyoscine	Hyoscine	Scopoderm	Transderm-scop/ Transderm-V (Canada)	Scop
Antimetics-Antinauseants/ Suxamethonium/ Succinyl chloride	Hysocine	Scoline	Scoline	Scoline
Antiseptic/Hexamine Mandelate	Hexamine Hippurate Methenamine (US) Mandelate (Aust)	Mandelamine	Mandelamine	Mandelamine
Diuretic/Ethacrynic Acid	Ethacrynic acid	Edecrin	Edecrin	Edecrin
Frusemide Furosemide (US)	Frusemide Furosemide (US)	Lasix	Lasix	Lasix
Hypnotic-Sedative/Barbiturates	Amylobarbitone Amobarbital (US)	Sodium amytal	Amytal	Amytal
" "	Pentobarbitone Pentobarbital (US)	Nembutal	Nembutal	Nembutal
Hyperacidity/Aluminium Salts			Basaljel	Neutralon
Immune Suppressants/ Cyclosporin	Cyclosporin	Sandimmun	Sandimmun	Sandimmun
Keratolyrics/Salicylic Acid	Salicylic Acid		Wartoff	Wartkil

Glossary

Absolute zero   Lowest temperature that is theoretically possible and is equal to 0 K or −273°C

Absorption   The uptake of substances into or across tissues

Acceleration   Change of velocity with time

Acellular   Non-cellular

Acetyl CoA   A substance that is composed of an acetyl group and coenzyme A and is involved in the production of energy

Acid   Any substance that releases hydrogen ions into water

Acidity   The relative number of free hydrogen ions in water; the greater the number of hydrogen ions the more acidic is that solution

Acidosis   Condition resulting from the accumulation of acid or the loss of base from the body

   Metabolic   Acidosis that results from either an increase in acidic metabolic products other than carbon dioxide or an excessive loss of base

   Respiratory   Acidosis resulting from excess retention of carbon dioxide in the body

Action potential   A wave of current that is conducted along a nerve fibre

Active process   Energy-dependent movement of substances across membranes

Active transport   An active process that moves substances across membranes by means of carriers

Adipose tissue   A specialized form of loose connective tissue which is involved in the production and storage of fat

Adrenergic nerve   Neuron that has norepinephrine (noradrenaline) as its transmitter

Adsorption   The holding of a substance to a surface

Aerobic   A process that occurs in the presence of oxygen

Aerosol   A colloid composed of liquids or solids dispersed in a gas

Alcohol   A molecule with an —OH functional group attached to a carbon atom

Aldehyde   A molecule that contains the functional group

$$-C-C\underset{}{\overset{\displaystyle O}{\diagup\!\!\!\diagdown}} H$$

Alkali   *See* Base

Alkalosis   Condition resulting from the accumulation of base or the excessive loss of acid from the body

   Metabolic   Alkalosis that results from either a decreased hydrogen ion concentration or an elevated base concentration

   Respiratory   Alkalosis resulting from the excess loss of carbon dioxide from the body

Alkanes   Hydrocarbons that have carbon atoms linked to each other by single bonds

Alkenes   Hydrocarbons that contain one or more carbon–carbon double bonds

Alkyl group   A saturated side chain which is derived from an alkane

Alkynes   Hydrocarbons that contain one or more carbon–carbon triple bonds

Alleles   Different forms of a particular gene

Allergen   An antigen that causes an allergy

Allergy   Oversensitivity of a person to a particular antigen

Alpha particle   A combination of two protons and two neutrons which is emitted from the nucleus of some radioactive isotopes

Amides   Organic compounds in which a carbonyl group is connected to a nitrogen atom

Amines   A group of organic compounds derived from ammonia (NH_3); the one, two or three hydrocarbon chains are attached to it according to the number of hydrogens that have been displaced

Amino acids   Organic acids that contain an amine group

    Essential   Amino acids that are unable to be produced by the body in sufficient quantities for normal metabolism

    Non-essential   Amino acids readily manufactured by the body

Amniocentesis   The collecting of amniotic fluid using a syringe and needle

Ampere   SI unit for electric current

Anabolism   Synthesis of a biochemical

Anaemia   A relative deficiency of haemoglobin

Anaerobic   A process that occurs in the absence of oxygen

Anaphylactic shock   A rapidly developed allergic reaction

Anion   An atom that has a relative excess of electrons and has a negative charge of at least 1

Anode   Positively charged electrode

Antagonism   A relationship between organisms where one microbial population adversely affects the growth of another

Antibiotic   A chemical produced by microbes which has the capacity in dilute solutions to kill or inhibit the growth of other microbes

Antibody   *See* Immunoglobulin

Anti-codon   Nucleotide triplet on tRNA

Antidiuretic hormone   A hormone secreted from the posterior pituitary that increases the reabsorption of water by the kidneys

Antigen   Any substance that induces the formation of antibodies or reacts with them

Antimicrobial   The suppression or destruction of any microorganism

Antiport   The movement of substances across membranes by carriers in opposite directions

Antiseptic   A substance applied to tissue that will inhibit the growth and multiplication of microbes without necessarily destroying them

APUD System   Diffuse neuroendocrine system consisting of special cells that have the property of amine precursor uptake and decarboxylation

Aqueous solution   Contains water as the solvent

Arteries   Vessels that carry blood from the heart to capillaries

Arteriole   Small artery, connects arterial system to a capillary

Asepsis   Absence of pathogenic microbes

    Medical   Condition excluding the infectious agents of a communicable disease

    Surgical   Exclusion of all microbes

Asymmetric carbon atom   Carbon atom with four different groups attached

Atheroma   A mass of material, usually fat, which accumulates on an arterial wall

Atom   Smallest structure of matter that represents an element; it consists of protons, neutrons and electrons

Atomic number   The number of protons in an atom

Atomic mass   The relative mass of an atom compared with an atom of carbon; it is approximately equal to the number of protons and neutrons in an atom

Atomic weight   *See* atomic mass

ATP   Adenosine triphosphate is a high-energy molecule that provides energy for cell functions

Atria   Filling chambers of the heart

Audiometry   Testing of hearing

Autoimmunity   The formation of an antigen within the body and the subsequent formation and reaction of antibodies to that antigen

Autonomic nervous system   The nervous system that connects the central nervous system to smooth muscle, cardiac muscle and glands

Axon   A long projection of the nerve cell body that transmits action potentials away from the cell body

Axoplasmic flow   Slow movement of substances down an axon

Bacilli   Rod-shaped bacteria

Bacteraemia   The presence of bacteria in the blood

Bactericide   An agent that kills bacteria

Bacteriostatic   Inhibiting the growth of bacteria without killing them

Barr body   A small dark staining area that occurs when more than one X chromosome is present in a cell

Basal ganglia   Aggregations of grey matter located within cerebal cortex

Basal metabolic rate   Rate of metabolism at rest

Base   A substance that donates hydroxyl ions (OH^-) into water or accepts hydrogen ions (H^+) from water

Base of support   The region of support for holding an object in a balanced position

Basophil   A type of white blood cell

B-Cells   Lymphocytes that are involved in the immune system and which originate from recognition lymphocytes; they are later transformed into plasma cells

Beta oxidation   The process of forming acetyl CoA by removing acetyl groups from a fatty acid

Beta particle   An electron emitted from the nucleus of an atom as a result of the breakdown of a neutron

Bile   A secretion of the gall bladder which has the ability to emulsify fat

Biofeedback   The process whereby a patient is taught to consciously control some actions of the autonomic nervous system

Biological value   Term relating to the content of essential amino acids in a protein

Blood pressure   Hydrostatic pressure that forces blood through the vascular system

   Diastolic   Pressure that occurs during filling of the ventricle

   Systolic   Pressure that results from contraction of heart ventricles; this pressure is greater than diastolic pressure

Bone tissue   A form of connective tissue in which the intercellular matrix is calcified

Boyle's Law   The volume of a gas varies inversely with pressure when the temperature is constant

Brownian movement   The constant motion of particles in random directions

Budding   Form of asexual reproduction in which a small new cell is pinched off from the parent cell

Buffer   Chemical that resists changes in pH on addition of acids or bases

Cancer   A cellular disease that is characterized by uncontrollable cellular multiplication

Capacitance   The property of a system to store an electric charge when a potential difference exists between a set of conductors. Charge which can be stored per unit volt of electrical potential

Capillary   Smallest blood vessel, site of nutrient and waste exchange between the blood and tissues

Capsid   The protective protein coat of a virus

Capsule   Slimy mucus-like coat surrounding the bacterial cell wall

Carbohydrate   An organic compound containing carbon, hydrogen and oxygen arranged into sugar molecules

Carbonic anhydrase   An enzyme that rapidly forms carbonic acid from water and carbon dioxide

Carcinogen   An agent that initiates the uncontrollable multiplication of cells, i.e. it initiates cancer

Cardiac arrhythmia   Abnormal rhythmic contraction of the heart

Cartilage   A form of connective tissue that consists of a gel-like matrix enclosed in a layer of dense connective tissue

Catabolism   The breakdown of biochemicals into simpler structures

Catalyst   Substance that alters the rate of a reaction without itself being permanently changed

Cathode   Negatively charged electrode

Cation   An atom with a positive charge of at least 1; the charge results from the loss of electrons

Cell   The smallest and simplest unit of matter that has the potential to duplicate itself

   Eucaryotic   Contains a highly organized internal structure

   Procaryotic   Contains a simple internal structure

Cell membrane   *See* Plasma membrane

Cell surface antigens   Antigens located on the surface of cells

Central nervous system   Comprises the brain and spinal cord

Centre of gravity   The point where the resultant gravitational force acts on an object

Centrioles   Small cylindrical cytoplasmic structures that play an important role in cell division

Cerebellum   Second largest region of the brain located over the medulla and pons; it is involved in subconscious coordination of skeletal muscle movements

Cerebral cortex   Region of grey matter in the cerebral hemispheres

Cerebral hemispheres   Two large lobes of the brain that are the site of conscious thought

Cerebrospinal fluid (CSF)   Fluid that surrounds the brain and spinal cord

Cerebrum   *See* Forebrain

Charles' Law   At constant pressure the volume of gas is directly proportional to its absolute temperature

Chemical energy   Energy required to bind atoms together

Cholesterol   A steroid that is an important component of cell membranes

Cholinergic nerve   Neuron that uses the neurotransmitter acetylcholine

Chromatin   Uncoiled DNA forming a diffuse thread-like network during interphase

Chromosome   Thick, thread-like structure found in the nucleus of a cell that contain the cell's hereditary information

Chylomicrons   Fat droplets that form an emulsion in lymph and blood

Cilia   Short, hair-like motile projections that occur in numerous quantities on the plasma membrane of some cells

Circadian rhythm   A twenty-four hour cycle

Cleaning   The removal of dust and dead organic matter, not microbial populations

Coagulation   Formation of suspended particles due to the combination of positively- and negatively-charged colloidal particles

Cocci   Spherical-shaped bacteria

Codon   Nucleotide triplet in mRNA

Coefficient of expansion   The response of a material to heating

Coefficient of friction   The ratio of the frictional force to the applied force

Coenzyme A   Coenzyme that acts as a carrier and assists enzyme function in the catabolism of carbohydrates and fats

Colloid   A fluid mixture in which the particles dispersed in the fluid are too large to be solutes and too small to form suspensions

Commensalism   An interrelationship between organisms in which one organism benefits from the association while the other is not affected

Communicability   The ability of a microbe to be communicated from an infected individual to another

Compensation   Return of pH towards normal due to body homeostatic mechanisms

Compound   A combination of atoms in a fixed proportion which confers definite physical and chemical properties to that compound

Inorganic Chemical compound that lacks carbon, with the exception of substances such as carbon dioxide

Metallic Chemical compound consisting of a lattice held together by metallic bonds

Organic Chemical compound that contains carbon, with the exception of substances such as carbon dioxide

Concentration The quantity of substance present in a given volume

Concentration gradient A difference in concentration between two regions

Conductivity Relative conducting ability of a material

Conformations Molecular shapes arising from rotations of atoms about bonds

Connective tissue Tissue that binds, supports and protects other tissue

Connective tissue proper A form of connective tissue that consists of cells and extracellular fibres embedded in a semi-fluid matrix

Covalent bond A linkage of atoms joined by sharing electrons

Covalent compound A compound formed of atoms linked by covalent bonds

Cranial nerves A set of twelve pairs of nerves that connect directly with the brain

Crystal Solid composed of a definite geometrical form

Cystinuria An inborn error which results in an inability to transport cysteine and similar structured amino acids across membranes

Cytochrome chain *See* Electron transport system

Cytology The study of cells

Cytoplasm General name for all the contents of a cell apart from the nucleus; it consists of organelles, inclusions and a cytoplasmic matrix

Cytoplasmic matrix Cellular fluid in which organelles and inclusions lie

Dalton's Law Each gas in a mixture of gases exerts its own pressure as if all other gases were not present

Deamination Removal of amine groups from the amino acid pool

Decibel Unit of loudness

Decimal reduction time The time taken to kill one-tenth of the microbial population

Decomposition Reaction involves the breakdown of one substance to form two or more products

Decontamination The process of removing all microbes from an object containing a heavy growth of microorganisms

Defibrillation Process whereby defibrillators apply strong electric shocks to the heart

Dehydration Excessive loss of water from the body resulting in a hypertonic extracellular fluid

Density The amount of a mass in a given volume

Depolarization A decrease in potential difference

Diabetes mellitus A chronic disorder due to a relative or absolute deficiency of insulin

Dialysate Bathing solution used in dialysis

Dialysis The separation of suspended particles and colloids from solutes by a membrane

Haemodialysis An artificial membrane is used to remove soluble toxic substances from the blood

Peritoneal The capillary network of the peritoneal cavity is used to remove toxic waste substances from the blood.

Diet The daily intake of food and drink

Diet therapy The use of a diet to manage and treat a specific medical condition

Differentiation The process whereby cells acquire specialized functions

Diffusion The net movement or flow of particles independent of metabolic energy from one region to another. Diffusion occurs down an electro chemical gradient

Dipole–Dipole interaction Linking of a polar molecule with other polar molecules as a result of the attraction of the slightly charged regions in each molecule

Disaccharide A compound consisting of two sugar molecules

Disinfection The process of destroying pathogens or rendering them inert on inanimate objects by chemical or physical agents

Dissociation Breakdown of a substance into ions when that substance is placed in a solvent

Dissolving The loose linking of solute molecules to solvent molecules

DNA Deoxyribonucleic acid; contains the genetic code

Doppler effect Apparent change in frequency of sound due to the relative motion between the source and the observer

Dorsal horn Point of entry of sensory neurons into the spinal cord

Droplet nuclei Airborne particles containing viable microbes

Earthing Process whereby the metal casing and other areas of a piece of equipment are connected to the earth

ECG *See* Electrocardiogram

Ecology The study of the relationship between organisms and their environment

Ectoparasite Parasite living on the skin or outer mucosal surfaces of the host

Elasticity The property of matter that returns it to its original shape after a force has altered the shape

Electric current The flow of positively charged ions in a liquid or the flow of electrons through a metal

Electrical conductor Substance that enables charged particles to move to their oppositely charged regions

Electrical energy Results from a flow of charged particles

Electrical gradient Difference in charge between two regions

Electrocardiogram A tracing made of various phases of the heart's electrical activity

by a machine known as an electrocardiograph

Electrochemical gradient The combined differences of chemical concentrations and electrical charges across a membrane

Electrolysis The movement of ions to oppositely charged electrodes in fluids

Electrolytes Substances that move to oppositely charged electrodes when placed in a liquid

Electromagnet Magnet associated with the movement of an electric current which can be turned off by stopping the current

Electromagnetic induction Generation of electricity in a loop of wire by a changing magnetic field

Electromagnetic radiation Waves or rays of energy that require no medium for propagation

Electron Subatomic particle with a small mass and a electrical charge of -1; located in orbits around the nucleus

Electron affinity The amount of energy released on gaining an electron.

Electron cloud Region of space surrounding a nucleus which is occupied by electrons. Also called electron shell

Electron transport system A system whereby the transfer of electrons along a chain of substances results in the release of energy that can be used to form ATP

Electrotherapy Range of therapeutic applications of electricity that are used in the treatment of pain, nerve damage, muscle injuries and soft tissue injuries

Element Matter that is composed of atoms with the same atomic number; it may be changed by physical means but usually not by chemical methods

Emulsion A colloid where one liquid in the shape of small droplets is dispersed throughout a second liquid

  Permanent The two liquids exist as a homogeneous mixture

  Temporary The two liquids form separate layers upon standing

Endocrine glands Secrete substances referred to as hormones directly into the bloodstream

Endoparasite Parasite living within the tissue or cells of the host

Endoplasmic reticulum Membranous network of canals that runs through the entire cytoplasm

  Rough Surface contains ribosomes

  Smooth Surface lacks ribosomes

Endoscopes Instruments that use optic fibres to examine hollow organs or internal cavities

Endospores Dormant cells within the cytoplasm of some bacteria

Endothermic reaction Reactions requiring a net input of energy

Energy Creates a potential to do work or enables matter to do work

Energy level Represents the energy within an electron cloud and is often used to describe an electron cloud

Energy sublevel Energy levels represented as s, p, d, f within an electron cloud. Each sublevel contains pairs of electrons spinning in opposite directions

Enzymes Proteins that affect the speed of chemical reactions

Eosinophil A type of white blood cell

Epithelial tissue Covers the surface of the body and organs, lines body cavities and organs as well as forming glands

Erythema Localized inflammatory response which is visible as a reddening of the skin

Erythrocytes Red blood cells

Erythropoiesis The production of erythrocytes (red blood cells)

ESR The erythrocyte sedimentation rate is a measure of the rate at which erythrocytes settle; used in the diagnosis of various pathological states

Ester Molecule that contains the functional group

$$-C-\overset{\overset{\textstyle O}{\|}}{C}-O-C$$

Excretion Process of removing unwanted substances from the organism

Exocrine glands Secrete substances via ducts into the body

Exothermic reaction Reactions involving a net release of energy

Extracellular fluid Body fluid located outside cells

Facilitated diffusion A process by which a lipid-insoluble substance is passively transported across a membrane by a carrier

Fats A group of lipids that consist of three fatty acids bonded to a glycerol molecule

Feedback, Negative Mechanism that results in a reversal of a physiological response back to the normal range following an imbalance

Fibrillation Asynchronous contraction and quivering of the atria or ventricles

Fibrinogen Plasma protein involved in the formation of blood clots

Flagella Long motile projections of the plasma membrane

Fluid A substance that takes the shape of its container and can be a liquid or a gas

Fomites Inanimate objects that carry viable pathogenic organisms

Force Any influence that either changes the position, the state of rest or the motion of an object. The SI unit of force is the newton

Forebrain Anterior region of the brain which contains the cerebral hemispheres, thalamus, hypothalamus and pineal gland

Formulae

  Molecular States the actual number of atoms of each element present

  Structural Shows the actual number of atoms of each element present and their structural arrangement

Friction Force that resists the movement of one object over another

Functional group An arrangement of atoms that has very similar chemical and physical properties wherever it is found in an organic molecule

Fungicide   An agent that kills fungi

Gamma rays   Electromagnetic radiation emitted from radioactive isotopes with a shorter wavelength than X-rays

Ganglion   Junction region where a mass of nerve cell bodies exist

Gas   The state of matter where molecules are able to move independently of each other; the molecules have a greater kinetic energy than those of liquids

Gastrostomy   Surgical placement of a tube into the stomach through the abdominal wall

Gel   A colloid composed of solid particles set in a semi-solid that has jelly-like properties

Gene   The smallest unit of heredity which represents a single physical characteristic

Genetics   The study of genes and their relationships to hereditary characteristics

Genetic code   The language that is used by a cell to transfer genetic information into chemical manufacture

Genetic predisposition   An individual that has a genetic potential for a specific disease but this potential is only realized when certain environmental conditions exist

Genome   The complete set of genetic material

Genotype   The genetic composition of an individual

Germicide   An agent that kills the growing microbial forms but not necessarily the resistant spore forms

Gluconeogenesis   The synthesis of glucose from the conversion of amino acids or the glycerol portions of fat

Glycerol   A three-carbon alcohol that combines with fatty acids to form fats

Glycogen   A polysaccharide that acts as a temporary storage of body carbohydrate; it is composed of chains of glucose molecules

Glycogen storage disease   A disease where glycogen is unable to be reconverted into glucose

Glycolipid   Lipid containing branched chains of sugar

Glycolysis   The first step in glucose catabolism whereby glucose is broken down to form pyruvic acid

Glycoprotein   Proteins with covalently bonded sugar units

Glycosuria   The appearance of glucose in urine

Golgi complex   Network of flattened tubes that act as the cell's storage and distribution centre

Gravity   The force of attraction between objects; it is often used to describe the attraction of objects to the earth

Grey matter   Regions of the brain and spinal cord that consist mainly of cell bodies

Ground state   Resting energy level of an electron which represents the lowest possible energy level for that electron

Growth   Increase in size or number of cells

Guthrie Test   Used to detect the presence of phenylalanine in the blood and urine

Haem group   A chemical structure that has iron located in its centre

Haemoglobin   A pigment that consists of the protein globin wrapped around four haem groups

   Oxygenated   The loss of hydrogen ions from haemoglobin or the addition of oxygen to haemoglobin

   Reduced   The addition of hydrogen ions to haemoglobin or the loss of oxygen

Haemophilia   A sex-linked genetic disorder that results in either the failure of blood to clot or the very slow clotting of blood following bleeding

Haemostasis   The arrest of bleeding

Half-life   Time taken for half a given number of radioactive atoms of an isotope to decay into a new element

Halogen   An element in group VIIA of the periodic table

Heat   Energy possessed by a substance as a result of vibration of atoms and molecules

Henry's Law   The amount of gas dissolved in a liquid varies proportionally with the partial pressure of the gas, when the temperature remains constant

Herpes Simplex   Virus responsible for the development of cold sores

Hertz   The SI unit of frequency which represents the number of waves per second

Heterocyclic compound   Cyclic organic compounds that contain another element within the carbon ring

Heterozygous   The presence of two different alleles of the same gene

Hindbrain   Contains three principal structures known as the cerebellum, pons and medulla oblongata. Also called the rhombencephalon

Homeostasis   A relative state of equilibrium between the internal environment of an organism and the changing external environment

Homologous series   An organic series in which each member differs from the member of next higher weight by a methylene group (CH_2)

Homozygous   The presence of a pair of chromosomes with the same allele

Hormone   Any substance that is released from a gland into the blood in small amounts and which on arrival at a particular tissue elicits a response

Hydrated diameter   The diameter of the combination of a solute and its attached water molecules

Hydrocarbon   Compounds composed of carbon and hydrogen

  Aromatic   A compound that contains a ring of six carbon atoms joined together in an alternating sequence of single and double bonds

Hydrogen bond   A dipole–dipole interaction involving hydrogen

Hydrophilic   Water attracting

Hydrophobic   Water repelling

Hydrostatic pressure   The pressure that results from the particles of a liquid colliding with the walls of a container

Hydroxyl ion   The radical OH^-

Hypertension   Persistently high blood pressure

Hypertonic solution   A solution that has a greater osmotic pressure than intercellular fluid; these solutions cause cells to shrink

Hyperventilation   A rate of breathing that is faster than normal

Hyphae   Threadlike structures in fungi formed of elongated cells

Hypothalamus   A major neuroendocrine connection located in the forebrain

Hypoventilation   A rate of breathing that is slower than normal

Hypoxaemia   An insufficient concentration of oxygen in the blood

Hypoxia   Diminished amount of oxygen in the tissues

Immiscible   A liquid which is insoluble in another liquid

Immunity

  Cell mediated   Specific defence mechanism that involves the production of specialized lymphocytes

  Humoral   Specific defence mechanism that involves the production of immunoglobulins

Immunoglobulins   Specific defence proteins produced by plasma cells

Inanimate   Without life, lacking in animation

Inclusions   A diverse group of structures found in cells

Incubation period   The time elapsing between exposure to infection and the appearance of disease symptoms

Inertia   The reluctance of a body to start moving after a force has been applied to it and the reluctance of the body to stop once it has begun to move

Infection   Invasion and multiplication of microorganisms in a host which results in a pathological condition

Infectious disease   Disease induced by an organism

Inflammation   The response of tissues to infection or injury which is characterized by localized dilation of blood vessels, the accumulation of fluid, pus formation and the formation of a clot

Inflammatory response   A body' response to harmful foreign material that involves the combined action of non-specific defence mechanisms and the repair of any damaged region

Infra-red rays   Electromagnetic radiation represented by waves that have a wavelength that ranges between microwaves and light rays

Insulator   Substance or medium incapable of carrying charged particles to oppositely charged regions, or a substance that is incapable of transmitting heat

Intercellular fluid   *See* Interstitial fluid

Interferon   Antiviral proteins formed by T-cells

Interphase   Period between cell divisions

Interstitial fluid   Extracellular fluid that surrounds tissue cells

Intracellular fluid   Fluid found within cells

Intravascular fluid   Extracellular fluid located in the vascular system; commonly referred to as blood

Invasiveness   The ability of a microbe to infect hosts, survive and multiply

Inverse square law   Intensity is inversely proportional of the square of the distance from the source

Ion   An atom or group of atoms that contains an electrical charge of at least $+1$ or -1

Ionic bond   A linkage that binds ions together as a result of the attraction of opposite charges

Ionic compound   A compound formed from the combination of ions

Ionization energy   The amount of energy that must be added to remove an electron

Ionizing radiation   Radiation which is capable of directly or indirectly causing ionization of atoms

Irritability   Ability to respond to a stimulus from the environment

Isomer   Substances that have the same molecular formula but different arrangements of atoms which form either structural, functional, geometric or optical isomers

Isosmotic solution   *See* Isotonic solution

Isotonic solution   Has the same osmotic pressure as the solution with which it is compared; cells neither shrink nor swell when placed in such a solution

Isotopes   Atoms of the same element that contain different mass numbers

Joule   The SI unit for energy

Karyotype   A formal arrangement of chromosomes used to identify chromosomal abnormalities and identify the sex of an individual

Kelvin   The SI unit for temperature

Ketone   Organic substances that contain the functional group

$$-\overset{|}{\underset{|}{C}}-\overset{|}{\underset{\parallel}{\underset{O}{C}}}-\overset{|}{\underset{|}{C}}$$

Ketone body   A group of ketones that are formed during fatty acid and amino acid catabolism; most ketone bodies are acids

Ketosis   A form of metabolic acidosis due to the excessive production of ketone bodies

Kilogram   The SI unit for weight

Kinematics   Descriptive study of motion used to describe the relative movement of body parts

Kinetic energy   Energy resulting from action or performing work

Kinetics   Study of the size and direction of forces

Krebs cycle   Aerobic catabolism of acetyl group to carbon dioxide and hydrogen

Lactose intolerance   A deficiency in the enzyme lactase which results in an inability to digest and absorb milk

Laser   Light amplification by stimulated emission of radiation. A beam of parallel rays consisting of the same wavelength

Latent heat   Heat involved in the breaking apart of particles to cause a change of state

Leucocyte   White blood cell

Leukaemia   A blood disease in which an uncontrolled production of white blood cells occurs

Lever   A bar which connects an object and a force

Light   Electromagnetic radiation that contains a smaller wavelength than infra-red rays but a greater wavelength than ultraviolet rays; it is able to stimulate the retina of the human eye to produce images in the brain

Lipids   A diverse group of organic substances which share the property of being relatively insoluble in water and readily soluble in organic solvents

Liquid   A state of matter in which molecules have limited movement; the molecules have a greater kinetic energy than those in solids

Litre   The SI unit for volume

Loose connective tissue   Consists of a loose network of collagen and elastic fibres

Lumbar puncture   The insertion of a needle into the CSF in the lumbar region of the spinal cord

Lymph   Extracellular fluid located in the lymph vessels

Lymphatic system   Composed of the spleen, tonsils and thymus, tissue called lymph nodes, and a network of lymphatic vessels

Lymphocyte   A type of white blood cell

Lysosomes   Small organelles that contain powerful digestive substances for the breaking down of unwanted material

Magnetic field   Region between the poles of a magnet where magnetic lines of force exist

Magnetic resonance imaging   An imaging scanner that focuses on a single element in a tissue to magnetism

Magnetism   Property of certain metals called magnets where metals such as iron are attracted to the magnet

Malnutrition   Any disorder of nutrition. It may be due to insufficient or unbalanced diet or to defective assimilation or utilization of foods

Maltose   A disaccharide formed in the mouth and small intestine

Mass   The quantity of matter of an object

Mass number   The number of protons and neutrons present in an atom

Matter   Anything that occupies space and has some mass

Mechanical advantage   Ratio of load to effort

Mechanical energy   Energy associated with moving parts

Medulla oblongata   Hindbrain structure that links the spinal cord and the remainder of the brain

Meiosis   A process that results in the formation of cells with half the number of chromosomes of the parent cell

Memory cells   Cells involved in the immune process; recognition lymphocytes that remain unchanged following an infection

Mesencephalon   *See* Midbrain

Metabolism   The manufacture and breakdown of body chemicals

Metallic bond   Linkage of cations by a highly mobile cloud of electrons

Metastasis   Transfer of disease from one organ or part of an organ to another not directly connected to it

Metre   The SI unit for length

Microtubules   Thin rigid-like tubular structures that consist mainly of the protein tubulin

Microvilli   Small cytoplasmic extensions that increase the surface area of cells

Microwaves   Electromagnetic radiation with wavelengths ranging from short radio waves to rays near the infra-red region

Micturition The process of expelling urine from the bladder; also known as urination or voiding

Midbrain Connects the forebrain to the hindbrain and is involved in the coordination of visual and auditory reflexes

Milliequivalent The amount of substance required to combine with, or displace, one milligram of hydrogen

Minerals Inorganic substances that function in the body in combination with other minerals or with organic substances

Miscible A liquid which is soluble in another liquid

Mitochondria Double-membraned organelles in which the inner membrane is folded to form cristae; site of aerobic respiration

Mitosis The stages by which a cell divides to form two cells that are identical with the parent cell

Mixture Contains two or more elements that are not bound to each other and which may exist in variable proportions

Mole The atomic or molecular weight of a substance in grams; one mole contains 6.023×10^{23} particles

Molecular weight The total weight of all the constituent atoms of a molecule

Molecule The simplest unit of a compound to retain the properties of that compound

Moment The measure of the tendency of a force to rotate an object about a point

Momentum Motion of a body as a result of its mass and velocity

Monera Organisms with a procaryotic cell

Monoclonal antibodies Homogeneous preparations of a specific antibody

Monocyte A type of white blood cell

Monosaccharide A single sugar molecule

Multiple alleles Two or more alleles that exist for the one gene

Muscle atrophy Muscle wasting

Muscular tissue Tissue that has the ability to contract

Mutualism A co-existence in which each organism benefits from the association

Mycelium A branched network of hyphae constituting the vegetative structure of a fungus

Myelinated axon Axon covered with sheaths of myelin

Myopathy Disorder of skeletal muscle

NAD A coenzyme that plays an important role in the transfer of hydrogen to the cytochrome chain

Nebulizer A device that uses either compressed air or ultrasonic waves to form an aerosol by dispersing liquids or solids into a gas

Nerve Combination of many bundles of nerve fibres

Nerve fibre Nerve axon and its surrounding sheaths

Nervous tissue Composed of neurons and neuroglia

Neuroglia A group of cells that support, protect and assist the function of neurones

Neuromuscular junction Region where a nerve and muscle make functional contact

Neuron Cell capable of conducting and transmitting impulses; it consists of a cell body with short protrusions called dendrites and a long projection called an axon

Neurotransmitter Chemicals released from presynaptic nerves that indirectly transfer a nerve impulse to postsynaptic nerves or muscle cells

Neutralism A completely independent association between organisms

Neutralization Process whereby acids and bases are combined until neither is in excess and the solution has a neutral pH

Neutron Uncharged subatomic particle of similar mass to a proton; located in the nucleus

Neutrophil A type of white blood cell

Nitrogen balance The amount of nitrogen in the urine compared with nitrogen intake over a period of time

Negative More nitrogen is being excreted than is being taken into the body

Positive Intake of nitrogen exceeds excretion

Non-disjunction The failure of chromatids to separate during cell division

Non-pathogen Non-disease producing microbe

Non-polar molecule A molecule that is composed of atoms that share their electrons approximately 50% of the time with other atoms

Nuclear emissions Particles ejected from a nucleus

Nuclear energy Energy released from interactions within the nucleus of an atom

Nucleolus Spherical body found in the nucleus of cells

Nucleotide A combination of a nitrogen base, a sugar and a phosphate group which acts as the building block of DNA and RNA

Nucleus

Atom Central part of an atom containing protons and neutrons

Cell A relatively large membrane-bound structure that controls and regulates cell multiplication and maintains cell function

Obesity A condition in which more kilojoules than the body requires are taken in over a period of time

Optic fibres Flexible glass rods that are capable of conducting light from one end to the other

Organ Group of tissues that act in a unique, coordinated and functional manner

Organelles Small membrane-bound functional structures found in cells

Osmol Unit of measurement that measures a solute's ability to induce osmosis and osmotic pressure; it is a measure of the total number of particles present in a solution

Osmolality The osmols of particles per kilogram of water

Osmolarity The osmols of particles per litre of solution

Osmosis The net movement of water through a semi-permeable membrane from an area of high water concentration to an area of low water concentration

Osmotic pressure The pressure required to exactly oppose the net movement of water by osmosis, that is, the resistance that is required to just stop the net flow of water

Oxaloacetic acid An important compound in the Krebs cycle involved in protein, carbohydrate and fat metabolism

Oxidation The process of either combining oxygen with a substance or removing hydrogen from a substance

process where a substance loses one or more electrons

–reduction reactions Reactions resulting in the transfer of electrons from one substance to another

number Number of electrons gained or lost with an increase in the number indicating the oxidizing of a substance

Oxidative phosphorylation A process whereby energy from the electron transport system is used to form ATP in the presence of oxygen

Oxidizing agent Substance that accepts electrons from another substance causing an oxidation of that substance. Also called oxidant

Parasitism A relationship between organisms in which one organism derives some degree of support from another at the latter's expense

Parasitology Study of the parasitic or disease-producing protozoa and other non-microbial parasitic organisms

Parasympathetic nervous system A division of the autonomic nervous system that generally acts as an inhibiting system

Parathyroid glands Tiny glands located on the thyroid gland that are involved in the regulation of calcium and phosphate concentrations in the blood

Parenteral Introduction of substances into

the body by a route other than the gastrointestinal tract

Nutrition The delivery of nutrients directly into the bloodstream via a catheter into a large vein

Partial pressure The pressure exerted by a particular gas in a mixture of gases

Particle Unit of matter consisting of one of the following: atoms, molecules, ions, electrons, positrons, protons, neutrons, helium nuclei

Pascal The SI unit for pressure

Pascal's Law Pressure exerted on a confined liquid is transmitted equally in all directions

Pathogen Disease-causing microbe

Pathogenicity Capacity to cause disease

Peptide bond A bond that links the amine group of one amino acid with the carboxyl group of an adjacent amino acid

Periodic group The atoms in a periodic group contain the same number of outer shell electrons and are found in the same vertical rows of the Periodic Table

Periodic period The elements in the same horizontal row of the Periodic Table

Peripheral nervous system Consists of the spinal nerves, cranial nerves and the autonomic nervous system

Peripheral resistance The resistance of small diameter blood vessels to blood flow

Peristalsis Rhythmic waves of smooth muscle contractions

Permeability The ease with which a substance passes across a membrane

pH A numerical scale that represents the powers of ten of hydrogen ions; it is a relative indicator of acidity and alkalinity

Phagocytosis The active ingestion of large particles by specialized cells

Phenol A molecule with a — OH functional group attached to a benzene ring

Phenotype Physical expression of the genotype

Phenylketonuria An inborn error of metabolism that results in an inability to convert phenylalanine into tyrosine; it can prevent normal development of the brain

Phospholipids A group of lipids that contain glycerol combined with two fatty acids and one phosphate group; a major constituent of membranes

Pineal gland An important neuroendocrine connection located in the forebrain; its function is linked with light and darkness and it is believed to play an important role in the biological clock and the control of the endocrine system

Pinocytosis The active movement of substances across a membrane by vesicles

Pitch Conscious perception of a particular frequency of sound wave

Pituitary gland A major endocrine gland that is linked to the hypothalamus

Pivot Point around which rotation occurs

Plasma The non-cellular component of blood

Plasma cells Involved in the immune reponse; transformed B-cells that have the ability to secrete immunoglobulins

Plasma membrane Membrane that separates the cell's internal contents from the extracellular environment

Platelets Tiny disc-shaped cells found in blood that lack a nucleus. Also called thrombocytes

Polar molecule A molecule that is composed of slightly-charged atoms due to unequal sharing of electrons between atoms

Polypeptide A chain of many amino acids

Polysaccharide A carbohydrate that consists of many sugar molecules

Pons Hindbrain structure that links the medulla oblongata and cerebellum to the midbrain

Pore A small hole in a membrane

Portals of entry Points of entry for a microorganism into a host

Portals of exit Routes of discharge of microbes from a host

Positron Postively charged nuclear particle

with the same mass as an electron and an equal but opposite charge to the electron

Postural hypotension A decreased blood pressure that results from the inability of the heart to force enough blood to the brain on sudden rising from a horizontal position

Potential difference The potential for electricity to flow due to a difference in charge between two regions; it is a form of potential energy

Potential energy The energy stored in an object as a result of its position or chemical composition

Power The rate of doing work; the SI units are joules per second or watts

Precipitate Undissolved solute that is found in saturated solutions

Pressure The force exerted by particles on a given surface area of matter

Negative Pressure lower than standard atmospheric pressure

Positive Pressure greater than standard atmospheric pressure

Prostaglandins A group of lipids that consist of twenty carbon fatty acids of which five of the carbon atoms are arranged in a ring; they are sometimes referred to as tissue hormones

Proteins An essential group of biochemicals composed of polypeptide chains

Fibrous Long helical chains of amino acids entwined with each other

Globular Considerably folded polypeptide chains

Integral Contains polar regions and located on both sides of plasma membranes

Peripheral Loosely bound to the surface of the membrane through binding with integral proteins or polar lipid ends

Protoplasm The matter contained in biological cells (consists mainly of water, macromolecules and inorganic substances)

Proton Subatomic particle which has an electrical charge of +1 located in the nucleus

Pulley A grooved wheel on an axle that is used to change the direction of a force

Purgative agent An agent which assists evacuation of the bowels

Qualitative measurement Descriptive signs used to record observations

Quantitative measurement Numbers used to express measurements recorded by an instrument

Radical A group of atoms which acts as a unit within a molecule, and when that molecule undergoes a chemical change the radical remains as an intact unit

Radioimmunoassay Diagnostic test that uses an antigen–istope complex to compete with unlabelled antigen for a particular antibody

Radioisotope An unstable isotope that emits radiation

Recognition lymphocyte Special lymphocytes that identify antigens

Reducing agent Substance that donates electrons to another substance causing a reduction. Also called reductant

Reduction Process of gaining electrons

Reflection Returning of electromagnetic waves after hitting a surface

Refraction Bending of electromagnetic waves when changing from one medium to another

Regulating hormones Hormones secreted by the hypothalamus that either stimulate the release or inhibit the release of specific hormones from the anterior pituitary

Relative humidity The relative amount of water vapour compared to the closed system

Renal calculi Precipitate found in the kidney that is composed of uric acid or calcium salts, commonly referred to as kidney stones

Replication The process by which viruses multiply. The duplication of DNA molecules

Repolarization A return of a potential difference towards the resting potential

Reprodution

Asexual One parent cell or organism gives rise to progeny

Sexual The combination of two nuclei of different cells in fertilization and the mixing of their genetic material

Resistance, Electrical Opposition to the flow of charges, measured in ohms

Resonance Occurs in molecules where several electron arrangements occur due to electrons moving around the entire molecule instead of forming pairs

Respirator Machine that assists breathing

Respiratory distress syndrome Results from a lack of pulmonary surfactant in newborn babies

Resting potential Potential difference between the inside and outside of a nerve or muscle cell prior to an electrical event

Reticuloendothelial system A functional system that consists of highly phagocytic cells broadly distributed throughout the body

Retina Layer of photoreceptive cells in the eye that convert light images into nerve impulses

Reversible reaction Products can unite to reform the original reactants thereby resulting in a two-way reaction

Rhombencephalon *See* Hindbrain

Ribosomes Small organelles that are either located on the endoplasmic reticulum or are dispersed throughout the cytoplasm

RNA Ribonucleic acid provides the means by which genetic information can be transformed into actions within the cell

mRNA Carries genetic information from the nucleus to the ribosomes

tRNA Carries amino acids to the ribosomes

Salt An ionic compound formed as a result of combining an acid with a base

Sanitization The removal of pathogens to an acceptable safe level from inanimate objects by mechanical or chemical cleaning

Saprophyte Organism that obtains its nutrients from non-living organic material produced by or derived from other organisms

Saturated compound Carbon atoms are linked by single bonds

Solution Contains the maximum quantity of dissolved solute

Scalar Any physical quantity that is described only in terms of magnitude

Semi-permeable membrane A membrane which allows the movement of water through it, but not other substances

Semi-qualitative measurement The use of relative scale, usually in the form of 'plus' or relative words

Sensitized Possession of a quantity of immunoglobulin along with a reserve of memory cells for a particular antigen

Septicaemia The presence and multiplication of bacteria in the blood resulting in an infection of the blood stream

Serum Fluid component of blood that differs from plasma in that it lacks clotting factors

Short wave diathermy Use of high frequency current to create an electrical field in tissue which results in the generation of heat through the movement of ions

Signs Evidence of a disease to an observer

Sol A colloid composed of solid particles dispersed in a liquid

Solid A state of matter in which atoms, ions and molecules are held in a relatively fixed position

Solubility A measure of the amount of solute that will dissolve in a specified volume of solvent

Solutes Substances dissolved in a solvent

Solution A fluid that consists of a homogeneous mixture of two or more substances

Solvent The greater quantity of substance in a solution

Sonic energy Vibration of particles in the form of wave through matter; sound waves require a medium for propagation

Species Organisms sharing the characteristic of interbreeding or the capacity to interbreed

Specific gravity The weight of a certain volume of substance compared with the weight of the same volume of water

Specific heat capacity The amount of heat required to raise 1 kg of a substance by 1°C

Sphygmomanometer An instrument that is used to measure arterial blood pressure

Spinal cord A long rod of nervous tissue that connects the brain with the nerves in the body

Spinal nerve Each nerve contains afferent nerve fibres that conduct information to the spinal cord and efferent nerve fibres that carry information to muscles or glands

Spinal reflex A localized reflex between the sensory and motor neurons of the same spinal cord segment

Spirilla Spiral-shaped bacteria

Spore A resistant body formed by certain microorganisms

Sporicide An agent that kills spores

Stability The ability of an object to resist falling

Statics Study of objects in equilibrium

Steatorrhoea The occurrence of large amounts of fat in faeces

Sterilization Measure which destroys or removes all living organisms

Steroids A group of lipids that contain four carbon rings arranged in a specific configuration; includes cholesterol, bile salts and adrenocortico hormones

Stress A condition of the body produced by injurious agents or stressors

Stressors Injurious agents or stimuli that initiate a condition of stress

Surface tension The pull of the surface particles of a liquid into the body of the liquid

Surfactant A substance that decreases the surface tension of a liquid

Suspension Non-homogenous fluid mixture that contains large particles that settle when the mixture is left to stand

Symbiosis A dependent association between two different organisms or populations of organisms

Sympathetic nervous system A division of the autonomic nervous system that prepares the body to respond to stress

Symport The transport of two different substances across a membrane in the same direction

Symptom Subjective evidence of a disease or of a patient's condition

Synapse A region where two neurons make close contact with each other

Synovial fluid A low friction substance found in cavities between bones

System A group of interacting organs that operate as a functional unit

Target gland A gland that is acted upon by a hormone

Target tissue Tissue acted upon by a hormone

T-Cell Specialized lymphocytes that combine directly with an antigen in a response referred to as cell mediated immunity

Telencephalon Cerebral hemispheres and basal ganglia located within them

Temperature A measure of heat intensity

Thalamus A giant relay system located in the forebrain that distributes sensory information to the cerebral cortex

Thermal death time The time it takes at a certain temperature to kill a stated number of organisms (or species) under specified conditions

Thermal expansion Results from increase in the size of vibrations with increasing heat

Thrombocyte *See* Platelet

Tincture A solution in which alcohol is used as the solvent

Tissue A combination of many cells that have a similar structure and function

Tissue rejection Immune response to the introduction of transplanted cells

Tomography The production of a series of cross-sectional images of a structure by means of an instrument

Toxigenicity The ability of a microbe to

produce substances that are toxic to the host

Traction Process whereby the fractured ends of a bone are kept in position by a system of pulleys and weights

Transamination Process by which an amine group is transferred from one amino acid to an organic compound to form another amino acid

Transcription Formation of RNA from DNA

Transformer Device consisting of a primary coil of wire which induces a current in a secondary coil of wire

Translation Mechanism of forming protein through the conversion of genetic information

Transport maximum (T_m) The flow rate for a substance that is carried across a membrane; it represents the concentration gradient when all carriers are occupied

Triglyceride Fat

Trisomy The presence of an additional chromosome due to an error in chromosome division

Trophic factors Substances that travel down nerves by axoplasmic flow to assist in the development, maintenance and regeneration of the nerve network

Tropic hormone A hormone that regulates the release of hormones from a target gland

Tumour A swelling due to the abnormal growth of tissue

Ultrasound Extremely high frequency sound waves used for diagnosis and therapy

Ultraviolet rays Electromagnetic radiation with wavelengths ranging in size between those of X-rays and light rays

Unit Standardized descriptive word which specifies the dimensions of a number

Unmyelinated Axon that lacks sheaths of myelin

Unsaturated

Compound A compound where some of the carbon atoms are linked to other carbon atoms by either double or triple bonds

Solution A solution that has the ability to dissolve additional solute

Urea A relatively non-toxic end product of protein catabolism

Urine Fluid that is secreted by the kidneys

Vaccination Artificial introduction of a small quantity of antigen which results in the recipient being immunized for that antigen

Vagus nerve Principal parasympathetic nerve

Valence The combining power of an atom

Vector Any physical quantity that has both magnitude and direction

Vegetative stage Stage of active growth of microbes, as opposed to resting or spore stages

Veins Vessels that return blood from capillaries to the heart

Velocity A vector describing the distance that something has travelled divided by the time taken

Ventral horn Point of exit of motor nerves from the spinal cord

Ventricles Large chambers from which blood is forced out of the heart

Venule Small vein, connects a capillary to the venous system

Viraemia The presence of viruses in the blood

Virion The entire virus particle

Virucide An agent that kills viruses

Virulence A term which describes the relative ability of a pathogen to produce a disease

Virus Small acellular structure that consists of hereditary material surrounded by protein

Viscosity The tendency of a liquid to resist flow; the SI unit of viscosity is the poise

Vitamins Organic substances that act in trace amounts to promote enzyme function

Volt SI unit for potential difference

Wavelength The distance between two identical points of adjacent waves.

EXAMPLE: The distance between the crest of two adjacent waves

Waxes   A group of lipids that are less greasy than fats

White matter   Regions of the brain and spinal cord that contain a predominance of axons

Wire

  Active   Carries current from the power source to an instrument or appliance; the wire is covered by brown or red insulating material

  Earth   A green/yellow or green covered wire that connects equipment directly to the earth

  Neutral   Blue or black covered wire that returns current from a piece of equipment to the power supply

Work   The transfer of energy from one object to another. It is the distance that an object is moved in the direction of a force multiplied by the magnitude of that force; the SI unit of work is the joule

X-rays   Electromagmetic radiation with a shorter wavelength than ultraviolet rays and a longer wavelength than gamma rays; capable of penetrating most matter including human tissue

Zwitterion   An ion that contains a region with a positive charge and another region with a negative charge

Bibliography

Chemistry

Baum, S. J. and Scaife, C. W. (1980) *Chemistry: A Life Science Approach*, second edition. Macmillan, New York.

Bettelheim, F. A. and March, J. (1984) *Introduction to General, Organic and Biochemistry*. Saunders College Publishing, Philadelphia.

Bloomfield, M. M. (1987) *Chemistry and the Living Organism*, fourth edition. John Wiley, New York.

Chang, R. (1981) *Physical Chemistry with Applications to Biological Systems*, second edition. Macmillan, New York.

Fessenden R. J. and Fessenden J. S. (1984) *Basic Chemistry for the Health Sciences*. Allyn and Bacon, Boston.

Holum, J. R. (1986) *Fundamentals of General, Organic, and Biological Chemistry*, third edition. John Wiley, New York.

Huheey, J. E. (1983) *Inorganic Chemistry: Principles of Structure and Reactivity*, third edition. Harper and Row, London.

Klaasen, C. D., Amdur M. O. and Doull, J. (eds) (1986) *Casarett and Doulls Toxicology, The Basic Science of Poisons*, third edition. Macmillan, New York.

Korolkovas, A. (1988) *Essentials of Medicinal Chemistry*, second edition. John Wiley, New York.

Liska, K. and Pryde, L. T. (1984) *Introductory Chemistry for Health Professionals*. Macmillan, New York.

Sackheim, G. I. and Lehman, D. D. (1990) *Chemistry for the Health Sciences*, sixth edition. Macmillan, New York.

Sears, C. T. and Stanitski, C. L. (1983) *Chemistry for Health-related Sciences: Concepts and Correlations*, second edition. Prentice-Hall, Englewood Cliffs, New Jersey.

Toon, E. R. and Ellis G. L. (1986) *Foundations of Chemistry*. Holt, Rinehart and Winston, Toronto.

Wolfe D. H. (1986) *Essentials of General Organic and Biological Chemistry*. McGraw Hill, New York.

Zilva, J. F. and Pannall, P. R. (1988) *Clinical Chemistry in Diagnosis and Treatment*, fifth edition. Lloyd-Luke, London.

Human Nutrition

Alberts, B., Bray, D., Lewis, J. et al. (1989) *Molecular Biology of the Cell*, second edition. Garland Publishing Inc., New York.

Brown, W. H. and Rogers, E. P. (1987) *General, Organic, and Biochemistry*, third edition. Brooks-Cole.

Cohn, R. M. and Roth, K. S. (1983) *Metabolic Disease: A Guide to Early Recognition*. W. B. Saunders, Philadelphia.

Darnell, J., Lodish, H. and Baltimore D. (1986) *Molecular Cell Biology*. Scientific American Books, New York.

Davidson, R. and Eastwood, M. A. (1986) *Davidson and Passmore Human Nutrition and Dietetics*, eighth edition. Churchill Livingstone, Edinburgh.

De Robertis, E. D. and De Robertis E. M. (1987) *Cell and Molecular Biology*, eighth edition. Lea & Febiger, Philadelphia.

Goldsby, R. A. (1977) *Cells and Energy*, second edition. Macmillan, New York.

Kornberg, A. (1980) *DNA Replication*. W. H. Freeman and Co., San Francisco.

Lehninger, A. L. (1982) *Principles of Biochemistry*. Worth Publishers, New York.

McGilvery, R. W. and Goldstein, G. W. (1983) *Biochemistry: A Functional Approach*, third edition. W. B. Saunders, Philadelphia.

Rodwell Williams, S. (1982) *Essentials of Nutrition and Diet Therapy*, third edition. The C. V. Mosby Company, St. Louis.

Stanbury, J. B., Wyngaarden, J. B. and Frederickson, O. S. (eds) (1983) *The Metabolic Basis of Inherited Disease*, fifth edition. McGraw-Hill, New York.

Stryer, L. (1988) *Biochemistry*, third edition. W. H. Freeman and Co., San Francisco.

Varley, H., Gowenlock, A. H. and Bell, M. (1987) *Practical Clinical Biochemistry, Vol. 2, Hormones, Vitamins, Drugs and Poisons*, sixth edition. Heinemann Medical Books, London.

Wahlqvist, M. L. (1988) *Food and Nutrition in Australia*. Thomas Nelson Australia Ltd., Sydney.

Yost, H. T. (1972) *Cellular Physiology*. Prentice-Hall, Englewood Cliffs, New Jersey.

Medical Microbiology

Boyd, R. F. (1984) *General Microbiology*. Times Mirror/Mosby College Publishing, St. Louis.

Boyd, R. F. and Hoerl, B. G. (1991) *Basic Medical Microbiology*, fourth edition. Little Brown & Co., Boston.

Brock, T. D. and Madigan, M. (1990) *Biology of Microorganisms*, sixth edition. Prentice-Hall, Englewood Cliffs, New Jersey.

Burton, G. R. W. (1992) *Microbiology for the Health Sciences*, fourth edition. J. B. Lippincott Co., Philadelphia.

Cano, R. J. and Colomé J. S. (1986) *Microbiology*. West Publishing Co., St. Paul.

Cronenberger, J. H. and Jennette J. C. (1988) *Immunology: Basic Concepts, Diseases and Laboratory Methods*. Appleton & Lange, Norwalk.

Frazier, W. C. and Westhoff, D. C. (1988) *Food Microbiology*, third edition (revised). McGraw-Hill, New York.

Jawetz, E., Melnick, J. L. and Adelberg, E. A. (1991) *Review of Medical Microbiology*, nineteenth edition. Prentice Hall, California.

Lowbury, E. J. L., Ayliffe, G. A. J., Geddes, A. M. et al. (1982) *Control of Hospital Infection*, second edition. Chapman and Hall, London.

Pelczar, M. J., Reid, R. D. and Chan, E. C. S. (1985) *Microbiology*, fifth edition. McGraw-Hill, New York.

Schmidt, G. D. and Roberts, L. S. (1985) *Foundations of Parasitology*, third edition. Times Mirror/Mosby College Publishing, St. Louis.

Tortora, G. S., Fuake, B. R. and Case, C. L. (1991) *Microbiology, An Introduction*, fourth edition. Benjamin Cummings Publishing Company, Redwood City.

Wilson, M. E., Mizer, H. E. and Morello, J. A. (1979) *Microbiology in Patient Care*, third edition. Macmillan, New York.

Winner, H. I. (1979) *Microbiology in Patient Care*, second edition. Hodder and Stoughton, London.

Youmans, G. P., Paterson, P. Y. and Sommers, H. M. (1980) *The Biologic and Clinical Basis of Infectious Diseases*, second edition. W. B. Saunders, Philadelphia.

Pathology

Anderson Price, S. and McCarty Wilson, L. (1991) *Pathophysiology Clinical Concepts of Disease Processes.* McGraw Hill, New York.

Bloom, W. and Fawcett, D. W. (1986) *A Textbook of Histology*, eleventh edition. W. B. Saunders, Philadelphia.

Groër, M. W. and Suekelton M. E. (1989) *Basic Pathophysiology: A Conceptual Approach.* C. V. Mosby, St. Louis.

Cormack, D. H. (1987) *Harris Histology*, ninth edition. J. B. Lippincott, Philadelphia.

Robbins, S. L., Cotran, R. S. and Kumar, V. (1989) *Pathologic Basis of Disease*, fourth edition. W. B. Saunders, Philadelphia.

Tighe, J. R. (1984) *Pathology*, fourth edition. Baillière Tindall, London.

Pharmacology

Bailey, R. E. (1983) *Pharmacology for Nurses*, fifth edition. Baillère Tindall, London.

Clark, W. G., Brater, D. C. and Johnson, A. C. (1988) *Goth's Medical Pharmacology*, twelfth edition. C. V. Mosby, St. Louis.

Hahn, A. B., Barkin, R. L. and Oestreich, S. J. (1985) *Pharmacology in Nursing*, sixteenth edition. The C. V. Mosby Co., St. Louis.

Society of Hospital Pharmacists of Australia. (1989) *Pharmacology and Drug Information for Nurses*, third edition. W. B. Saunders, Sydney.

Physics

Benedek, G. B. and Villars, F. M. (1974) *Physics with Illustrative Examples from Medicine and Biology, Volume 3, Electricity and Magnetism.* Addison-Wesley, Reading.

Duncan, G. (1990) *Physics in the Life Sciences*, second edition. Blackwell, Oxford.

Gray, H. J. and Isaacs, A. (eds) (1990) *Dictionary of Physics*, third edition. Longman, London.

Greenberg, L. H. (1978) *Physics for Biology and Pre-med Students.* W. B. Saunders, Toronto.

Greenberg, L. H. (1978) *Physics with Modern Applications.* W. B. Saunders, Toronto.

Gustafson, D. R. (1980) *Physics: Health and the Human Body.* Wadsworth Publishing Co., Belmont, California.

Halliday, D. and Resnick, R. (1981) *Physics, Parts 1 and 2*, third edition. John Wiley, New York.

Hilyard, N. C. and Biggin H. C. (1977) *Physics for Applied Biologists.* Edward Arnold, London.

Horsfield, R. S. (1978) *Biomechanics.* Science Press, Sydney.

Horsfield, R., Solomons, S. and Ward, A. (1978) *Physics and Chemistry for the Health Sciences.* Science Press, Sydney.

Kilgour, O. F. G. (1978) *An Introduction to the Physical Aspects of Nursing Science*, third edition. W. Heinemann Medical Books, London.

Kane, J. W. and Sternheim, M. M. (1988) *Physics*, third edition. John Wiley, New York.

Marshall, S. V. and Skitek, G. G. (1990) *Electromagnetic Concepts and Applications*, third edition. Prentice-Hall.

Morley, A. and Huge, S. E. (1986) *Principles of Electricity*, fourth edition. Longman Scientific & Technical, Harlow.

Nave, C. R. and Nave, B. C. (1985) *Physics for the Health Sciences*, third edition. W. B. Saunders, Philadelphia.

Snow, T. P. and Shull, J. M. (1986) *Physics.* West Publishing Co., St. Paul.

Physiology and Biology

Anderson Price, S. and McCarthy Wilson, L. (1982) *Pathophysiology: Clinical Concepts of Disease Processes*, second edition. McGraw-Hill, New York.

Anthony, C. P. and Thibodeau, G. A. (1987) *Textbook of Anatomy and Physiology*, twelfth edition. Times Mirror/Mosby, St. Louis.

Arms, K. and Camp, P. (1987) *Biology*, third edition. W. B. Saunders, Philadelphia.

Bell, G. H., Emslie-Smith, D. and Paterson, C. R. (1988) *Textbook of Physiology and Biochemistry*, eleventh edition. Churchill Livingstone, Edinburgh.

Bennett, A. and Sanger, G. J. (1979) Prostanoids and their relationship to the non-pregnant uterus. *Research and Clinical Forums* 1(2), 21–5.

Burns, G. W. and Bottino, P. J. (1989) *The Science of Genetics*, sixth edition. Macmillan, New York.

Cioffi, D. (1979) The fundamentals of blood gases. *The Lamp*, August, 5–12.

Creager, J. G. (1992) *Human Anatomy and Physiology*. Wadsworth Publishing Co., Belmont, California.

Groër, M. W. and Shekleton, M. E. (1989) *Basic Pathophysiology: A Conceptual Approach*, second edition. C. V. Mosby, St. Louis.

Grollman, S. (1978) *The Human Body: Its Structure and Physiology*, fourth edition. Macmillan, New York.

Guyton, A. C. (1985) *Anatomy and Physiology*. W. B. Saunders, Philadelphia.

Guyton, A. C. (1984) *Physiology of the Human Body*, sixth edition. W. B. Saunders, Philadelphia.

Guyton, A. C. (1990) *Textbook of Medical Physiology*, eighth edition. W. B. Saunders, Philadelphia.

Hardisty, R. M. and Weatherall, D. J. (eds) (1974) *Blood and Its Disorders*. Blackwell Scientific Publications, Oxford.

Hinchliff, S. M. and Montague, S. E. (1988) *Physiology for Nursing Practice*, Baillière Tindall, London.

Iveson-Iveson, J. (1979) The nervous system 1. *Nursing Mirror*, 25 January, 20–3.

Iveson-Iveson, J. (1979) The nervous system 2. *Nursing Mirror*, 1 February, 26–8.

Iveson-Iveson, J. (1979) The nervous system 3. *Nursing Mirror*, 8 February, 32–3.

Kappers, J. and Ariens Pevet, P. (eds) (1979) *The Pineal Gland of Vertebrates Including Man*, Progress in Brain Research, Vol. 52. Elsevier/North Holland Biomedical Press, Amsterdam.

Keele, C. A., Neil, E. and Joels, N. (1982) *Samson Wrights Applied Physiology*, thirteenth edition. Oxford University Press, Oxford.

Luft, R. (1979) Diabetes: The outlook is bright. *World Health*, May, 3–7.

Memmler, R. L., Cohen, B. J. and Wood, D. L. (1992) *The Human Body in Health and Disease*, seventh edition, Lippincott.

Mountcastle, V. B. (1980) *Medical Physiology*, Volumes 1 and 2, fourteenth edition. C. V. Mosby, St. Louis.

Pearce, E. (1975) *Anatomy and Physiology for Nurses*, sixteenth edition. Faber and Faber, London.

Robinson, J. R. (1975) *Fundamentals of Acid–Base Regulation*, fifth edition. Blackwell Scientific Publications, Oxford.

Ross, J. S. and Wilson, K. J. (1990) *Anatomy and Physiology in Health and Illness*, seventh edition. Churchill Livingstone.

Silverstein, A. (1988) *Human Anatomy and Physiology*, second edition. John Wiley, New York.

Smith, L. H. and Thier, S. O. (1981) *Pathophysiology: The Biological Principles of Disease*. W. B. Saunders, Philadelphia.

Sodeman, W. A. and Sodeman, T. M. (1985) *Pathologic Physiology. Mechanisms of Disease*, seventh edition. W. B. Saunders, Philadelphia.

Strand, F. L. (1978) *Physiology: A Regulatory*

Systems Approach. Macmillan, New York.

Tortora, G. J. and Anagnostakos, N. P. (1990) *Principles of Anatomy and Physiology*, sixth edition. Harper Row, New York.

Vander, A. J. and Luciano, D. S. (1990) *Human Physiology: The Mechanisms of Body Function*, fifth edition. McGraw-Hill, New York.

Watson, J. E. (1979) *Medical Surgical Nursing and Related Physiology*. W. B. Saunders, Toronto.

Williams, R. H. (ed.) (1981) *Textbook of Endocrinology*, sixth edition. W. B. Saunders, Philadelphia.

Williams, S. (1979) Physiological aspects of stress, *Australian Nurses Journal*, **9**(1), 45–8.

General

Brooks, S. M. (1979) *Integrated Basic Science*, fourth edition. C. V. Mosby, St. Louis.

Carter, C. O. (1979) Recent advances in genetic counselling. *Nursing Times*, 18 October, 1795–8.

Champney, B. and Smiddy, F. G. (1979) *Symptoms, Signs and Syndromes: A Medical Glossary*. Ballière Tindall, London.

Clarke, M. and Montague, S. (eds) (1980) Stress. *Nursing*, February.

Cochaud, G. A. M. and Cochaud, J. E. (1978) *Basic Science for the Health Team*. Pitman Medical, Melbourne.

Commonwealth Department of Health (1977) *Metric Tables of Composition of Australian Foods*. Australian Government Publishing Service, Camberra.

de Gruyter, W. (1983) *Concise Encyclopedia of Biochemistry*. Walter de Gruyter, Berlin.

(1988) *Dorland's Illustrated Medical Dictionary*, twenty-seventh edition. W. B. Saunders, Philadelphia.

Health Commission of N.S.W. (1977) *S. I. Units in Clinical Pathology*, Sydney.

Kilgour, O. F. G. (1978) *An Introduction to the Biological Aspects of Nursing Science*. Heinemann Medical Books, London.

Lankford, T. Randall (1984) *Integrated Science for Health Students*, third edition. Reston Publishing Company, Reston, Virginia.

Middleton, D. (1984) *Baillière's Ward Information*, fourteenth edition. Baillière Tindall, London.

Mims Annual, 1992 Incorporating the Australian Drug Compendium, Australian edition. Intercontinental Medical Statistics, Sydney.

Neller, B. F. and Wells, R. (eds) (1990) *Baillière's Nurses' Dictionary*, twenty-first edition. Baillière Tindall, London.

Walker, F. W., Kirovac, G. J. and Rourke, F. M. (1977) *Chart of the Nuclides*, twelfth edition. General Electric Company, San Jose, California.

Uvarov, E. B., Chapman, D. R. and Isaacs, A. (1986) *The Penguin Dictionary of Science*, sixth edition. Penguin Books, Harmondsworth, Middlesex.

Index

Page numbers in **bold** refer to applications, those in *italic* refer to tables.

Periodic Table of Elements

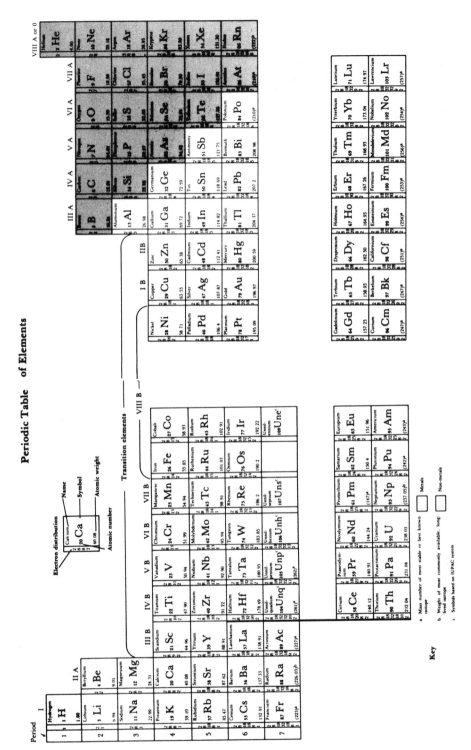

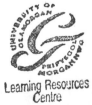

Learning Resources Centre